MEDICAL ENCOUNTERS

A VOLUME IN THE SERIES
Native Americans of the Northeast

EDITED BY
Colin G. Calloway
Jean M. O'Brien, and
Barry O'Connell

MEDICAL ENCOUNTERS

Knowledge and Identity in Early American Literatures

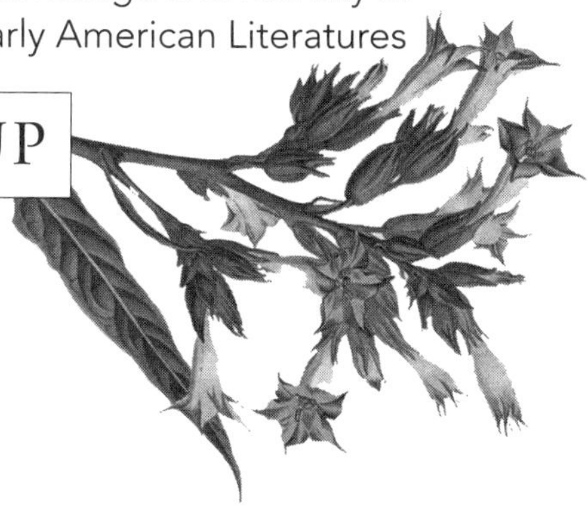

KELLY WISECUP

University of Massachusetts Press
Amherst and Boston

Printed in the United States of America

ISBN 978-62534-057-3 (paper); 056-6 (cloth)

Designed by Sally Nichols
Set in Arno Pro
Printed and bound by IBT/Hamilton, Inc.

Library of Congress Cataloging-in-Publication Data

Wisecup, Kelly, 1981– author.
Medical encounters : knowledge and identity in early American literatures / Kelly Wisecup.
pages cm. — (Native Americans of the Northeast)
Includes bibliographical references and index.
ISBN 978-1-62534-056-6 (hardcover : alk. paper) — ISBN 978-1-62534-057-3 (pbk. : alk. paper)
1. Medicine—United States—History. 2. Medicine in literature—United States. 3. American literature—History and criticism. I. Title.
R151.W57 2013
610—dc23

2013028727

British Library Cataloguing-in-Publication Data
A catalogue record for this book is available from the British Library.

To Wayne

CONTENTS

ACKNOWLEDGMENTS

THIS BOOK WOULD not have come into being but for the wise guidance and inspiration of my teachers and colleagues. Thanks go to Leslie Babcox, James Bell, David Dalton, William Horrell, and Stephen Kneeshaw for encouraging my early attempts at scholarship; this book owes much to their direction and intellectual curiosity. I thank my master's committee members at Texas Tech University: Marjean Purinton and Yuan Shu encouraged my interest in literature and medicine and offered expert advice, and Cristobal Silva's graduate class on early American literature and epidemiology made me want to keep reading colonial texts. At the University of Maryland, Ralph Bauer, Robert S. Levine, Vincent Carretta, Tita Chico, and Heather Nathans were ideal committee members and model scholars. Particular thanks go to Ralph Bauer, who after directing my dissertation has continued to read and support my work; his generosity and guidance helped transform the book into its current state. Conversations with faculty and graduate student colleagues at the University of Maryland shaped my interests and the earliest manifestations of the book, and I'm grateful to Kandice Chuh, Theresa Coletti, Neil Fraistat, Peter Mallios, Orrin Wang, Mary Frances Jimenez, Tasos Lazarides, Rebecca Lush, Chris Maffuccio, Jason Payton, Joanne Roby, and Elizabeth Veisz.

I owe much to the vibrant community of early Americanists, whose willingness to share writing, critiques, conference panels, and dinners made working on this book a pleasure. Angela Calcaterra, Katy Chiles, Matt Cohen, Matt Crawford, Kathleen Donegan, Joy Howard, Toni Wall Jaudon, Julie Kim, Cassie Smith, Dan Walden, Joanne van der Woude, and Maria Windell all read or heard parts of the book and asked perceptive questions.

I thank Neilesh Bose, Claire Gherini, Katie Paugh, Chris Parsons, and Mac Test for very helpful conversations about science, empire, and the Atlantic World. Dan Richter, Christina Snyder, Scott Manning Stevens, and Coll Thrush offered helpful comments that, while focused on various versions of chapter 1, helped me understand the larger argument of the book. Joanna Brooks, Elizabeth Maddock Dillon, Mary Fuller, Karen Ordahl Kupperman, Steven Mentz, Susan Scott Parrish, Ivy Schweitzer, and Hilary Wyss offered advice on individual chapters and support along the way. Theresa Strouth Gaul and Desiree Henderson made me feel welcome in north Texas and shared advice and long drives to Society for the Study of Women Writers study groups. David Fletcher's work as my research assistant was very useful to chapter 1. I thank the many conference participants who engaged with the project, including but not limited to the attendees at the Newberry Library's Early American History and Culture Seminar (especially Betsy Erkkila, Robert Michael Morrissey, Eric Slauter, and Abram van Engen); the Early Caribbean Society Symposiums (especially Tom Krise); the NEH Summer Seminar "English Encounters with the Americas, 1550–1610"; the 2009 Atlantic History Seminar; and the McNeil Center for Early American Studies Works-in-Progress Series. For friendships that, in some cases, extend across the country and that have provided enjoyable and much-needed respites from writing, I'm grateful to Heather Brown, Toni Jensen, Gretchen Hoffman, Lisa Vining, and Jennifer Wallach. Finally, the following colleagues at the University of North Texas have supported my work: Kevin Curran, Ian Finseth, Jacqueline Foertsch, Stephanie Hawkins, David Holdeman, Kyle Jensen, Jack Peters, Alexander Pettit, and Jacqueline Vanhoutte.

At the University of Massachusetts Press, I have been very fortunate to work with Clark Dougan, whose support and professionalism are everything one could ask for. I thank Bruce Wilcox, Carol Betsch, Mary Bellino, and Kay Scheuer as well as the editors for the Native Americans of the Northeast series, Colin G. Calloway, Jean M. O'Brien, and Barry O'Connell. I am very grateful to Kristina Bross, Jim Egan, and an anonymous reader for their incisive and productive readings of the manuscript; the book benefited immensely from their expertise and from Kris's and Jim's ongoing support.

Several grants and fellowships have supported research for this book: two Junior Faculty Summer Research Fellowships, a Research Initiation Grant, and a Small Grant from the University of North Texas provided time for writing and support for travel to examine Samson Occom's papers. A Newberry Library Short-Term Fellowship and a Newberry Renaissance Consortium Grant (from UNT's Medieval-Renaissance Colloquium) facilitated work at the Newberry Library. A Barbara S. Mosbacher Fellowship from the John Carter Brown Library supported research on chapters 2 and 4, and a Cosmos Club Foundation Young Scholars Award supported initial research on chapter 3. I'm very grateful to the staff at various research libraries and archives for making my research both productive and a great pleasure, especially Scott Manning Stevens, Carla Zecher, and Diane Dillon at the Newberry Library; Peter Carini at Rauner Library at Dartmouth College; Trisha Royston at the New London County Historical Society; Diana McCain at the Connecticut Historical Society; and Val Andrews, Kim Nusco, Leslie Tobias Olson, Ken Ward, and the rest of the staff at the John Carter Brown Library.

An altered version of chapter 3, "African Medical Knowledge, the Plain Style, and Satire in the 1721 Boston Inoculation Controversy," appeared in and is reprinted from *Early American Literature*, vol. 46, no. 1 (2011). I thank *Early American Literature* for the permission to reprint this essay, and Sandra M. Gustafson for her perceptive comments on the essay.

Finally, I thank my family for their ongoing support and interest in my work. My grandparents, parents, and siblings have provided meals, dogs, and rest that undoubtedly improved the book. Wayne Marko has always provided remarkable support for this project; his patience, love, and humor saw it to completion.

Introduction

Medicine and Writing in Early American Colonial Encounters

In 1761, Samson Occom, a Mohegan Indian and a Presbyterian minister, wrote an "Account of the Montauk Indians, on Long Island" in which he described several aspects of Montaukett culture. Occom had lived at Montauk since 1749, during which time he founded a school for Montaukett students, married and established a family with Mary Fowler (Montaukett), and studied herbal medicine with a Montaukett man named Ocus. Occom adopted the form of an ethnographic account: a report, usually written by European travelers, that included information regarding political, domestic, religious, and medical practices belonging to exotic cultures. He employed this perspective, however, not to highlight the unfamiliar nature of Montaukett cultural practices, as European and colonial writers often did, but to speak from his position as an insider. He pointed out the similarities between New and Old World peoples, particularly their medical practices. He wrote:

> I have heard some [Montaukett people] say, that have been poisoned, it puts them into great pain, and when a powaw [medical practitioner] takes out the poison they have found immediate relief; at other times they feel no manner of pain, but feel

> strangely by degrees, till they are senseless, and then they will run mad. Some-times they would run into the water; sometimes into the fire; and at other times run up to the top of high trees and tumble down headlong to the ground, yet receive no hurt by all these. And I don't see for my part, why it is not as true, as the English or other nation's witchcraft, but is a great mystery of darkness, &c.[1]

Unlike most British American writers who described Native American medical practices in the eighteenth century, Occom did not express skepticism regarding powaws' ability to make patients pass unharmed through water and fire and to survive great falls, nor did he discount such healing practices as diabolic or irrational. Instead, he emphasized similarities between Montaukett and English "witchcraft" by describing practitioners' use of herbs viewed as "poison," their ability to make patients "feel strangely by degrees," and their power to control the effects of fire, water, and gravity.[2] Occom's account highlighted the fact that Montaukett and English peoples alike credited medical practitioners' capacity to influence disease using material and metaphysical means and to perform a variety of services, from removing poison to influencing patients' minds. Finally, Occom insisted that Montaukett "witchcraft" was "as true" as that practiced by the English and other nations, thus highlighting the fact that European colonists categorized Native medical practices as witchcraft while failing to recognize that their own medicine shared similar elements.[3] In this way, Occom's "Account" exposed the distance that British American colonists had constructed between their own, allegedly more rational and Christian medical practices and those belonging to Native Americans.

Furthermore, Occom's "Account" reminded readers that Euro-American colonists had not always been convinced of the differences between their medical knowledge and the medical traditions belonging to Native Americans —and to Africans as well. To be sure, the European, Native American, and African medical knowledges that met in the New World possessed long, divergent histories, and they proceeded along different tracks during the colonization and settlement of the Americas. However, for much of the sixteenth, seventeenth, and eighteenth centuries, European colonists, Native Americans, and Africans employed medical knowledge that included a belief in connections between natural and supernatural realms as well as in the power of special rituals or ceremonies to influence the body. In their cosmologies, the supernatural did not belong to another realm but interacted with and influenced the natural world.[4] For British Americans, the connections between the body and supernatural realms went back as far as classical traditions, in which Apollo, the Greek god of poetry and medicine, healed disease by providing instructions for its cure and music to soothe the mind and soul. Apollo's powers depended on an understanding of the body as a physical entity that was also susceptible to influences from metaphysical realms, such as divine arrows of disease or healing words.[5] Classical understandings of Apollo's powers were later adapted for Protestant contexts, so that for British colonists diseases had their origin in divine words, that is, God's judgment on his people for individual or national sin, and illness could be ameliorated by words, from the comforting message of a minister or poet or patients' own words of repentance.[6]

Thus colonists, Natives, and Africans alike understood disease both as a physical state and as a moral or spiritual condition that indicated an imbalanced relationship to other-than-human powers, who were responsible for illness. Medical knowledge and practice included petitions to these non-human forces as well as applications of medicinal remedies, which were expected to be efficacious once prayer and penitence had healed patients' "diseased" relationship to the forces who sent illness.[7] Although Native, African, and Euro-colonial medical experts possessed knowledge of curative remedies, they also taught individuals how to maintain or recover a proper relation to metaphysical forces. These duties were performed in colonial contexts by minister-physicians—including Michael Wigglesworth, Edward Taylor, Thomas Thacher, and Cotton Mather—who attended to their communities' bodies and souls, much as Native *powahs* and African healers appealed to divine forces to cure disease.[8] Meanwhile, in the eighteenth century, colonial physicians such as James Grainger, Alexander Hamilton, and James Kirkpatrick revived classical traditions by presenting medical knowledge in genteel, witty language that healed the body even as it entertained the mind.[9] The same words that soothed and pleased the mind also brought healing to the body by providing specific instructions for its cure or by soothing a mental disturbance.

As a result of these shared beliefs, colonists, Natives, and Africans drew on medical knowledge and practices as a shared form of communication, in order to adapt to the new conditions brought about by colonization. In the new world that was created by unfamiliar medicines and devastating maladies, Native Americans, Africans, and colonists signaled their relation to supernatural forces, to the natural world, and to other people for audiences throughout the Americas and, in the colonists' case, in Europe as well by presenting interpretations of illness and healing. Medical communications—such as explanations of diseases and their causes, healing ceremonies or rituals, and decisions to rely on certain medical authorities—established one's spiritual and sociopolitical status in several contexts. In cross-cultural encounters, one could present an explanation or a cure for illness to indicate that he or she possessed a special relationship to the non-human forces that caused disease; in this way, one could signal a corresponding ability to influence the course of disease. In transatlantic publication contexts and medical networks, colonists countered metropolitan biases regarding knowledge produced in the colonies by offering their accounts of New World medical knowledge as evidence that the American environment had not altered their bodies and minds.

This book examines the ways in which colonists, Native Americans, and Africans communicated medical knowledge in colonial encounters throughout the British Americas, and it investigates as well representations of these communications in early American literatures. It studies medical communications in both transatlantic and intercultural contexts that include not only exchanges between colonists and their European counterparts but also encounters among colonists, Natives, and Africans. In this way, the book contributes to recent scholarly efforts to broaden the geohistorical horizons of early American studies from proto-national and North American contexts.[10] However, *Medical Encounters* also expands transatlantic, transnational, and hemispheric approaches by examining how the Native American and African medical knowledge and practices that circulated in cross-cultural encounters shaped colonial literatures and by investigating how Natives and Africans, as well as colonists, employed such medical knowledge to react to encounters. The book shows that early American medical writing—the textual manifestation of the medical knowledge communicated in cross-cultural encounters—was shaped by Native, African, and colonial responses to medicines and diseases in the New World.

Medical Encounters builds on previous studies of exchanges of illness in the colonial Americas while also reorienting the epistemological and geographic frameworks of this previous scholarship. Historical and literary studies published in the past fifty years have established the significant role that diseases and medicines played in the colonization of the Americas. As Alfred Crosby pointed out in his now classic work, the "Columbian Exchange" of diseases, plants, and medicines between Europe and the Americas resulted in the depopulation of Native peoples and the rise of a transatlantic medicinal trade. Devastating illnesses to which Native Americans lacked immunity swept throughout North and South America, emptying Native villages and enabling European colonists to claim and settle land in the New World. Meanwhile, starting in the fifteenth century, diseases such as syphilis, which allegedly originated in the Americas, spread rapidly throughout Europe. At the same time, American herbs, such as tobacco, that Native Americans employed for a variety of ceremonial purposes quickly became desirable medicinal commodities throughout Europe. Colonists likewise relied on Native informants to locate and harvest herbs such as sassafras, which Europeans employed in the Old World and in the Americas as a treatment for syphilis.[11]

More recent studies of colonization and medicine have shifted Crosby's focus on the biological and ecological consequences of imperialism in Spanish America to examine the ways in which contact-era epidemics in New England not only allowed English settlements to take root but also influenced colonists' conceptions of their biological and cultural identities. Joyce Chaplin has pointed out that early modern natural philosophies—which included medical knowledge—shaped British colonists' understanding of America's natural environment and of their relationship to Native Americans. Natural philosophies provided analytical and rhetorical tools with which colonists contrasted their increasing population with Native mortality. Constructing conceptions of their own bodily superiority on the basis of these observations, colonists argued that their bodies were best suited to improve and possess New England. At the same time, British Americans described their bodies as more refined than those of Africans, a view that subsequently supported arguments for slavery. Ultimately, Chaplin argues, colonists developed a "racial idiom" in which they used "theories of nature to explain their own physical suitability to America" and to posit their bodies and minds as superior to those of Native Americans and Africans.[12] In order to support their arguments about nature and bodies, colonists sometimes engaged in "ventriloquism," in which they put words in Natives' mouths that "made more sense within English debates over nature than they did within the conceivable field of Indian opinions."[13] Chaplin concludes that colonial literatures do not offer insight into Natives' or Africans' responses to the new diseases and medicines that circulated throughout the Americas as a result of colonization, for she argues that if colonists did actually record Native statements, they did so accidentally, because colonists "believed them too ridiculous (absurd) to comment on."[14]

In addition, Cristobal Silva has examined the ways in which accounts of colonial epidemics justified the dispossession of Natives in New England while also making the "notion of [colonial] community formation transparent as a function of illness and health."[15] Silva shows that colonists represented the epidemics as signs of divine approval by suggesting that the land had been providentially cleared for their settlement; colonists aligned Natives' "wasted" bodies with the wasted land in order to argue that the newcomers were better suited to use the land.[16] He revises Chaplin's use of the term "ventriloquism" by analyzing "counter-epidemiologies" that "offer alternative readings of how and why epidemics spread as they did in the wake of colonial encounters" and that, he allows, may accurately represent Native and African voices.[17] But, Silva argues, colonists ultimately appropriated Natives' and Africans' accounts of disease to "establish the moral, technological, and biological superiority of their bodies in the New World, to reify the narrative conventions of epidemiology for colonial ends, and to help secure the settlers' lawful rights to property in New England."[18] These acts of ventriloquism and appropriation subsequently circumscribe what scholars may glean from counter-epidemiologies: "Ultimately, this [appropriation] means that from a narrative perspective, the figure we encounter in these counter-epidemiologies is not Tisquantum the Wampanoag, but 'Tisquantum' the rhetorical figure who echoes the economic strategies behind early English epidemiology, and makes the genre's colonialist function transparent."[19]

Many insights are to be gained from understanding the ways in which western discourses such as natural philosophy and epidemiology acted as colonial strategies for defining and reinforcing difference and identity. Furthermore, these prior studies compellingly elucidate the role that the New England colonies played in the construction and development of the modern scientific methods with which Anglo-Americans delineated cultural differences. *Medical Encounters* opens a new area of inquiry in early American literary studies by shifting the focus on New England, on European or colonial responses to disease, and on western, European medical philosophies. This book broadens the analytical framework through which colonial diseases and medical knowledge are viewed, and it consequently presents an alternate trajectory for the formation of early American literary strategies and for colonial conceptions of identity throughout the British Americas. With illnesses such as AIDS, SARS, and influenza spreading rapidly across the globe and inspiring the proliferation of print discourses that debate various cultural approaches to medical technology and responses to the trans- and inter-national travel of pathogens and persons, it seems an opportune time to reconsider the literatures of medical encounters which responded to transatlantic, transnational, and intercultural medicinal exchanges as well as to cross-cultural communications of medical knowledge.

I consider colonists' reports of medicine and illness in the context of Native American and African, as well as colonial, medical knowledge, in order to illuminate the multiple accounts—both corresponding and conflicting—of illness and healing that circulated in colonial encounters and that shaped early American medical writing. I focus on moments when colonists did not or could not, for a variety of reasons, employ European medical philosophies to justify colonization or to take possession, with the goal of accounting for the shared beliefs, intercultural communications, and the mutually intelligible medical practices that sometimes characterized colonial encounters. As Colin Calloway has explained of Native Americans' responses to the cultural upheaval brought about by contact-era epidemics: "Medicine was power, and Indian people needed to draw on all the power available to them as they struggled to survive in the disease-ridden land that was their world."[20] Indeed, medicine was a form of power for many of the people who encountered one another in the New World, and medical knowledge and practices offered a system with which these individuals situated themselves in challenging new natural, spiritual, and sociopolitical worlds.

Native American and African Medical Knowledge in the Literatures of Encounter

Despite the central role that communicating medical knowledge played for all the participants in colonial encounters, scholars have overlooked the importance of cross-cultural exchanges of such knowledge for early American literatures. This oversight may be traced to methodological frameworks established in studies of the literatures of colonization inspired by the 1992 quincentennial commemorations of Christopher Columbus's first voyage to the Americas.[21] New historicist and postcolonial studies revised earlier views of colonial reports as histories of encounter that could be read straightforwardly;

they emphasized instead the connections between Europeans' representations of Natives and their acts of possession and appropriation.[22] Colonial reports, in this view, offer neither an empirical view of encounter nor a window into Natives' actions and communications, but rather insight into the literary practices that enacted colonial power dynamics. As Ed White has pointed out, scholars did not deny that Natives and Africans possessed cultures that were influenced by colonization, but they held that attempts to recover these cultures would reenact the colonizing process.[23] For example, Stephen Greenblatt and Anthony Pagden have argued that colonial literatures themselves foreclose an investigation of Native responses to colonization, for immense, incommensurable differences separated colonists from the peoples they met in the New World. Colonists sought to overcome these differences by invoking familiar contexts, that is, by describing New World phenomena with words and concepts recognizable to audiences in Europe. As a consequence, Europeans' interpretations of encounter were performed "*for a world elsewhere*," the only world that could comprehend such linguistic acts.[24] These literary strategies familiarized the Americas for Old World audiences: colonists placed New World entities into European categories, subsequently representing the Americas in the terms of the Old World. Such strategies of "attachment" allowed travelers to name and subsequently to take cognitive possession of the unfamiliar objects and actions they observed.[25] Accordingly, scholars examined colonial literatures in the context of European imperialism and its genres in order to understand the ways in which literary and epistemological practices allowed "large parts of the non-European world [to be] *produced* for Europe."[26]

Although new historicist and postcolonial approaches provided a useful caution against reading colonial texts transparently and against ignoring the effects of European power in colonial writing, they rest not only on an "overstated skepticism" of colonial accounts of Natives and Africans but also on reductive views of cross-cultural relations and of colonial literatures.[27] In particular, analyses of the literatures of encounter as reflecting solely European perspectives and desires have reproduced the incommensurability allegedly governing colonial encounters. In these readings, European literary strategies offered tools that colonists employed to create knowledge of the "other" but not to engage this "other."[28] Such viewpoints prevent analyses of moments when Natives and Africans directed the outcome of encounters, when colonists were uncertain how to respond to or represent their experiences, or when colonists, Natives, and Africans held knowledge in common. Furthermore, colonists could not always make Natives and Africans into objects of study, for as I explain below, travel to the New World was believed to alter Europeans' bodies and minds, meaning that colonists could not identify unproblematically with Europeans in the Old World after they had traveled to the Americas. As a consequence, they did not automatically assume positions as distanced, superior observers but had to construct and maintain those positions in their writings—and even then, colonists were viewed as having altered or degenerated as a result of their exposure to New World environments.

Finally, studies of colonial discourse rest on a view of European representational strategies as remaining stable in colonial encounters. Colonial accounts of encounter are said to mistranslate, ventriloquize, and appropriate Native and African words, actions, and knowledge to advance colonial agendas without being influenced by Natives and Africans themselves.[29] If any exchanges did occur, colonists effaced such interchanges by placing familiar words and frameworks onto unfamiliar situations, an act that allowed them to retain interpretive control of the encounter. As a consequence of this focus on colonists' strategies of familiarization and manipulation, the question of how early American literatures register Native and African perspectives not only remains unanswered but has also been categorized as unanswerable.

But colonists did sometimes depart from familiar European literary strategies when they came into contact with Native and African medical knowledge. In particular, they altered conventional narrative strategies of describing illness and healing that constituted forms called *historia.* Possessing a classical history going back to Herodotus and Aristotle, *historia* documented both human experience and natural phenomena by placing them into a temporal sequence that connected events to an authoritative conclusion.[30] As scholars such as Andrew Wear and Nancy Siraisi have pointed out, medicine is "in fundamental ways a narrative discipline," for diseases mirror the temporal movement of narrative: illness has a beginning, middle, and end, even if not all of these elements are equally apparent to an observer.[31] As a consequence, the narrative forms of *historia* lent authority to accounts of illness by providing a temporal structure through which to consider an illness, its course, and its cure. As Wear points out, narrative accounts of disease had great credibility "because [narrative] is in the logical form of 'because something happened then something else occurred.' The fit between cause and symptom also creates belief."[32] Indeed, *historia* provided a rhetorical strategy with which medical practitioners traditionally explored the final causes of medical phenomena.[33]

In early modern Europe, *historia* were a popular form utilized by lay and elite practitioners alike, with the goals of identifying and describing the course of diseases in individual patients and throughout communities and of recommending or defending treatments. Medical practitioners from the Spanish physician Nicolás Monardes to English physicians Hans Sloane and Thomas Sydenham employed the strategies of *historia* to give shape and authority to their case studies of healing and, sometimes, of fatal illnesses; they created "descriptive accounts of the nature and course of diseases, parts of the body . . . , the spread of epidemics . . . and the cases of individual patients."[34] Furthermore, unlicensed practitioners, lay people, and patients themselves drew on *historia* to describe their own and others' illnesses and cures; such accounts of disease appeared in various genres, from reports of illness or case studies to letters, *belles lettres,* and accounts of miracles or preternatural events.[35] The narrative forms of *historia* provided strategies with which to connect visible effects or symptoms to invisible physical states and in this way to identify a cause and cure for the illness. These strategies consequently allowed accounts of illness to be brought to satisfying, authoritative conclusions, even in cases when treatment did not end in a return to health. Finally, narrative forms authorized practitioners' accounts of disease by shifting the focus from the patient to the practitioner, so that his medical authority and ability to diagnose the illness verified the text.[36]

Most colonists in the British Americas would have been familiar with *historia,* thanks to their widespread use among people with various levels of medical training. Moreover, as detailed in the chapters that follow, the colonists studied in *Medical Encounters* had specific opportunities to learn the literary strategies of *historia,* whether through formal education, often in medicine, or through encounters with popular medical texts in their libraries or in others' collections. Colonists in the British Americas drew on the rhetorical strategies of *historia* by employing narrative frameworks to describe New World medicines and diseases and to connect visible symptoms or events with invisible causes. For example, as I explain in chapter 1, Thomas Harriot began his description of a mysterious epidemic that infected the Roanoke Algonquians but not the English colonists by establishing a narrative in which the disease appeared after the colonists had visited a village. Similarly, Pilgrim Edward Winslow described his cure of the Wampanoag sachem Massasoit in narrative forms that attributed Massasoit's return to health to Winslow's ministrations. However, colonists did not complete their *historia,* for they broke off their narratives by omitting conclusions. They shifted their rhetorical strategies to alternate, non-narrative literary forms, including lists, recipes, satires, and footnotes. Colonists presented the Native and African medical knowledge they encountered in these non-narrative forms: for instance, by listing Native theories of disease, by providing the recipe for a Native medicinal concoction, and by detailing African medical practices in footnotes or satirical forms. Harriot, for example, did not complete his narrative but instead listed the Algonquians' theories regarding the disease's origin. Winslow likewise explained that he drew on Wampanoag medical expertise and local herbs to make a concoction for Massasoit; he modified his narrative by providing a recipe that detailed the Wampanoags' medicinal knowledge. Colonists' incomplete narratives indicate that Native and African medical practices disrupted and altered conventional narrative strategies for representing illness and healing.

Medical Encounters proposes the concept of "texture" to read colonists' fragmented narratives as rhetorical signs of encounters with Natives' and Africans' medical knowledge and of the influence of that knowledge on colonists' medical writing. The anthropologist Neil L. Whitehead has defined "texture" as "any syntactical anomaly, semantic contradiction or logical inconsistency, as well as the physical properties of the document, including alterations, margin notes, format and the existence of multiple editions."[37] As Whitehead argues, texture is one of the "potential indicators of the relations between text and testimony," that is, between European literary practices and expectations, on the one hand, and events or experiences in the New World, on the other.[38] It points to moments when Natives and Africans transmitted their knowledge, for a number of reasons, to colonists in the context of encounter and when colonists incorporated that knowledge into their accounts. Studying the texture of colonial writing can elucidate how Native and African sociocultural forms and practices are registered in the rhetorical features of colonial texts and indeed formed an "inseparable part of the production of colonial text."[39] Moreover, as Myra Jehlen points out of textual ruptures in the literatures of encounter more generally, these "lapses and incoherencies, their redundancies and paradoxes" constitute moments when alternative interpretations and conclusions to narratives of encounter are possible; they consequently provide opportunities to consider the multiple perspectives on and responses to colonial encounters.[40] Texture does not provide an occasion to read colonial texts transparently; instead, it points to the contexts that colonists, Natives, and Africans shared and to the ways in which these people responded to colonial encounters. In the case of medical writing, colonists' incomplete narratives expose the ways in which Native and African medical knowledge shaped descriptions of New World medicines and illnesses.

Texture requires an analysis of Native, African, and colonial sociocultural and historical contexts as well as of these peoples' modes of communication in order to illuminate the source and significance of narrative ruptures. In this way, texture is distinguished from the "stutters" or "rifts" that postcolonial and new historicist scholars have examined in colonial literatures. Peter Hulme argues, for example, that textual stutters "can therefore be used as levers to open out the ideology of colonial discourse,"[41] while Greenblatt reads the "cracking apart of contextual understanding" as characteristic of the experience of wonder.[42] For both scholars, textual inconsistencies expose the operations of colonialism and provide insight into the ways in which colonists rhetorically enacted and justified imperialism. But the turn to examine the "ideology of colonial discourse" limits these studies to European contexts while ignoring the Native and African knowledge and practices that gave rise to textual inconsistencies in the literatures of encounter.[43] Indeed, Greenblatt states emphatically that he has "resisted as much as I can the temptation to speak for or about the native cultures as if the mediation of European representations were an incidental consideration, easily corrected for."[44] Yet although Greenblatt's insistence that scholars take seriously the work colonial literatures performed as tools of empire is well taken, his conclusion that "We can be certain only that European representations of the New World tell us something about the European practice of representation" overlooks the knowledge that Natives, Africans, and colonists held in common and the ways in which colonial literatures manifest, in both their content and their form, the strategies that participants in colonial encounters employed to debate the meaning of medical phenomena.[45]

Thus while Hulme's and Greenblatt's studies certainly advanced our knowledge of colonial discourses, one repercussion of their turn to European contexts to understand textual stutters or cracks is that the Native or African presence hinted at by rhetorical inconsistencies is already constituted as the "other," while colonists maintain a position of cultural and epistemological primacy. The practice of reading accounts of Native and African knowledge only in the context of colonial epistemologies and rhetorical strategies subordinates Native and African histories and voices to colonial ones. In this way, analyses of textual stutters and rifts have solidified views of Native, African, and colonial knowledges as incommensurable and have foreclosed an investigation of the Native and African knowledge represented in colonial texts.

Medical Encounters departs from these prior studies by viewing colonial writing as shaped not only by colonists' medical practices and European literary traditions but also by Native and African medical knowledge. This perspective does not ignore the presence and effects of power in colonial encounters but rather acknowledges that taking stock of power relations does not preclude examining the ways in which colonial texts were constructed out of "entangled" meanings and practices that circulated in exchanges and encounters.[46] Neither a manifestation wholly of cross-cultural understanding or of European imperialism, texture registers the mutual attempts by Natives, Africans, and colonists to interpret unfamiliar illnesses and medicines as well as the ideas and practices that circulated in such meetings and their implications for participants' identities and relationships.[47]

Texture counters the idea that colonial encounters were characterized by incommensurable boundaries among colonial, Native, and African knowledges that motivated colonists to turn to familiar European contexts. Instead, the texture of colonists' medical writing manifests their efforts to explain previously unknown maladies, their causes, and their cures, and it indicates the significant role that Native and African knowledge played in these efforts. The conceptions of disease and healing shared by the people who encountered one another in the New World made Native and African knowledge a compelling, sensible resource on which colonists could draw to describe and explain unfamiliar medical phenomena. Colonists' descriptions of Native and African medical practices reflect not a projection or ventriloquism of English knowledge onto Natives or Africans but rather a transcription, however partial or incomplete, of medical knowledge and practices from cross-cultural encounters. The texture of colonists' medical writing thus manifests not only encounters among colonial, Native, and African medical knowledge but also attempts, by all the participants in colonial encounters, to describe and explain unfamiliar medicines, medical knowledge, and illnesses by drawing on available resources.

Colonists' medical writing represents one permutation of these exchanges, appropriations, and translations, a textual representation of the ideas and practices that were exchanged in colonial encounters. But texture also offers the opportunity to consider the multiple forms of communication employed in colonial encounters: as the syntactical anomalies of colonists' printed texts indicate the presence of additional voices and forms of knowledge, they also require attention to the various media—oral, inscriptive, performative, or material—in which that knowledge was transmitted. In this way, my focus on texture maintains the attention to textual details that characterizes strategies of close reading even as it attends to specific cultural and historical contexts and to various modes of communication. *Medical Encounters* considers the range of communicating practices that constituted colonial medical writing by following new efforts in early American studies to expand the focus on printed texts that has traditionally characterized the field. I draw on the insights of recent studies of communication and literacy in colonial New England, which have reconceptualized "literature" and "writing" in the early Americas to include a range of interdependent oral, inscriptive, and performative practices. These studies have critiqued the prestige traditionally accorded to printed forms of communication by showing that colonists, Natives, and Africans perceived printed, spoken, and non-alphabetic modes of expression as having rhetorical authority in different moments and contexts.[48] These modes of communication did not merely coexist but rather, as Sandra M. Gustafson explains, interacted with and profoundly shaped one another.[49] In addition, scholars have challenged the use of the terms "oral" and "literate" as cultural categories by showing that European, African, and Native peoples employed both oral and inscribing modes of communication and that, as a consequence, they "constituted each others' audiences."[50] The European, Native American, and African participants in New World medical encounters variously employed oral, performative, and written modes of communication to signal their interpretations of illness and healing and subsequently to claim positions of medical authority. *Medical Encounters* investigates the range of communicating practices with which medical knowledge was transmitted by reading colonists' printed texts alongside accounts of conversations, testimony, and medical ceremonies and rituals. As it helps to redefine what counted as a "text" in the British Americas, *Medical Encounters* opens up a new area for the study of early American medicine and literature.[51]

Instances of texture in the literatures of medical encounter provide insight into the medical knowledge communicated in colonial encounters as well as into the ways in which these communications informed oral, written, and performative reactions to encounters. In *Medical Encounters,* I account for the Native and African medical knowledge, practices, and perspectives that colonists met with by placing colonial literatures in the context of anthropological, ethnohistorical, and linguistic studies of Native and African medical systems. Moreover, I read contemporary studies of Native and African medicine alongside early modern and eighteenth-century accounts of this medical knowledge in order to discover how Natives and Africans may have employed and adapted their medical knowledge in contexts of encounter. This interdisciplinary method allows me to shift the focus from European historical and literary contexts and to avoid reading colonists' transcriptions of Native and African knowledge back into Euro-colonial contexts. As I show, elements of Native, African, and colonial medical practices shaped one another, and they subsequently assumed new forms: for example, new strategies of describing illness, composed of Native images and English words; conceptions of healing that included the practices of Native *powahs* and colonial ministers; and practices of preventing or curing disease imported from Africa and mixed with Africans' knowledge of Caribbean herbs. Pre-contact medical knowledge was not completely effaced in medical encounters but rather accrued different meanings and purposes as Natives and Africans translated it for use in the unstable world of epidemics, depopulation, and enslavement. The new forms of knowledge that circulated in colonial encounters, far from being incommensurable, held related, interconnected meanings for British Americans, Natives, and Africans.

Just as colonists altered their narrative rhetorical strategies and descriptions of illness in acknowledgment of cross-cultural encounters, so Natives and Africans responded to the unfamiliar medical phenomena they came upon as a result of colonization, forced migration, and enslavement. In these responses, Natives and Africans both drew on their traditional medical knowledge and incorporated some elements of colonial medicine into pre-existing systems. In particular, Native Americans employed their medical knowledge to articulate the apparent connections between their illnesses and the colonists' arrival and to engage colonists' claims to their land and bodies. For example, Carolina Algonquians and New England Wampanoags responded to the nearly simultaneous arrival of mysterious epidemics and unfamiliar peoples by incorporating colonists into their stories of disease and by employing these stories to seek positions of authority in the new sociopolitical contexts created by colonization. In New England, the Patuxet Indian Tisquantum (or Squanto, as he is often called) suggested that the Plimouth colonists (also called Pilgrims) were to blame for diseases that killed thousands of southern New England Algonquians; the colonists, he suggested, kept the disease in their storehouse for gunpowder. Recognizing Tisquantum's ability to interpret and, by extension, to control the causes of disease, the Wampanoags gave him gifts that showed their respect for his power. Indeed, contact-era epidemics significantly altered Native power structures, for Natives observed that colonists remained healthy during contact-era epidemics and that their own *powahs,* or medical practitioners, were unable to cure their illnesses. Consequently, many Natives concluded that colonists possessed special powers over disease or connections to the powers who sent disease, and they transferred to colonists some of the respect traditionally accorded *powahs.*[52] Some Natives incorporated Christian religious beliefs into traditional healing practices as they sought to restore spiritual and physical health to themselves and their communities. At Montauk, Samson Occom obtained medical knowledge from a Native man named Ocus, and Occom added Christian religious practices to this knowledge by offering both physical and spiritual "medicine" to invalids he met on his preaching tours. In these instances, adopting elements of Christianity did not mean that Natives turned away from pre-contact beliefs and practices; instead, they used Christianity and colonial medical knowledge to strengthen their indigenous religious systems and social relationships.[53]

Just as Natives' relation to their land and the plants they traditionally employed in healing ceremonies were altered by European illnesses and religious beliefs, New World Africans also experienced great cultural and geographic upheaval as they traveled across the Atlantic and throughout the colonies. Enslaved Africans were inflicted with unfamiliar diseases on the Middle Passage and in the colonies, but they also brought with them knowledge of Old World African healing practices, and they adapted these practices to the exigencies of the Americas. Preventive treatments for smallpox, which colonists called inoculation, were one of these practices, and enslaved Africans practiced inoculation quietly, in their own communities, and sometimes shared this knowledge with colonists. For example, an African whose master, the Boston minister Cotton Mather, named him Onesimus, informed Mather that he had been inoculated in Africa and showed Mather the scar he had received. Although Onesimus's testimony has not been the focus of histories of inoculation or smallpox, his communications with Mather endowed him with medical authority, if only temporarily. Indeed, colonists frequently acknowledged Africans' medical expertise and their knowledge of unfamiliar herbs and diseases, especially before the mid-eighteenth century, when there were still few licensed physicians in the colonies. This authority allowed enslaved African medical practitioners to operate relatively independently of their colonial masters. Africans throughout the Americas also employed medical knowledge to resist and rebel against enslavement, and they developed secret strategies for transmitting their medical knowledge throughout their communities without colonists' knowledge. By replicating and adapting Old World practices to the Americas, African healers could restore individual and communal health and could maintain interpersonal relationships and links with their ancestors.[54]

Investigating the texture of colonial medical writing opens the way for examining these accounts as intercultural texts that manifest colonists' engagement with Native and African ideas and practices as well as colonists', Natives', and Africans' endeavors to interpret the strange new worlds created by colonization. Joshua David Bellin has proposed an intercultural literary criticism of American literature in which, he argues, "it is precisely through intimate, rich, dynamic interactions among multiple peoples that American literature exists at all."[55] I expand Bellin's insights into American texts and the "mutual acculturation" they reflect by showing that, rather than being denied by American literatures, as Bellin argues, intercultural encounters were manifested and acknowledged in colonial medical writing.[56]

Mary Louise Pratt's concepts of the "contact zone" and "transculturation" offer additional possible frameworks for studying the relation between cross-cultural encounters and colonial writing. For Pratt, the term "contact" emphasizes the "interactive, improvisational dimensions of colonial encounters so easily ignored or suppressed by diffusionist accounts of conquest and domination."[57] Yet despite Pratt's acknowledgment throughout *Imperial Eyes* that European travel writing must have been influenced by indigenous interlocutors, she laments that there is no "systematic way to address the extent to which this is so."[58] Her book thus focuses on the ways that Europeans' rhetorical strategies transformed Native and African interlocutors into objects of study and defined European observers as a "self-sufficient, monadic source[s] of knowledge."[59] Pratt writes that the "interactional history of the representation [of Natives or Africans] will turn up only as traces," and she explores transculturation in detail only in the writings of Spanish American creoles.[60] In choosing the term "intercultural" over "transculturation," then, I mean to emphasize the centrality of cross-cultural encounters to medical writing and the fact that Native and African knowledge shaped the very structure of colonial writing rather than appearing only as traces.

Furthermore, I draw on the concept of "interculturalism" as employed in performance studies, in order to emphasize the range of media and forms in which medical knowledge was communicated. In this context, "interculturalism" refers to the "cultural borrowing" that often occurs in the context of unequal power relations and that results in the reconfiguration or translation, by all parties involved in an encounter, of pre-existing concepts in order to explain new contexts.[61] Intercultural processes are neither unifying nor apolitical but involve negotiation on unequal terms; appropriation as well as acculturation; and claims to power alongside the destabilization of that power. As Julie Stone Peters has argued, translation is a necessary condition of communication in the context of cross-cultural encounters, such that "what is lost in translation may be gained in communication."[62] Thus although intercultural processes in the British Americas did take place in contexts of inequality, new meanings were produced by the range of voices speaking from different locations and perspectives.[63] In colonial medical encounters, intercultural texts were created as words, actions, and objects were appropriated from one context into others and as they were endowed with new meanings that were layered over previous significances.

Identifying Difference in Colonial Medical Encounters

The commensurability characterizing medical encounters in the British Americas had not only epistemological but also corporeal foundations. In addition to sharing similar medical cosmologies with Natives and Africans, colonists believed that the New World climate would alter their bodies and minds, making them resemble those of the people indigenous to the Americas and to places characterized by similar climates. As Daniel Carey points out, the "English diagnosed themselves as peculiarly susceptible to change . . . a fact that made travel a social threat."[64] For colonists who traveled to or were born in the Americas, this physical and mental alteration meant that they were likely to process information and produce knowledge in the same ways that Natives and Africans did. From the perspective of Europeans in the Old World, such transformations stood as a sign of colonists' degeneration and of the untrustworthy nature of colonial medical writing. In the sections that follow, I delineate why colonists were so concerned to authorize their medical writing by defining their relation to Natives and Africans in the colonies and to Europeans in the Old World. As I explain, colonists added classificatory literary forms to their medical writing as they explored various ways of differentiating themselves from Natives and Africans and of defending their medical knowledge to European audiences.

Colonists' concerns that their bodies and minds would change in the New World have formed a key part of scholarly discussions on the history of race. Studies of the "dispute of the New World" have shown that colonists in the British and Spanish Americas developed theories of biological difference with the goal of countering European natural philosophers' accusations that colonists degenerated in the New World's environment.[65] Writing of the British context, scholars have posited a key shift at the end of the eighteenth century whereby inherent characteristics and biology replaced environmental and social factors as a cause of difference. Colonists claimed whiteness as a unique trait that set them apart from Natives and Africans and aligned them with Europeans in the Old World. By attending to colonists' sociopolitical motivations for developing theories of difference, these studies have revised older explanations of race as responses to the alleged peculiarity of Natives' and Africans' skin color, behavior, and religion. Instead, early modern conceptions of difference developed as Europeans and colonists revised existing conceptions of bodies and of identity in order to define some traits and physical features as unnatural and others as natural so as to privilege their own identities. Before the end of the eighteenth century, these views of bodies and of skin color originated in ideas about the environment and its influence on the body and on cultural practices, rather than in biological theories of difference as inherent. In the Americas, theories of difference that privileged people of European origin and, eventually, whiteness were thus not responses to empirical observations of Africans' blackness or Natives' tawny skin but a strategy calculated to defend colonists' identities.[66]

The following sections expand these prior studies of the history of race in the Americas by focusing on colonists' concerns regarding the possibility that their mental faculties would change in the New World. In particular, I bring to light colonists' concerns about hot climates, which were believed to characterize the Americas, and anxieties about those climates' effect on colonists' intellectual faculties, especially the imagination. Furthermore, I offer a new analysis of colonists' characterization of Native and African knowledge as witchcraft by showing that such characterizations were motivated by colonists' awareness that they might share mental qualities with Natives and Africans and by their desire to defend their medical knowledge. Although British and U.S. Americans would eventually employ binary conceptions of difference to separate themselves from Natives and Africans, before the end of the eighteenth century colonists employed a triangulated notion of identity by comparing themselves to Natives and Africans on the one hand and to Europeans on the other. Rather than moving in a teleological fashion toward the biological theories of race that would characterize the nineteenth century, theories of difference remained flexible and interchangeable throughout the eighteenth century.[67]

Colonists' concerns that biases regarding knowledge from the British Americas would affect the reception their medical writing received in England were rooted in theories that America's environmental features degenerated Europeans' bodies and minds, subsequently rendering colonial medical knowledge untrustworthy. Europeans believed that travel to and birth in the New World's environment would alter the particular physical and psychological features that defined colonists' identities as English (or Spanish, Portuguese, French, and so on).[68] Such anxieties were authorized by Galenic conceptions of the body as a system whose inner parts were influenced by the environment and by one's management of the non-naturals: air, diet, sleep, movement and rest, retention and evacuation, and the emotions.[69] Early modern medical philosophies usually followed Galenic theories by holding that the environment also determined one's temperament, or the mixture of qualities—hot, cold, moist, and dry—that predominated in the body and that defined physiological and psychological characteristics shared by people inhabiting a specific place. Travel to a different climate would reorder the humors, endowing travelers' temperaments with new, place-specific characteristics. As Jim Egan writes in his study of the implications of travel to the New World, "Losing your place meant, quite literally, losing your identity."[70] Transatlantic travel thus held sobering consequences for English colonists by posing the possibility not only of illness but also of physical and intellectual alteration so significant that one would "remaine at home a stranger."[71]

The humors determined not only physical characteristics but also intellectual strengths and weaknesses, with the result that travel to an unfamiliar climate could alter the form of knowledge one produced. The three intellectual faculties—imagination, memory, and understanding—were each supported by different humors, meaning that people with dissimilar temperaments were thought to "frame different notions of the same things, according as they are conformable or disagreeing to their natures."[72] The imagination collected and gave shape to sensory knowledge, while the memory acted as a storehouse of this knowledge, and the understanding transformed such sensory information into reportable knowledge.[73] The temperament, or one's combination of humors, suited people for expertise in one of these activities. As the Spanish physician Juan Huarte wrote in his well-known and frequently translated treatise on the wits: "*Galen* writ a booke, wherein he prooueth, That the maners of the soule, follow the temperature of the body, in which it keepes residence, and that by reason of the heat, the coldnesse, the moisture, and the drouth, of the territorie where men inhabit, of the meats which they feed on, of the waters which they drinke, and of the aire which they breath: some are blockish, and some wise."[74] The correspondence between the temperament and the mental faculties ensured that climatological and dietary alterations would alter the "maners" of one's mind and, by extension, the knowledge one was capable of producing.[75]

The humoral basis of mental faculties also meant that some temperaments led people to produce irrational, untrustworthy knowledge while others would excel at producing rational knowledge. As Steven Shapin points out:

> environmental theories of human nature occasionally touched upon the coarsening or refining effects of ways of life on the nervous system, and, hence, upon perceptual sensitivity. In addition, there was an even more diffuse sensibility that delusionary tendencies might be differentially distributed among types of human being. Sensations might need to be processed by higher intellectual faculties before they were rendered into properly reportable perceptions.[76]

In such instances, scientific and medical knowledge could be authorized only once it was "processed" by practitioners whose geographic location and corresponding temperament had endowed them with rational intellectual faculties.[77]

According to early modern tripartite geographies, people shaped by the extreme cold temperatures of the north lacked understanding or reason, while those shaped by the extreme heat of the south possessed intelligence but lacked the vigor with which to act on their wisdom. Only people with mental faculties influenced by the temperate regions between the northern and southern extremes possessed both reason and the ability to put it to use.[78] America's place within tripartite geographies was unstable, for theories regarding the nature of the New World's climate were revised several times from the sixteenth to the eighteenth century. One line of argument, going back to classical geographies, posited that the New World lay in the Torrid Zone, the region between the Tropic of Cancer and the Tropic of Capricorn, and as such was uninhabitable. Columbus and the Spanish natural historians who traveled to the New World after him carefully revised this theory to argue that the Americas were both habitable and fertile, but they continued to describe people indigenous to the Caribbean and Spanish America, more broadly, as possessing traits shaped by tropical regions. As a consequence, Columbus could argue not only that "he was about to venture into the most sizable and wealthiest lands of the globe but also that the peoples he would encounter in those latitudes were bound to possess a nature—ranging from 'childish' to 'monstrous'—that seemed to justify rendering them Europe's subjects or slaves."[79]

By the time English colonial ventures began in the late sixteenth century, English colonists feared that the Americas' hot climates would be particularly detrimental to their health and their temperaments. As Mary Floyd-Wilson has explained, English natural philosophers had redefined their cool northern climate as ideal for producing moderate, rational people by contrasting England with tropical locations such as Africa and by arguing that northern rather than Mediterranean climates supported advanced civilizations.[80] This revision placed England in the temperate middle zone, the region that had traditionally been seen as ideal for producing rational intellectual faculties. However, these new geographic hierarchies also raised serious concerns for English colonists traveling to or born in the British Americas, all of which lay in latitudes south of England and which colonists thus expected to be warmer than England. As Karen Ordahl Kupperman notes, "The fear of hot climates was exaggerated in the early years of colonization because Europeans did not realize that the climate of eastern North America was quite different from what their knowledge of climates in comparable latitudes in western Europe led them to expect. Since Newfoundland lies south of London, and Virginia is at the latitude of Spain, promoters expected colonists to face extreme heat in almost all plantations."[81] Colonists even characterized New England's climate as hotter than England's, notwithstanding its name and promotional writers' efforts to assure potential colonists that the climate was similar to England's. For example, the colonist Edward Winslow observed that accounts of New England's climate as similar to England's were contradictory, since New England was located in a lower latitude than England: "Some object, because our Plantation lieth in the latitude of 42 [degrees], it must needs be much hotter."[82] Indeed, promoters went to great lengths to convince their audiences not only that America was habitable but also that its climate would not harm English bodies and minds.[83]

Concerns about hot climates were not quickly resolved but continued to shape British Americans' conceptions of their identities throughout the eighteenth century. By then, it was widely believed that traveling to America would degenerate English colonists' rational mental faculties, although explanations for this degeneration varied. Several conflicting arguments about America's degenerative effects coexisted: one version, popularized by Georges LeClerc, Comte de Buffon, in his *Historie naturelle,* held that America's climate was colder and wetter than Europe's. However, other theories continued the older tradition postulating that the Americas were hotter than Europe, and some writers continued to identify America, along with Asia and Africa, as part of the "Torrid Zone."[84] As a result, as Martin Brückner has explained, eighteenth-century colonists had to "confront the idea, popularized by natural historians and physiocrats, according to which the American continent's southern geographic position (relative to Europe) subjected its occupants to a generally labile environment in which the warmer climate, summers of excessive heat, coastal swamps, and so forth fostered biological and cultural decay."[85]

Descriptions of Native Americans, whose bodies were thought to reflect the long-term effects of America's environmental features, supported theories that the Americas were characterized by hot climates and that these climates would roughen colonists' bodies and alter their minds. Europeans initially believed Natives to be born white and to take on their "tawny" color as a result of their exposure to the elements and their practices of dyeing their bodies.[86] Dionyse Settle, an English gentleman and explorer, reported in 1577 that the Natives' "color is not much unlike the Sunne burnte Countrie man, who laboureth daily in the Sunne for his liuing."[87] Although Settle was traveling in Arctic waters in search of a Northwest Passage, his description of Natives' tawny bodies confirmed expectations that North America's people would reflect the influence of a hot climate. Writing of southern New England

Natives, William Wood explained: "Their swarthiness is the Sun's livery, for they are borne faire."[88] The Natives' transformation from "faire" to "swarth[y]" modeled the physical changes that similarly fair English colonists could expect to undergo.

Colonists also analyzed Natives' religious practices as an indication of the mental faculties that characterized people indigenous to the Americas. The Spanish historian Gonzalo Fernández de Oviedo y Valdés described indigenous people in Spanish America as having weak faculties of the understanding, writing that they were "symple and ignorant people whiche hath smaule defence" against so great an "adversarie as the deuell."[89] Oviedo explained that the Indians were deceived into honoring the devil's powers with blood and human sacrifices because:

> the deuyll beinge so auncient an Astronomer, knowethe the tymes of thynges and seeth howe they are naturally directed and inclined. And makethe theym beleue that they come so to passe by his ordynaunce, as though he were the lorde and mouer of all that is and shall be: And that he gyueth the day lyght and rayne: causeth tempest and ruleth the stations of tymes, gyuying lyfe or takynge awaye at his pleasure.[90]

Natives' "symple" minds, as Nicolás Wey-Gómez has pointed out, justified Europeans' enslavement of Native Americans. These mental traits also marked Natives as lacking the rational faculties that would allow them to resist the devil's deception. Superstition was traditionally a trait of people from southern climates, as Pierre Charron explained when he wrote: "The temperature of the imagination is hot, from whence it commeth that franticke men, and such as are sicke of burning maladies, are excellent in that that belongs to imagination, as *Poetry,* [and] *Divination*"; he further identified "superstitious" as one of the characteristics of people living in southern areas.[91] Colonists' descriptions of Natives' diabolic religious practices thus suggested that their temperaments were influenced by hot environments and, accordingly, that their minds were ruled by fancy and superstition.

Such accounts of Natives' bodies and minds served as mirrors that indicated how colonists might look and think once they had acclimated to America's environment. Indeed, colonists and promotional writers alike admitted that the British American climate changed English travelers' minds along with their bodies. Wood invoked theories of the wits to discuss the "strange" ways that English bodies responded to New England's extreme temperatures, which were both hotter and colder than England's temperatures in the same seasons.[92] He described the mental alteration of a colonist who was "something distracted, [and] broke away from his Keeper" and ran into the woods.[93] After four days of exposure to the elements, however, the man returned and was "in minde much better."[94] Wood's story was consistent with Huarte's account of the mental faculties, according to which humoral alteration—whether due to illness or environmental factors—could reverse one's mental faculties, such that wise men could become foolish, and "simple" people could become wise.[95] The New England environment had so transformed the man's mind that he returned from the woods with completely altered mental faculties—a boon for the distracted, that is, mentally unstable or deranged, man but a sobering fact for colonists traveling to the Americas with rational mental faculties that could be reversed by the hot climate. Similarly, the physician William Vaughan cautioned that an American diet could affect the mind, writing in his book of medical advice for travelers, *The Newlander's Cure,* "Wee must consider, that out of the abundance of meates, which wee receiue into our Bodies, there will arise Vapours from the Stomacke up to the Head, which will darken the Understanding; and also store of Humours and Blood ingendred in the Liver, Melt, and Veines, which will inflame upwards, and helpe with the former Vapours to overcloud the cleare Rayes of Reason and Wisdom."[96] As Ruth Harvey has pointed out, classical medical philosophies posited that when moist humors rose to the brain, they interfered with the reason's ability to control the mind and thus gave the imagination free rein to "make new shapes and forms by combining and separating the images."[97] In this way, vapors gave rise to thoughts that seemed real but were in fact products of the imagination. For colonists, who subsisted on local resources once supplies from Europe were exhausted, the act of eating and drinking American food and water carried the possibility that vapors from the stomach would rise to cloud their faculties of understanding, or reason, thus rendering their medical knowledge irrational and untrustworthy.

Vapors were a source of great concern in the Caribbean: Hans Sloane, a physician and fellow of the Royal Society, described opinions that the air in the West Indies had altered colonists' minds. He explained: "it is thought by some Men, that they are bewitch'd or charm'd by the Air; by others that desire in Women by this heat is Augmented."[98] Although Sloane claimed to be uncertain whether the air actually caused people to become "bewitch'd," he did explain that "The Passions of the Mind have a very great power on Mankind here, especially Hysterical Women, and Hypochondriacal Men. These cannot but have a great share in the cause of several Diseases, some of the People living here being in such Circumstances, as not to be able, to live easily elsewhere."[99] Sloane's comment on the connections between the "Passions of the Mind" and being "bewitch'd or charm'd by the Air" manifested concerns that transatlantic travel or an American birth would alter colonists' minds by degrading their reason and strengthening the faculties of the imagination.[100] As a result, colonists' mental faculties could compromise their medical writing by leaving it open to influence from fancies, irrational ideas, and even diabolic knowledge masquerading as insight into the causes of unfamiliar events. As the Dutch philosopher Cornelius de Pauw wrote of people native or seasoned to America: "climate has governed them full as much as reason."[101] As the climate came to "govern" colonists' mental faculties, their medical knowledge would come to resemble information produced by simple minds and by faculties of the imagination rather than by the rational faculties associated with English climates.[102] Environmental theories of the wits thus made describing New World medicines, cures, and diseases a potentially hazardous enterprise for colonists, one that could raise questions about their intellectual faculties and the reliability of their knowledge.

Climate and Classification

Geographic understandings of colonists' intellectual traits positioned them in a marginal, subordinate position and constrained their ability to speak as equals to British subjects in England. Indeed, British Americans could not always identify with their counterparts in Europe, for colonists were culturally and often geographically positioned between the Native and African peoples they encountered in the New World and Europeans in the Old World.[103] Colonists thus possessed a different relation to western medical knowledge and its production than their counterparts in Europe did. As Michel de Certeau has written, western knowledge is constituted by its relationship to a silenced yet decoded body, "born almost simultaneously from the rift between a subject that is supposedly literate and an object that is supposedly written in an unknown language. The latter always remains to be decoded."[104] In the context of medicine, this object is represented by the patient's body; in the production of western historiography, by the "other," who may be "the Indian, the past, the people, the mad, the child, [or] the Third World."[105] Although colonists in the Americas certainly sought to maintain their identification with their European origins, they could not be certain that their bodies and knowledge, altered by New World climates, would not become the silent, unknown object of study on which philosophers in Europe founded their medical knowledge. Categories of cultural difference in the early Americas were thus not occupied solely by Native and African peoples, for colonists could also occupy these categories. Colonists certainly did not experience these categories and their consequences in the same ways that Natives and Africans did, but they did face the possibility that they would be seen as resembling the people with whom they shared the New World's climate.

Colonists' writing consequently held great importance as a demonstration of whether their humors and intellectual faculties had degenerated. For both colonists and their European audiences, communicating had medical significance. Oral, written, and printed rhetorical strategies all represented the state of the writer's wits, for both speech and actions were considered to be manifestations of the humors. As Thomas Wright explained, just as "leaues, floures, and fruit declare the vertues of trees, so wordes and actions the qualities of minds."[106] Writing, speaking, and acting signaled one's predominant intellectual faculty, thus indicating as well any humoral imbalance or alteration. Thomas Walkington described the rhetorical styles expected of people with various wits: people from the "frozen zone" had "gyantly bodies and yet dwarfish wits" that were "intimated by a vulgar speech,"[107] while people with sanguine temperatures were "very affable in speech, and have a gracious faculty in their delivery, much addicted to witty conceits."[108] "Wordes and actions" acted as signs of the temperament and wits; rhetorical practices were symptoms that visibly reflected inner, hidden characteristics located in the body and mind.[109] Finally, both literary form and style indicated the status of one's wits. For example, colorful or fanciful language could suggest that one's style of writing and speaking had been produced by a strong imagination and that the writer was prone to inflate sensory information.

Colonists thus had to ensure that their literary strategies reflected rational intellectual faculties and that their writing did not indicate that their bodies and minds had degenerated. They responded to metropolitan biases regarding their mental faculties and medical knowledge by revising their accounts of medical encounters. Specifically, they added sections to their fractured *historia* in which they categorized Native and African knowledge as witchcraft. Colonists appended classificatory forms to their texts, and they relocated Native and African medical knowledge from the body of the text to these forms, from catalogs to natural and moral (or cultural) histories. These forms of classification created rhetorical spaces in which colonists could present Native and African knowledge as objects for scrutiny and comparison with colonial medical knowledge.[110] As colonists identified Natives' and Africans' medical knowledge as witchcraft, they defined their own knowledge as Christian and as founded on faculties of the understanding rather than as diabolic knowledge or irrational ideas arising from the imagination. At the same time that they absorbed Native and African knowledge in order to dominate it, classificatory forms ultimately distanced colonists from cross-cultural encounters as well as from the experiences of unfamiliar illness and of the environment that they shared with Natives and Africans.

In the seventeenth century, colonists attributed Natives' medical and religious practices to communications with the devil that, while admittedly effective, were founded in inappropriate, diabolic knowledge that the devil put into Natives' minds. For example, missionary John Wilson stated in one of his tracts promoting Indian missions in New England that the Natives' "*Pawwaws* are great witches having fellowship with the old Serpent, to whom they pray, and by whose means they heale sicke persons."[111] Wilson, like most colonists, noted that *pawwaws* could heal the sick, but he attributed their knowledge of healing strategies to their direct communication with the devil. In this way, colonists made the religious beliefs that they held in common with Europeans across the Atlantic, rather than the environmental factors or illnesses they shared with Natives, key markers of identity. Colonists did not question whether the *pawwaws'* powers were effective but instead marked Native medical knowledge as diabolic and inappropriate.

In the eighteenth century, colonists revised their acknowledgment of witchcraft's efficacy, and they began to attribute both Natives' and Africans' claims that their medical ceremonies were powerful entirely to Natives' and Africans' imaginations in order to deny that they had investigated or credited witchcraft. Moreover, colonists began to describe Natives' and Africans' mental faculties as possessing qualities specific to each group across time and space. They raised the possibility that features specific to Natives and Africans, rather than the environment they shared with colonists, shaped their bodies and minds. For example, the Moravian missionary John

Heckewelder transcribed a conversation he had with a Delaware sachem, "Killbuck," who stated: "'Had the white people sorcerers among them as the Indians have, they would find it necessary to adopt our practice and apply our remedies in the same manner that our doctors do. They would find it necessary to take strong measures to counteract and destroy the dreadful effects of witchcraft.' Heckew: 'The sorcerers you speak of exist only in your imagination; rid yourselves of this, and you will hear no more of them.'"[112] As Heckewelder's comment suggests, colonists attributed "sorcerers'" powers to Natives' and Africans' minds rather than to the diabolic communications of Native or African doctors.[113] Nonetheless, Heckewelder still admitted that "The *Materia Medica* of the Indians consists of various roots and plants known to themselves, the properties of which they are not fond of disclosing to strangers."[114] Even as they argued that some of Natives' and Africans' medical practices originated in the imagination, colonists continued to credit Natives' and Africans' knowledge of natural medicines and healing practices.

Colonists employed classificatory forms to define and maintain the status of Native and African knowledge as irrational and dangerous and in this way to construct differences between colonial medical knowledge and mental faculties, on the one hand, and those belonging to Natives and Africans, on the other. These strategies notwithstanding, British Americans' process of subordinating the knowledge of colonized peoples was ongoing and always incomplete. Colonists were constantly working to maintain the status of Native and African knowledge as superstitious and dangerous, meaning that they had to engage this knowledge, often on its own terms, and that subordinating Native and African knowledge was never inevitable.

Medicine and Magic: Reconsidering Native and African Witchcraft

Colonists' use of classificatory forms to define Native and African knowledge as witchcraft and to respond to metropolitan biases must complicate our understanding of the relationship among colonists and Native and African peoples and of theories of cultural difference in the early Americas. In their influential studies of science and empire in the British Americas, Joyce Chaplin and Susan Scott Parrish have posed answers to the question of why colonists denied parallels between Old and New World medical knowledge by categorizing Native and African knowledge as diabolically informed.[115] In these scholarly accounts, the influence of the British Royal Society and emergent mechanical philosophies, which posited that all natural phenomena were the result of natural causes, acted as key factors that motivated colonists to revise their initial descriptions of Native and African knowledge and to locate differences among colonists, Natives, and Africans. Chaplin argues that New England colonists repudiated Native American knowledge because Natives did not distinguish between matter and spirit and thus appeared to possess "improper views of nature" to colonists who had adopted the Royal Society's view that supernatural forces would not intervene in the natural world.[116] Parrish revised Chaplin's argument that colonists disregarded Native knowledge by showing that "elites in America associated . . . power to manipulate the inspirited natural world with Indians and New World Africans."[117] As a consequence, Parrish argues, both Natives and Africans were seen as valuable resources who could obtain knowledge for colonists, who themselves desired to collect exotic curiosities for their sources in Europe without tainting their transatlantic identities as trustworthy observers. Parrish concludes that colonists associated Natives and Africans with realms of the natural world "deemed 'hidden' or 'secret'" and that they maintained distinctions between colonial and Native or African views of the natural world by refusing to venture into such realms.[118]

But as several historians of science have shown, natural magic and natural philosophy were not opposed forms of knowledge throughout the sixteenth and much of the seventeenth century, even after the formation of the British Royal Society. Far from being routed by the skepticism and materialism associated with the Enlightenment, so-called magical worldviews—such as the acceptance of the existence of demons, of the connections between microcosm and macrocosm, and of harmony in nature—coexisted with and indeed influenced medical philosophies.[119] Magical and natural knowledge were less contrasting viewpoints or "mentalities" than compatible ways of investigating and explaining the world; many philosophers in Europe did not perceive them as opposing or even as separate.[120] Magical worldviews continued to exist on a continuum with so-called scientific practices and to possess authority for colonists in the British Americas, just as they did for Europeans in metropolitan centers of knowledge production.[121]

Consequently, it was not the case that colonists described Native and African medical knowledge as witchcraft because they embraced and imported natural philosophies emanating from Europe or because they found Native and African knowledge to be incompatible with a focus on natural causes and mechanical theories. Instead, colonists classified Native and African knowledge as diabolic, inappropriate magic as part of a defensive strategy with which they hoped to counter metropolitan biases against colonial minds and medical knowledge. This defensive posture, rather than an inability to understand Native and African medical knowledge or a rationalist rejection of those perspectives, was responsible for colonists' descriptions of Native and African medical knowledge as witchcraft.[122] The connections between Native and African knowledge and witchcraft were thus less the result of the "decline of magic,"[123] the triumph of mechanical philosophies, or a "racial idiom" than the consequence of colonists' attempts to interpret Native and African medical knowledge in cross-cultural encounters and simultaneously to avoid accusations that their mental faculties had degenerated in the New World environment.[124] Colonists employed classificatory forms to make religion and learning, rather than the environment, the foundation of identity, in order to reshape the cultural categories into which the American environment placed them. Distancing themselves from encounters with Native and African knowledge allowed colonists to create cultural connections and categories that extended across the Atlantic and that increasingly excluded Natives and Africans.

Colonists' concern regarding their relation both to Natives and Africans and to Europeans in the metropolis thus points to the ways in which categories of cultural difference were unstable and transformable in the early modern Atlantic world. As Roxann Wheeler has noted in her study of race in the eighteenth century, "Skin color was not the only—or even primary—register of human difference for much of the eighteenth century, and climate was not the only factor believed to shape appearance and influence behavior."[125] The following chapters trace the ways in which ideas about intellectual faculties and their transformation due to environmental influences were the site of debates about cultural difference before skin color and biological theories of race became standard explanations of identity. Categories of difference based on origin and allegedly innate characteristics developed unevenly and sometimes coexisted with environmental theories of difference as colonists sought to reshape the cultural categories they occupied as a consequence of their exposure to or birth in the American environment. Distancing themselves from encounters with Native and African knowledge allowed colonists to create cultural connections and categories that highlighted relations between colonial and European medical knowledge and mental faculties, regardless of environmental factors.

Finally, *Medical Encounters* attests to the importance of considering colonial conceptions of identity from the sixteenth to the eighteenth century. This long historical view foregrounds the commensurability that often characterized colonial encounters and that colonists only slowly and unevenly denied. It avoids reading accounts of Native and African knowledge as witchcraft as characteristic of colonists' views of Native and African medicine by instead showing the process whereby these conceptions were standardized. Moreover, this perspective highlights the fact that theories of difference were not stable and that they did not move in a teleological fashion toward recognizably modern biological articulations of race, as shown in chapter 5's discussion of the coexistence of environmental and biological theories of cultural difference. These theories developed in a peripatetic fashion, as colonists experimented with various strategies for understanding their bodies and identities in relation to the American climate and to the other peoples who shared that same environment. This is not to suggest that environmental theories of difference were kinder to Natives and Africans than biological theories of race but rather to stress that unique communications and exchanges were possible when colonists shared an environment with Natives and Africans that, they believed, would transform their minds and bodies to resemble those of Natives and Africans. The idea that identity was flexible and alterable was built into environmental theories of identity, and this flexibility meant that colonists, Natives, and Africans could possess the same mental faculties and, consequently, the same medical knowledge.

As *Medical Encounters* shows, colonial medical writing is characterized by rhetorical discontinuities: shifts from *historia* to non-narrative literary strategies and finally to classificatory forms. These formal irregularities indicate the ways in which experiences of cross-cultural encounter were incorporated into the rhetorical strategies of colonial texts. Just as important, the "texture" that distinguishes colonial medical writing points beyond the printed, published versions of colonial texts to the spoken and performative exchanges of medical knowledge among colonists, Natives, and Africans—exchanges that shaped colonists' printed texts.[126] As intercultural texts, colonial medical writing manifests medical knowledge belonging not only to colonists but also to Natives and Africans, and it suggests the ways in which people employed medical knowledge to address challenging, unfamiliar situations that arose in the New World. Colonial medical writing consequently points to the dangers of reducing Natives and Africans to rhetorical figures within colonial texts or to representations of colonial strategies of appropriation and dispossession. By seeing accounts of Natives and Africans primarily as the repercussion of colonial strategies, we overlook colonists' acknowledgments of the intercultural encounters that shaped their writing. I would not presume to speak for the Natives and Africans (or for colonists, for that matter) who transmitted their medical knowledge in the sixteenth, seventeenth, and eighteenth centuries, but I would argue that we cannot view colonial medical writing solely as the product of Euro-American discourses. Instead, *Medical Encounters* draws on textual analysis as well as on ethnohistorical and anthropological studies to examine the ways in which colonial medical writing was constituted by medical knowledge from multiple sources and perspectives.

The chapters that follow trace the ways in which early American medical writing represented encounters among Natives, Africans, and colonists and their medical knowledges. In addition, they examine colonists' attempts to efface the experiences of encounter they shared with Natives and Africans by categorizing their medical knowledge in classificatory forms. Chapter 1 analyzes Thomas Harriot's 1588 description of disease as "invisible bullets" during a mysterious 1586 epidemic that affected the Roanoke but spared the English. I depart from previous scholars' focus on Harriot's European influences to explain his representation of the illness; instead, I examine heretofore overlooked linguistic and ethnohistorical evidence, which suggests that Roanoke theories of disease contributed to the content and form of Harriot's *Briefe and True Report of the New Found Land of Virginia*. First, Native theories that supernatural entities, sometimes called thunder-beings, shot diseases into people and linguistic connections between Algonquian words for shooting a gun and shooting thunderbolts show how the Roanoke employed pre-existing medical knowledge to attribute their illness to the colonists' military technology. Second, although he has been virtually ignored by literary scholars, Harriot's fellow colonist Ralph Lane also reported that the Roanoke characterized the disease as bullets, a fact that suggests both men recorded Roanoke medical knowledge. While Lane subordinated Roanoke knowledge to foreground a providential theory of disease familiar to his readers, Harriot, by contrast, presented the Roanokes' invisible-bullets theory as a strategy for understanding the illness. Harriot's alchemical interests and knowledge of Paracelsian medical philosophies, which conceptualized disease as the result of chemical explosions similar to gunshots, provided a foundation for understanding the Algonquians' "invisible bullets" theory, yet also suggested that he had investigated New World medical knowledge to control the secret causes of disease. Harriot addressed such concerns by cataloging Virginian medicines, in this way transforming his observations of the Algonquians' medical knowledge into descriptions of useful commodities.

As the Roanoke Algonquians drew connections among colonization, guns, and illness, so in New England the Patuxet Indian and translator Tisquantum attributed contact-era epidemics to the Pilgrims, stating that they kept disease in their storehouse for gunpowder. This claim positioned Tisquantum as a *powah,* a man with significant powers as a healer and a political mediator. The Pilgrim Edward Winslow also assumed this position when he cured the Wampanoag sachem Massasoit of an apparently fatal illness. In an account of these healing practices in *Good Newes from New England* (1624), Winslow initially employed narrative forms to link his administration of English medicine to Massasoit's improved state. However, he transformed this narrative into a recipe when he turned to Wampanoag medical knowledge in order to concoct a broth that healed Massasoit. Ultimately, however, Winslow distanced himself from the repercussions of imitating *powahs'* medical practices by classifying Algonquian medical knowledge as witchcraft in a moral (or cultural) history of New England Natives.

Chapters 3 and 4 consider eighteenth-century encounters between colonists and Africans, in which colonists adapted the rhetorical practices they had previously employed to incorporate and classify Native knowledge. The physicians William Douglass and James Grainger drew on and developed earlier accounts of Natives' faculties of the imagination as inclining them to accept knowledge from diabolic sources in order to argue that Africans' similarly strong imaginations inclined them to give supernatural forces credit for mysterious medical phenomena that, in reality, had hidden natural causes. Furthermore, these chapters trace how colonists began to define difference as rooted in mental characteristics traceable to one's place of origin, rather than in religious practices. Chapter 3 examines the status of African medical knowledge during the 1721 Boston inoculation controversy, a debate regarding the safety of the preventive treatment for smallpox. Enslaved Africans brought knowledge of inoculation from Africa to the Americas, where some of them informed colonists of the treatment, as minister Cotton Mather's slave Onesimus did. As many studies have shown, Mather and William Douglass hotly disputed the efficacy of inoculation. As this chapter points out, however, the men shared a position of cultural and epistemological distance from metropolitan medical and philosophical societies: Mather because he was born in the colonies and Douglass because as a Scot who immigrated to Boston, he was doubly distanced from European centers of knowledge production. And—an important point—both men attempted to determine how medical communications—both the transmission of smallpox virus during inoculations and African testimony about inoculation—circulated in Boston. Mather presented Onesimus as a simple, yet wise witness, and he promoted Africans' testimony as evidence that inoculation was a providential gift to colonists. By contrast, Douglass attempted to control what he saw as unruly medical communications by tracking them in a history of the epidemic and by defining African knowledge as witchcraft. Later, in his 1749 history of the colonies, Douglass revised his earlier description of African medical knowledge by classifying it not as witchcraft but as poisonous herbal knowledge in order to display his ability to locate rational causes for unusual medical phenomena. Yet Mather and Douglass did not entirely control African testimony: as this chapter shows, communicating information about inoculation could have endowed Onesimus with medical authority and brought about his manumission.

Just as Africans in Boston developed methods for surreptitiously communicating knowledge of inoculation, enslaved Africans in the Caribbean employed secret medical practices to resist slavery and foster rebellion, as I show by reading James Grainger's 1764 georgic poem *The Sugar-Cane* in the context of a 1760 slave revolt inspired by obeah, interconnected medical and religious practices. The poem manifested colonists' fear and anxiety regarding rebellion, for Grainger departed from the georgic's traditional agricultural narrative of planting, cultivation, and harvest by substituting images of African bodies and medical practices for the conventional account of peaceful estates. Although Grainger poetically described the frightening effects obeah had on both Africans and colonists, in a footnote to these verses he acknowledged that obeah men could serve a useful role on plantations. Yet he ultimately attributed trust in obeah's power to Africans' underdeveloped mental faculties and finally to their Old World African environments. In this way, he posited that colonists and Africans possessed different mental capacities, despite the fact that they were both exposed to the Caribbean environment. Shortly thereafter, Grainger rewrote his georgic as a natural history of disease, in which he erased African knowledge from his descriptions of tropical diseases.

Chapter 5 concludes the book by considering medical exchanges in a global context that connects New England and the South Seas. It departs from prior chapters by foregrounding texts written by Native Americans, particularly Samson Occom, the Mohegan Indian and Presbyterian minister, and by showing how Occom contested colonists' classifications of indigenous peoples as irrational and heathen. Occom revised the differences that colonists had created between their own behavior and that of Native Americans by rewriting contemporary accounts of James Cook's 1768–1771 travels to Tahiti and a subsequent outbreak of syphilis, which colonists blamed on the Tahitians' licentious actions. As Occom showed, colonists' sexual behavior could be included in the same categories they employed to describe the Tahitians' allegedly lascivious customs. By participating in debates regarding the American origins of syphilis, Occom defended the behavior and intellectual faculties of peoples born in places believed to have hot climates, from Tahiti to the Americas. In this way, he also showed that Natives in New England were not inherently prone to drink alcohol to excess but, like colonists, became drunk by making a series of decisions. Finally, he suggested a cure of love for intemperate behavior and the moral and physical diseases it caused; this cure healed both bodies and minds by requiring people to transform their behavior. Occom's medical writing ultimately restored colonists to narratives of encounter, and his global perspective required new ways of acting and of interacting with others on the part of Natives and colonists alike.

CHAPTER 1

Epidemic, Encounter, and Colonial Promotion in Virginia

Invisible Bullets and Early American Colonization

IN 1585, SIR Walter Ralegh sent an expedition to the "new found land of Virginia" with Queen Elizabeth's nominal support and the use of her pinnace.[1] The colony of several hundred men was England's first attempt to establish a permanent settlement in the Americas, although Ralegh also directed the men to search for gold and a northwest passage that would provide a western route to East Indian ports. After a stop in the West Indies, where some of the men picked up sugar cane and plantains they hoped to cultivate in Virginia, the colonists landed in present-day North Carolina, or, as the Carolina Algonquians called their land, Ossomocomuck.[2] There the English colonists established trading relations with the Roanoke Algonquians and their *werowance,* or leader, Wingina.[3] Several colonists also observed the land and the Roanoke peoples, for Ralegh had commissioned the mathematician Thomas Harriot and the painter John White to map Virginia's coastline and to survey local resources.[4] Harriot published some of his findings in 1588: his *Briefe and True Report of the New Found Land of Virginia* presented some of the earliest descriptions of the Carolina Algonquians and of Virginia's natural resources.[5]

The *Report* is best known today for its description of the Roanoke Algonquians' explanation of a mysterious illness, which broke out among the Natives but left the colonists unscathed. As Harriot wrote, the Roanokes attributed the disease to "invisible bullets," and, he explained, "Those that were immediately to come after vs they imagined to be in the aire, yet inuisible & without bodies, & that they by our intreaty & for the loue of vs did make the people to die in that sort as they did by shooting inuisible bullets into them" (29). Both literary scholars and historians have observed that Harriot's description of the Roanokes' theory of disease as caused by "invisible bullets" was at odds with prevailing Galenic medical philosophies, which conceptualized illnesses not as discrete entities that entered and diseased the body but rather as interior conditions or imbalances stimulated by the environment.[6] To explain this incompatibility, scholars have identified alternative contexts that could have shaped Harriot's description of disease as "bullets." Stephen Greenblatt argues that Harriot described the epidemic and the Roanokes' responses in order to test theories about the political uses of religious power, theories seen as heterodox in England. Greenblatt suggests that Harriot recorded "alien voices" in order to document potentially subversive perspectives that justified the deployment of colonial power, and that attested to the superiority of English culture.[7] This recording ultimately solidified Harriot's "hypothesis about the origin and nature of European culture and belief," in this way allowing him to produce knowledge about European beliefs for European readers.[8]

Joyce Chaplin has revised Greenblatt's analysis by placing Harriot's account of the "invisible bullets" in the context of early modern natural philosophy (29). She focuses in particular on Harriot's interest in atomism, a controversial theory that "matter was composed of discrete, durable particles," similar to bullets.[9] Chaplin argues that Harriot placed a description of "natural phenomena being formed of distinct particles" in the Roanoke Algonquians' mouths in order to explore such ideas without being directly associated with them.[10] Rather than reporting actual Native ideas or words, Harriot attributed his own ideas to Native sources in order to avoid accusations of impiety and to contribute to scientific conversations among Europeans.

Both of these previous studies show how European religious and scientific debates, respectively, informed Harriot's account of the Carolina Algonquians' illness, but they occlude the cross-cultural contexts in which Harriot's *Report* was produced.[11] Philosophical and religious theories from Europe were not the only concepts available to Harriot to describe the mysterious epidemic, nor were Algonquian voices "alien" to Harriot by the time he wrote the *Report*.[12] He had observed the Carolina Algonquians' medical knowledge and practices during his time in Ossomocomuck, as he and colonist John White traveled throughout the area to document its peoples, flora, and fauna. Given their ignorance of the geography prior to 1585, it is extremely unlikely that Harriot and White traveled alone; Roanoke guides probably accompanied the men and determined where they went and what they observed on their expeditions. Harriot also reported having "special familiarity" (26) with the Roanoke priests, and as I discuss in more detail below, he smoked tobacco after the Roanokes' "maner" [*sic*] (16).

Furthermore, Harriot and representatives of the Roanoke Algonquians had multiple occasions to encounter one another's medical knowledge even before Harriot arrived in Ossomocomuck. Two of Ralegh's men, Arthur Barlowe and Philip Amadas, had made a reconnaissance voyage to Ossomocomuck in 1584; they returned with two Algonquian men, whom the English identified as Wanchese and Manteo. It is probable that the Roanoke *werowance* Wingina sent Manteo, son of the *weroansqua* (or female leader) on Croatoan Island, and Wanchese, probably an advisor to Wingina, to London as envoys and as intelligence gatherers.[13] Manteo and Wanchese lived at Durham House, Ralegh's house on the Strand, where they worked with Harriot to learn English and where he created a phonetic alphabet for Algonquian.[14] The men also provided information to Harriot and Ralegh useful for planning the 1585 voyage to Virginia, and they were displayed throughout London as a means of eliciting support for Ralegh's voyages.

Finally, even before the Roanoke voyages, the English had encountered indigenous representatives from the New World and had observed or heard about their illnesses and deaths. By the time Barlow returned with Manteo and Wanchese, several Inuit people from Baffin Island had already traveled to England with the Arctic explorer Martin Frobisher in 1576 and 1577. All the Inuit people died within a few weeks of reaching England, one from a disease apparently contracted on the transatlantic voyage; another, a man given the name Calichough, from a wounds caused by a "Cornishe tricke" (or wrestling move) one of the colonists used to capture him; and a woman and child, given the names Egnock and Nutioc, possibly from measles.[15] European audiences across the social spectrum would have been familiar with the Inuit visitors, their bodies, sicknesses, and responses to death as a result of widely circulating images of the captives. John White painted several images of Calichough, Egnock, and Nutioc, while the Flemish painter Cornelis Ketel produced a postmortem painting of the Inuit man who returned with Frobisher's 1576 voyage and five paintings of Calichough, including one of him naked. In addition, the physician Edward Dodding performed an autopsy on Calichough; he made Egnock observe this investigation before including her response in his report. By 1585, then, just ten years after the first Inuit man had visited London, the English public—and certainly someone like Harriot, who had trained navigators for Ralegh's New World ventures and who was well read in the narratives of New World travels—were not strangers to Native peoples' bodies, knowledge, and languages, especially those of the Roanoke Algonquians.[16]

Debates over Harriot's European sources have overlooked both his preexisting awareness of Algonquian peoples, languages, and knowledge and the shared medical knowledge that circulated in cross-cultural encounters and contributed to the account of invisible bullets in the *Report.* Conceptions of disease as an ontological entity were already circulating throughout both America and Europe before contact in Virginia, as I show by examining Native theories that disease originated outside the body, in bullet-like objects sent by divine beings, and by investigating Harriot's interest in Paracelsian medical philosophies, which included a "gunpowder theory" of disease.[17] While Harriot's, Manteo's, and Wanchese's respective knowledge of one another's languages and cultures was unlikely to have been perfect or exhaustive, their sustained conversations and their shared conceptions of disease made it possible for communication about illness and its causes to take place.

Descriptions of the illness as bullets originated in encounters with the Roanoke Algonquians and possibly developed in conversations between colonists, as this chapter shows by comparing the *Report* with a second, but often overlooked, description of the epidemic by Ralph Lane, governor of the colony, in his "Account of the Particularities of the Imployments of the English Men Left in Virginia." Lane wrote the preface to the 1588 publication of Harriot's *Report,* a fact that suggests at least some exchange between the men about their reports. A professional soldier with experience fighting in England's campaigns to control Ireland, Lane did not share Harriot's philosophical interests, but his description of the epidemic is nonetheless quite similar to Harriot's. As I detail below, Lane's and Harriot's accounts both fractured as a result of their encounters with the Roanoke Algonquians, but they did so for different reasons. Lane presented the Algonquians' theories of disease as evidence of the colony's potential by attempting to insert these theories into his narrative of discovery, only to find that Wingina controlled what the colonists discovered and how area Algonquians treated them. Meanwhile, Harriot departed from his narrative of disease by listing the invisible bullets-theory among other possible explanations of the illness. His apparent uncertainty regarding the disease's cause manifested his desire to promote colonization in Virginia and to assure readers that the New World environment had not degenerated colonists' bodies. Yet because Harriot's observation of and participation in Roanoke medical and religious practices threatened to alter his mental faculties and support his reputation for investigating heterodox knowledge, he ultimately employed his catalog of commodities to distance himself from his observation of and participation in the Roanokes' medical practices.

Providential Bullets

Initially a private report for Ralegh, Lane's "Account" defended his failure to find either a northwest passage or gold as well as his decision that the colonists should abandon the settlement and return to England with Sir Francis Drake.[18] Lane argued that he had fulfilled his duties as well as possible in difficult circumstances, which included Spanish threats, insufficient food supplies, and, he believed, a conspiracy against the English and false information about the location of gold mines from the Algonquians. He mitigated his own and the colony's failures by employing a narrative form to give undesired events purpose and meaning as signs of future success. The narrative records Lane's movement from "discovery" to "departure," but it is at times structured less by actual experiences than by Ralegh's instructions and expectations of Virginia.[19] Finding gold elusive and Virginia's geography and inhabitants different from his expectations, Lane nevertheless attempted to construct a narrative of discovery by imagining how he would have found a northwest passage and mine if circumstances had been different. He employed a conditional tense that made discovery hover on the horizon, requiring only support from England to be realized: he wrote that if only Ralegh "had" sent necessary supplies, the expedition "would have" set off.[20] Even the Roanokes were incorporated into the narrative; they stood ready to supply guides with whom Lane "would have gone up to the head of the river."[21] Lane's narrative gave real and imagined experiences in Virginia meaning as promise of future discovery. In his "Account," attaching narrative forms to disappointing or confusing experiences transformed them into signs of future satisfaction, in this way rhetorically fulfilling Ralegh's instructions.

Lane presented the Algonquians' medical knowledge as supporting his narrative of English discovery, just as he portrayed Algonquian guides as willing to direct the colonists to gold mines. He explained that an elderly and influential Roanoke advisor, Ensenore, said that the English were "the seruants of God, and that wee were not subject to bee destroyed by them: but contrariwise, that they amongst them that sought our destruction, shoulde finde their owne, [and] that they have bene in the night, being 100 miles from any of us, in the ayre shot at, and stroken by some men of ours, that by sicknesse had dyed among them."[22] Like Harriot, Lane described the Algonquians' belief that the colonists were powerful beings with the authority to send disease, and he, too, reported that the Roanokes perceived disease as an entity separate from bodies, which affected people by traveling from place to place and spreading when the English shot at them.

Lane located his account of the epidemic in the context of tensions between the colonists and Wingina, tensions that disrupted his narrative and that exposed Lane's lack of control over area politics, food supplies, and communication. The disease broke out in the midst of a debate among the Roanoke regarding the nature of the colonists' intentions and whether to allow them to stay in the area. Both Manteo and Wanchese seem to have concluded that the colonists had significant power on the basis of their experiences in England, but they came to different answers to the question of how to respond to that power. Manteo seems to have decided that the Roanoke Algonquians could make use of English power and an alliance with the colonists, while Wanchese came to the opposite conclusion, one that motivated him to counsel Wingina to refuse the colonists sustenance and assistance.[23] At the same time, Lane himself was mired in considerable confusion regarding which of the Algonquian leaders—and their accounts of friendly or hostile groups—he could trust. When he traveled inland, he found that Wingina had already sent word that the colonists had malevolent intentions to the Choanists and Mangoaks, who were "dismay[ed]" at Lane's arrival.[24] He further discovered that he could not tell signs of welcome from those of aggression: he explained that while on his journey, "certaine Savages . . . presently began a song, as we thought, in token of our welcome to them: but Manteo presently betooke him to his piece, and tolde mee that they meant to fight with us."[25] Finally, as Lane explained, while he was delayed on an expedition, Wingina circulated rumors that Lane had died of starvation and that the English god was consequently not powerful. Lane's attempts to create a narrative of success were disrupted by Wingina's superior control of local politics and of Native communication networks.

In Lane's "Account," Ensenore's explanation of the epidemic as "destruction" on the Algonquians for disobeying "the servants of God" refuted Wingina's rumors regarding Lane and the English god, and Lane's subsequent return further supported this interpretation of the colonists.[26] Furthermore, Lane concluded his account of the Algonquians' illness by calling the disease the "good prouidence of the Almightie for the sauing of us."[27] Citing a providential cause allowed Lane to position both the illness and Ensenore's invisible-bullets theory as evidence of the colonists' connection to powerful spiritual beings who supported their endeavors. Within Lane's narrative, the Algonquians' disease and medical knowledge pointed readers toward a satisfying conclusion in which English colonists, protected by providence, would overcome hardships to establish the colony. The narrative provided a familiar providential explanation for unfamiliar illnesses, in this way assuring readers of the colonists' moral and cultural superiority.

Yet while Lane returned to his narrative to conclude his account of the Roanokes' illness and to regain rhetorical authority, his "Account" continued to be riddled with confusion and disorder. Ensenore seems to have employed the theory of disease to emphasize his interpretation of the colonists to other Roanokes, particularly Wingina, who was beginning to adopt an unsympathetic stance toward the colonists. But as subsequent events proved, neither Ensenore nor Lane controlled phenomena and their interpretations: Ensenore died shortly after describing the illness, and Wingina successfully created a pan-tribal alliance that opposed the English. And, after initially providing the colonists with corn and fish, Wingina removed his people from Roanoke Island to an inland camp where he prepared to plant corn but refused to supply the colonists, in this way foiling their appropriation of the Algonquians' food supply and all but dooming them to starvation.[28] When Lane, fearing starvation and an attack, decided to attack the Roanokes preemptively, Wingina even eluded execution for a time: Lane explained that Wingina was "shot thorow" with a pistol and appeared dead before "he started up, and ran away as though he had not bene touched, insomuch as he overran all the companie."[29] Lane and a few other men ran after Wingina, only to lose him in the woods before

Lane's "Irish boy," Edward Nugent, managed to behead the *werowance*.[30] Lane added his providential explanation in an attempt to present the Roanokes' illness as evidence of the colonists' future success, but his narrative further degenerates into chaos, miscommunication, and violence before concluding with an account of why the colonists finally abandoned the colony. Thus while Lane did attempt to "attach" his narrative of success to unfamiliar and disappointing experiences, studies that focus only on colonists' use of familiar literary forms in the New World do not account for the moments when Natives' actions thwarted colonists' attempts to provide order to their experiences.[31] Lane's narrative offers insight into the Algonquians' responses to the colonists and into both parties' attempts to decipher rumors and determine the other's intent.

Lane's "Account" shows that the invisible-bullets theory was neither unique nor produced solely by Harriot's heterodox philosophical interests; instead, this medical knowledge may be traced to encounters in the New World. At the same time, comparing Lane's and Harriot's writings attests to the fact that not all colonists interpreted their encounters with Native or African medical knowledge in the same way: as I explain below, Harriot's interest in theories of disease as originating outside the body endowed the invisible-bullets theory with significance for different reasons from those that motivated Lane to include the theory in his "Account." In addition, Lane's aggressive behavior seems also to have at least partially influenced how the Roanoke treated him, and his military background, his experiences in Ireland, and his duties as governor in Virginia informed his response to and analysis of encounters in Ossomocomuck. By contrast, as I explain below, Harriot's medical and natural philosophical interests not only inclined him to consult with Roanoke priests but also meant that he understood the invisible-bullets theory in a different context than Lane did, a context that made the Roanokes' explanation of disease a paradoxically viable yet dangerous explanation for disease in Virginia and for defending English bodies that came into close contact with Virginia's environment.

A "disease so strange": Illness and Narrative in Harriot's Report

While Harriot's and Lane's accounts of the Algonquians' medical knowledge share similar content, Harriot structured his *Report* quite differently from Lane's "Account." The *Report*'s first two sections consist of lists of natural resources and the commodities into which colonists would transform them; they promoted the colony's flora and fauna to potential investors and settlers. In 1588, when the first edition of the *Report* was published, the list of commodities was still a relatively new form with which to describe and promote the New World, and Harriot's *Report* was one of the first English promotional texts to employ a list in this way. His third section is more characteristic of the travel narratives and ethnographic descriptions that often appeared in early modern writing about the New World. The third section departs from the catalog of commodities to offer descriptions of the Roanokes' "nature and manners," from their clothing, to their towns, houses, political structure, and religious beliefs (22). While he focused solely on descriptions of objects in the first two sections, Harriot altered his perspective and the *Report*'s form in the third section, for he represented conversations and interactions with the Roanoke in which he obtained information about their culture. For example, he presented their beliefs and practices as dialogue by repeating the phrase "they say," and he detailed his attempts to explain English technology and religion to the Roanokes (25).

In this third section, Harriot employed the narrative strategies of *historia* to relate information about the Roanokes' illness, specifically, to construct connections between the Algonquians' illness and colonial encounters. *Historia* were frequently employed in Europe to connect symptoms of disease with a cause by establishing temporal or logical relations between illness and cause. Harriot was educated at Oxford in the 1570s, and although he was trained as a mathematician, he had wide-ranging interests that included medicine; his familiarity with Nicolás Monardes's *Historia medicinal,* which Harriot cited in the *Report,* and other medical texts meant that he had already encountered the form of the *historia* before traveling to Ossomocomuck.[32] Harriot drew on *historia* to connect the Roanokes' disease with a cause when he explained, "There was no towne where we had any subtile deuice practised against vs, we leauing it vnpunished or not reuenged (because wee sought by all meanes possible to win them by gentlenesse) but that within a few dayes after our departure from euerie such towne, the people began to die very fast" (28). In this description, he placed the colonists' visits to Algonquian towns in a narrative sequence with the Algonquians' illness, in this way connecting the visits with the subsequent deaths. The *historia* positions the colonists' arrivals and the Algonquians' "subtile deuice" as causes for the illness (28).[33] But unlike Lane, Harriot did not conclude his narrative by incorporating a familiar cause of disease such as providence or climatological factors. He left his narrative of encounter and illness incomplete, for he did not identify one cause for the epidemic. Instead, he admitted that both the colonists and the Algonquians found the disease "so strange" and unprecedented that they were mutually uncertain regarding how to explain it (28). Rather than concluding with an identification of the disease's cause, he listed the Algonquians' various explanations of the disease, including the invisible-bullets theory. He wrote:

> Some therefore were of opinion that wee were not borne of women, and therefore not mortall, but that wee were men of an old generation many yeeres past then risen againe to immortalitie.
>
> Some woulde likewise seeme to prophesie that there were more of our generation yet to come, to kill theirs and take their places, as some thought the purpose was by that which was already done.
>
> Those that were immediately to come after vs they imagined to be in the aire, yet inuisible & without bodies, & that they by our intreaty & for the loue of vs did make the people to die in that sort as they did by shooting inuisible bullets into them. . . .
>
> Some also thought that we shot them ourselues out of our pieces from the place where we dwelt, and killed the people in any such towne that had offended vs as we listed, how farre distant from vs soeuer it were.
>
> And some other saide that it was the speciall woorke of God for our sakes, as wee ourselves have cause in some sorte to think no lesse. (29) (Figure 1)

Harriot had earlier called the disease an "accident," in this way designating it as an event that lacked an apparent or known cause, and his list of the Algonquians' multiple explanations for the disease reflects the confusion that both he and they seem to have felt (28).[34] The form of the list frustrates any attempt to connect the disease to a cause, for the list accumulates numerous theories of disease without authorizing any one. Harriot neither drew causal connections among the listed theories nor privileged his own conclusion at the end of the list, unlike Lane, who had attached a providential explanation to Ensenore's explanation of the Algonquians' disease. Harriot only noted tentatively that the colonists had some reason to agree with the Algonquians' suggestion that the disease might have a metaphysical cause. His list of possible explanations for disease thus represented the Algonquians' conception of the English as unusual, powerful people, and it

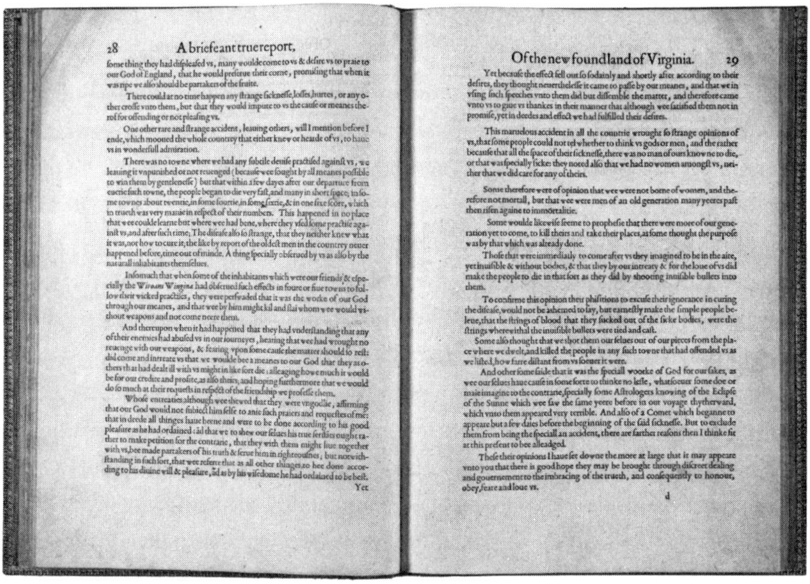

28 A briefe and true report,

ſome thing they had diſpleaſed vs, many woulde come to vs & deſire vs to praie to our God of England, that he would preſerue their corne, promiſing that when it was ripe we alſo ſhould be partakers of the fruite.

There could at no time happen any ſtrange ſickneſſe, loſſes, hurtes, or any other croſſe vnto them, but that they would impute to vs the cauſe or meanes therof for offending or not pleaſing vs.

One other rare and ſtrange accident, leauing others, will I mention before I ende, which mooued the whole countrey that either knew or hearde of vs, to haue vs in wonderfull admiration.

There was no towne where we had any ſubtile deuiſe practiſed againſt vs, we leauing it vnpuniſhed or not reuenged (becauſe wee ſought by all meanes poſſible to win them by gentleneſſe) but that within a few dayes after our departure from euerie ſuch towne, the people began to die very faſt, and many in ſhort ſpace; in ſome townes about twentie, in ſome fourtie, in ſome ſixtie, & in one ſixe ſcore, which in trueth was very manie in reſpect of their numbers. This happened in no place that wee coulde learne but where wee had bene, where they vſed ſome practiſe againſt vs, and after ſuch time; The diſeaſe alſo ſo ſtrange, that they neither knew what it was, nor how to cure it; the like by report of the oldeſt men in the countrey neuer happened before, time out of minde. A thing ſpecially obſerued by vs as alſo by the naturall inhabitants themſelues.

Inſomuch that when ſome of the inhabitants which were our friends & eſpecially the *Wiroans Wingina* had obſerued ſuch effects in foure or fiue towns to follow their wicked practiſes, they were perſwaded that it was the worke of our God through our meanes, and that wee by him might kil and ſlai whom wee would without weapons and not come neere them.

And thereupon when it had happened that they had vnderſtanding that any of their enemies had abuſed vs in our iourneyes, hearing that wee had wrought no reuenge with our weapons, & fearing vpon ſome cauſe the matter ſhould ſo reſt: did come and intreate vs that we woulde bee a meanes to our God that they as others that had dealt ill with vs might in like ſort die; alleaging howe much it would be for our credite and profite, as alſo theirs; and hoping furthermore that we would do ſo much at their requeſts in reſpect of the friendship we profeſſe them.

Whoſe entreaties although wee ſhewed that they were vngodlie, affirming that our God would not ſubiect him ſelfe to anie ſuch praiers and requeſtes of mē: that in deede all thinges haue beene and were to be done according to his good pleaſure as he had ordained: ād that we to ſhew our ſelues his true ſeruãts ought rather to make petition for the contrarie, that they with them might liue together with vs, bee made partakers of his truth & ſerue him in righteouſnes; but notwithſtanding in ſuch ſort, that wee referre that as all other thinges, to bee done according to his diuine will & pleaſure, ād as by his wiſedome he had ordained to be beſt.

Yet

Of the new found land of Virginia. 29

Yet becauſe the effect fell out ſo ſodainly and ſhortly after according to their deſires, they thought neuertheleſſe it came to paſſe by our meanes, and that we in vſing ſuch ſpeeches vnto them did but diſſemble the matter, and therefore came vnto vs to giue vs thankes in their manner that although wee ſatiſfied them not in promiſe, yet in deedes and effect we had fulfilled their deſires.

This marueilous accident in all the countrie wrought ſo ſtrange opinions of vs, that ſome people could not tel whether to think vs gods or men, and the rather becauſe that all the ſpace of their ſickneſſe, there was no man of ours knowne to die, or that was ſpecially ſicke: they noted alſo that we had no women amongſt vs, neither that we did care for any of theirs.

Some therefore were of opinion that wee were not borne of women, and therefore not mortall, but that wee were men of an old generation many yeeres paſt then riſen againe to immortalitie.

Some woulde likewiſe ſeeme to propheſie that there were more of our generation yet to come, to kill theirs and take their places, as ſome thought the purpoſe was by that which was already done.

Thoſe that were immediatly to come after vs they imagined to be in the aire, yet inuiſible & without bodies, & that they by our intreaty & for the loue of vs did make the people to die in that ſort as they did by ſhooting inuiſible bullets into them.

To confirme this opinion their phiſitions to excuſe their ignorance in curing the diſeaſe, would not be aſhamed to ſay, but earneſtly make the ſimple people beleue, that the ſtrings of blood that they ſucked out of the ſicke bodies, were the ſtrings wherewithal the inuiſible bullets were tied and caſt.

Some alſo thought that we ſhot them our ſelues out of our pieces from the place where we dwelt, and killed the people in any ſuch towne that had offended vs as we liſted, how farre diſtant from vs ſoeuer it were.

And other ſome ſaide that it was the ſpeciall woorke of God for our ſakes, as wee our ſelues haue cauſe in ſome ſorte to thinke no leſſe, whatſoeuer ſome doe or maie imagine to the contrarie, ſpecially ſome Aſtrologers knowing of the Eclipſe of the Sunne which wee ſaw the ſame yeere before in our voyage thytherward, which vnto them appeared very terrible. And alſo of a Comet which beganne to appeare but a few daies before the beginning of the ſaid ſickneſſe. But to exclude them from being the ſpeciall an accident, there are farther reaſons then I thinke fit at this preſent to bee alleadged.

Theſe their opinions I haue ſet downe the more at large that it may appeare vnto you that there is good hope they may be brought through diſcreet dealing and gouernement to the imbracing of the trueth, and conſequently to honour, obey, feare and loue vs.

d

Figure 1. Thomas Harriot, *A Briefe and True Report of the New Found Land of Virginia* (Frankfurt, 1590). Courtesy of the John Carter Brown Library at Brown University.

manifested questions and concerns regarding how the colonists would use this power in Ossomocomuck.

In Lane's "Account" the invisible-bullets theory advanced a narrative of English colonization, albeit a tenuous one; by contrast, in Harriot's *Report,* describing the Algonquians' multiple interpretations of the illness fractured his narrative and facilitated a rhetorical shift from narrative to list form. The textual anomalies in Harriot's *Report* reflect both his and the Algonquians' attempts to explain the relationships among illness, colonization, and the non-human causes of disease, including the Algonquians' theories of and cures for their illness as well as Harriot's own hesitation to cite a cause for the epidemic. In the sections that follow, I first discuss the ways in which the invisible-bullets theory provided strategies with which the Algonquians could have responded to colonization and illness. Then I explain how Harriot employed the invisible-bullets theory to respond to concerns regarding colonists' health after travel to Virginia, even as describing the Roanokes' medical knowledge threatened to undercut his rhetorical authority. For both Harriot and the Roanoke Algonquians, communicating the invisible-bullets theory signaled their relation both to other people and to non-human forces.

"Invisible Bullets" in Ossomocomuck

It may not be possible to determine precisely which medical practices circulated in encounters at Roanoke, for Harriot and Lane remain the primary sources on coastal Algonquian peoples throughout the sixteenth and seventeenth centuries. Yet while they did depict Native medical practices from English perspectives, this fact does not rule out the possibility that they also recorded the Algonquians' medical knowledge. Harriot shared several conceptions of disease causation with the Algonquians, and these shared beliefs could have facilitated exchanges of medical knowledge in Ossomocomuck. Moreover, colonial and contemporary observers have described Native medical practices and theories quite similar to those Harriot and Lane recorded, making it possible to consider the invisible-bullets theory in the context of Algonquian strategies of explaining and curing illness.

Carolina Algonquian medical philosophies conceptualized illness as an entity that, like "invisible bullets," originated outside the body, and the Roanokes seem to have employed and adapted these theories in order to make sense both of their illness and of the colonists' presence (29).[35] Many Carolina Algonquians and southeastern Indians held that an intruding object, sometimes an evil spirit or an object evoked by a shaman, entered the body if the patient had offended the spirit or if a shaman had bewitched the individual.[36] Similarly, an animal could penetrate the body and cause disease, for animals were often endowed with spiritual powers in Algonquian cosmologies.[37] Other theories attributed illness to witches who had transformed themselves "into other shapes, particularly into the guise of a purplish ball of fire, a wolf, a raven, a cat, or an owl."[38] Furthermore, as Harriot explained, the Roanoke held that the invisible bullets were shot by "Those that were immediately to come after vs [whom] they imagined to be in the aire, yet inuisible & without bodies" (29). Virginia Algonquians, or Powhatans, living in present-day Virginia, reported that supernatural beings with special powers sometimes appeared to priests before returning to the air. English colonial promoter Samuel Purchas recorded a conversation with a Powhatan religious practitioner or priest named Uttamatomakkin, in which the Powhatan man stated that the deity Okkeeus appeared to Powhatan priests after they spoke "words of a strange language."[39] After informing the priests of his will, Okkeeus "departeth vp into the aire whence he came."[40] It is unlikely that the Roanoke believed the colonists to be deities, but their description of colonists being "in the air" suggests that the Roanoke drew on existing strategies for describing the actions of non-human or powerful entities in order to speculate about the nature of the colonists' power and that of the beings responsible for their illness.[41]

Carolina Algonquians described disease as originating with non-human forces, and guns were sometimes identified as a source of such power after colonization. John Lawson reported that the Carolina Natives told a story about two men who "had been conversing with the white Man above, (meaning God Almighty) how they were very kindly entertain'd by that Great Being; he being much pleas'd with their Ways, and had promis'd to make their Capacities equal with the white People in making Guns, Ammunition, &c. in Retalliation [*sic*] of which, they had given him their Noses."[42] Later in Lawson's *New Voyage to Carolina,* he named venereal disease as the cause of losing one's nose.[43] In Lawson's account, the bodies of the two men who encountered the "white Man above" manifested the medical consequences of encounters with beings whose powers were represented by technology such as guns. It is unlikely that the Carolina Algonquians perceived the colonists as "God Almighty" in either the sixteenth or eighteenth centuries, but Lawson's comment attests to the ways that the Algonquians aligned the English and their new technologies with supernatural power. As Oberg states, "No evidence exists to suggest that the natives saw the English themselves as gods or as morally superior to them in any way. They did, however, view the English as powerful people bearing magical and perhaps otherworldly items permeated with *mantoac,*" a power or category of beings capable of performing actions that humans could not.[44]

For the Carolina Algonquians, the colonists' guns probably signaled their extraordinary abilities as well as their status as people who possessed desirable trade goods.[45] The Roanokes had already expressed interest in the colonists' "gunnes," which they had heard fired in 1584, when Barlowe and his men "discharged our harquebushot."[46] Moreover, the Roanokes seem to have understood their illness as a manifestation of the *mantoac* represented by such technology: their attribution of the illness to "invisible bullets" could have suggested that the disease emanated from metaphysical forces that shot bullets of illness, much as a witch might shoot a ball of fire. Linking the colonists' bullets with pre-existing conceptions of disease as caused by fiery objects would have allowed the Algonquians to explain the relation between the epidemic and the newcomers' powers.

Native and English etymologies for the word "bullet" suggest that, in the context of encounter, both Harriot and the Roanokes attributed the illness's origin to a bullet- or ball-like entity. The English word for "bullet" had recently developed out of "ball," meaning that Harriot may have translated the Algonquians' description of their illness as witch balls by employing the new word "bullet."[47] It is unlikely that the Algonquians possessed a word for "bullet" in 1588, but thunder, balls, and illness are linguistically connected in closely related languages. The Narragansett verb for firing a gun (*peskhómmin*) was originally used to mean "*to shoot thunderbolts*," or "*struck him with lightning*," possibly referencing "thunder beings" or birds, powerful deities who were reported to control and sometimes to send illness.[48] Furthermore, Virginia Algonquians, who lived north of the Roanoke and who shared similar religious and medical practices, identified thunder with their deity Okeeus, who was also responsible for illness. Colonist Robert Beverly reported a conversation about Okeeus and thunder with an Algonquian man who lodged with Beverly at another colonist's house to escape cold weather. When Beverly inquired into the Natives' gods, the man explained that Okeeus was a malevolent spirit who, if he was not pacified and obeyed, would punish people by "ruin[ing] their Health, their Peace, and their Plenty, by sending War, Plague, and Famine among them."[49] The man explained that Okeeus was "frequently visiting us, being present in the Air, in the Thunder, and in the Storms."[50] Identifying the colonists with thunder-beings thus allowed the Roanoke Algonquians to provide a familiar explanation for their illness, one that acknowledged the great power and potentially malevolent intent of the non-human beings who sent their disease.

Moreover, linguistic comparisons between guns and thunder allowed Natives to explain the spiritual power that colonists and their technologies appeared to possess. As the historian John Reed Swanton reported, a Creek Indian "stated that it used to be said that the thunder was a person who possessed missiles (li, the word employed here, may mean an arrow, a bullet, a sting, or a thunderbolt) and would dart them out toward the earth with great noise."[51] In New England, Roger Williams reported that the Narragansetts linguistically connected guns with thunder. He wrote, "Neimpâuog peskhómwock. *Thunderbolts are shot. Obs.* From this the Natives conceiving a consimilitude between our Guns and Thunder, they call a Gune *Peskunck,* and to discharge *Peskhómmin* that is to thunder."[52] Williams noted that the Narragansetts had words for "gun" (*Péskcunck*), "powder" (*Saûpuck*),[53] and "shot"

(*Shottash*); he writes that "shot" is a "made word from us, though their Gunnes they have from the *French*."[54] The Roanoke Algonquians seem to have developed the "consimilitude between our Guns and Thunder" that Williams observed among the Narragansett in the seventeenth century: in Virginia, the Roanoke adapted the meaning of words for "thunder" and "ball" to include the beings who were "invisible & without bodies" and who shot "invisible bullets" at them (29).[55]

Native Americans throughout the hemisphere employed similar associations between thunder and bullets or guns in order to characterize Europeans and their technologies. The Inca Titu Cusi Yupanqui wrote in his account of the conquest that the Spanish who invaded Peru used "*yllapas,* which is the word we use for 'thunder' and by which they meant their 'guns'; for they thought that the thunder they made came from the sky."[56] These links between guns and thunder seem to have taken visual form in Andean "mestizo baroque" paintings of angels carrying arquebuses, or guns (Figure 2).[57] The angels are attired in elegant fabric and lace, and their costumes contain both European and American elements; however, the angels themselves appear to be European. The connections between European technology and divine beings shown in the paintings could display Natives' conceptions of the unfamiliar peoples and spiritual forces responsible for colonization.

The medical cures with which the Roanoke treated their illness corresponded to conceptions of disease as "invisible bullets," a detail that elevates the invisible-bullets theory over the competing explanations in Harriot's list. Harriot explained that "their phisitions to excuse their ignorance in curing the disease, would not be ashamed to say, but earnestly make the simple people beleue, that the strings of blood that they sucked out of the sicke bodies, were the strings wherewithal the inuisible bullets were tied and cast" (29). Writing later than Harriot, John Lawson nonetheless reported a similar practice among the Carolina Algonquians; he wrote that the "Doctor begins, and utters some few Words very softly; afterwards he smells of the Patient's Navel and Belly, and sometimes scarifies him a little with a Flint, or an Instrument made of Rattle-Snakes Teeth for that purpose; then he sucks the Patient, and gets out a Mouthful of Blood and *Serum,* but *Serum* chiefly, which, perhaps, may be a better Method in many Cases, than to take away great Quantities of Blood, as is commonly practis'd."[58] In such ceremonies, medical practitioners localized and then extracted the offending object by employing a purgative or by sucking the object out of the body, sometimes using a hollow object

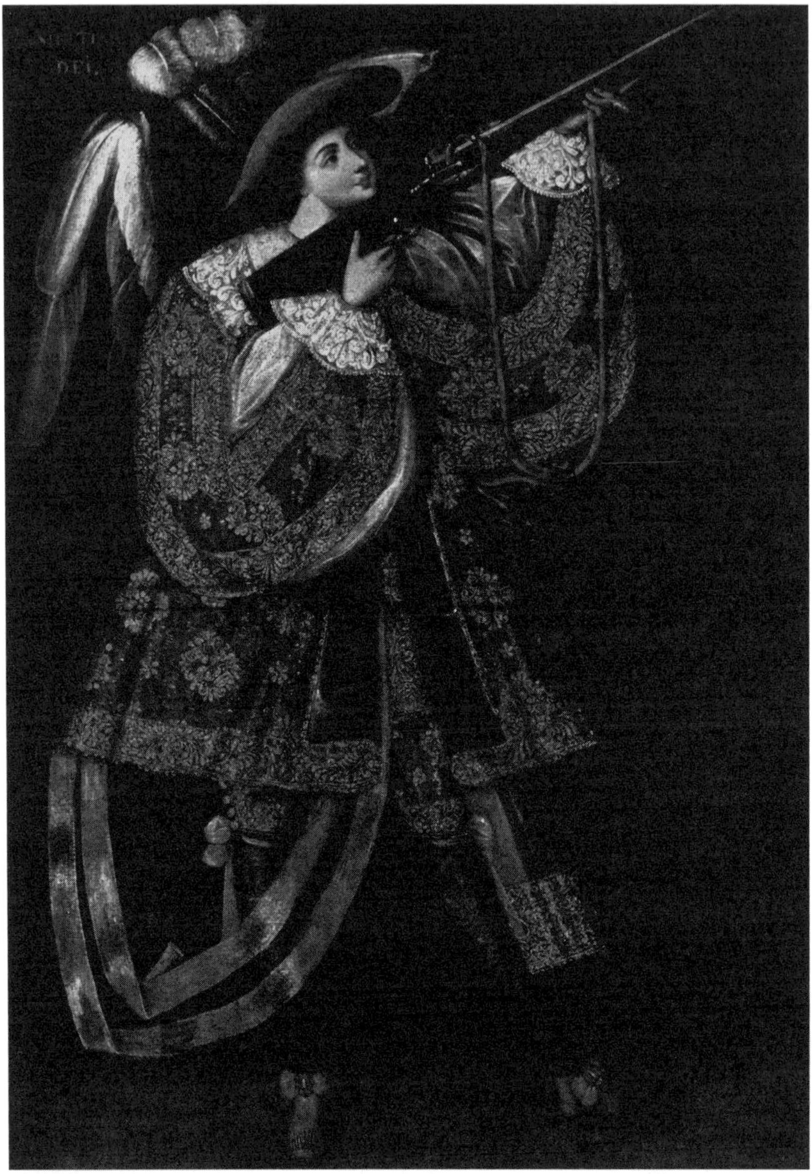

Figure 2. *Angel Arcabucero* (oil on canvas), Master of Calamarca (17th century). Museo Nacional de Arte, La Paz, Bolivia / © Paul Maeyaert / The Bridgeman Art Library.

such as a bone to form a suction over the afflicted part.[59] The use of sucking treatments suggests that the Carolina Algonquians conceptualized disease as a discrete foreign entity, similar to invisible bullets, that had to be extracted from the body.

Sucking treatments seem to have been applied especially in cases when a metaphysical source had shot, or injected, disease into the body. Swanton reports that southeastern Indians "sometimes believed that they had been supernaturally shot by enemies hundreds of miles away and would then consult a doctress . . . 'In these cases, scratching or cupping is the remedy.'"[60] The Carolina Algonquians might have drawn on knowledge regarding the non-human causes of disease to explain the unfamiliar illness as shot by powerful beings and subsequently to determine how to treat the disease. However, in contrast to the successful sucking treatments that Lawson observed, Harriot reported that the Algonquian medical practitioners employed sucking treatments primarily to enact their ability to treat the disease. The physicians' performance of sucking treatments manifests the ways in which contact-era epidemics frequently thwarted Native healing practices and destabilized shamans' position as powerful healers.[61]

Yet even if the Roanoke medical practitioners found that sucking treatments did not stop the epidemic that was devastating their population, such sucking treatments did not fall out of use. Instead, Native medical practitioners continued to employ them to cure illnesses, including those caused by literal bullets. In 1687, Minister John Clayton noted that Natives in Virginia were "exquisite at Cupping," or drawing blood out of a patient by forming a vacuum over a small part of the body, much as the Roanoke medical practitioners sucked "strings of blood" out of afflicted bodies (29).[62] Jean Bossu noted in 1771, "When the *Indians* are wounded with a bullet or an arrow, the doctors or jugglers begin with sucking the wound of the patient, and spitting out the blood . . . they have the powder of a root, which they blow into the wound, to accelerate its suppuration, and they make use of another which dries and heals it; they preserve wounds from mortification, by bathing them with a decoction of some roots, which they know."[63] Similarly, another colonist in Louisiana, Antoine-Simone Le Page Du Pratz, wrote that a Native medical practitioner employed sucking treatments to cure successfully his own "distemper."[64] Whether the bullets appeared in material form or whether their presence was manifested by illness inside Native or European bodies, Native sucking treatments continued to provide viable cures for such maladies.

The Carolina Algonquians' medical treatments and linguistic adaptations seem to have identified relationships among their illness; the colonists and their military technologies; and the non-human forces ultimately responsible for disease. The invisible-bullets theory also manifested the presence of a new disease that the Roanokes' medical practitioners found confusing and difficult to cure, and it reflected as well strategies with which the Carolina Algonquians sought to incorporate the disease and the colonists into their medical knowledge. The image of disease as "invisible bullets" designated the Europeans as beings who, similar to the Thunder-birds, possessed potent weapons and powers that had horrifying effects on the Roanokes' health. In this way, the invisible-bullets theory addressed the dramatic social and spiritual changes wrought by contact-era epidemics, and it communicated the Roanokes' altered spiritual relations with divine forces by interpreting the disease as a punishment for actions against the colonists.

Epidemic and Colonial Promotion

Just as the invisible-bullets theory allowed the Roanoke Algonquians to define the connections between the colonists and the mysterious illness, so reporting the theory allowed Harriot to define the colonists' relationship to both environmental and metaphysical causes of disease. In particular, he addressed anxieties regarding the relationship between transatlantic travel and British colonists' health with the rhetorical strategies he used to present the Algonquians' medical knowledge. The list of possible explanations allowed Harriot to evade the question of whether the Roanokes' illness was caused by environmental factors, which he had already invoked by referencing concerns that Virginia's environment was unhealthy.

In the *Report*'s introduction, Harriot described Virginia as a fertile land containing commodities that England had previously obtained by trading with its rival, Spain; he suggested that colonizing Virginia posed an opportunity to relieve England from dependence on Spain. He supported this argument by comparing Virginia's environment with hot climates known for desirable commodities and by drawing on theories that climate was consistent along lines of latitude. For example, Harriot wrote that Persia "is in the selfe same climate as Virginia," and he concluded that Virginia possessed silk grass and other commodities similar to those found in Persia (7). In addition, Harriot compared Virginia with other places that, while located in different latitudes, also enjoyed a warm climate. He further invoked Iberian contexts by citing the Spanish physician Nicolás Monardes's well-known herbal to promote Virginia's medicinal commodities. For example, when describing sassafras, a bark desirable for its virtues as a cure for syphilis, Harriot wrote: "For the description, the manner of vsing and the manifolde vertues thereof, I referre you to the booke of *Monardus*, translated and entituled in English, *The joyfull newes from the West Indies*" (9).[65] While Monardes's herbal presented information regarding medicines and plants from New Spain, Harriot's frequent references to the herbal were consistent with theories that New Spain and Virginia, sharing warm climates, would share flora and fauna as well.[66]

Yet while comparing Virginia with Persia and Spanish America allowed Harriot to present the English colony as a place of medicinal, mineral, and natural wealth, such comparisons also raised questions regarding the medical consequences of travel to hot southern climates for English colonists. While England's cool climate was alleged to endow its peoples with moderate temperaments and ideal rational intellectual faculties, Spain's warmer environment supported sanguine temperaments, supposedly making its people passionate and unstable. For colonists accustomed to England's cool climate, travel to and settlement in Virginia's allegedly hot climate threatened to alter their humors, subsequently causing illness and altering their English temperaments.[67]

Harriot acknowledged Virginia's environmental hazards, for he admitted that the colonists had eaten foods that "were very straunge unto us and might haue bene thought to haue altered our temperatures in such sort as to haue brought vs into some greeuous and dangerous diseases" (31). Indeed, by the time the epidemic occurred, the colonists had shared food, water, and a climate with the Algonquians for nearly a year and would have been expected to be affected by the same environmental influences and, presumably, the same diseases. In this context, shifting the narrative of disease to a list of the Algonquians' theories of disease avoided questions regarding whether Virginia's environment was unhealthy, for humoral alteration does not appear in the list as a possible cause. Moreover, Harriot's list effaced information regarding the Algonquian bodies that suffered from contact-era epidemics and the English bodies that observed and collected the Roanokes' medical knowledge. In this way, the list covered over the fact that the Algonquians and colonists shared the same environment and instead focused attention on metaphysical causes of disease. Recording the Algonquians' medical knowledge in the form of a list advanced Harriot's promotion of Virginia by allowing him to present non-environmental explanations for disease.

Invisible Explosions: Paracelsian Medical Philosophy and Disease Causation

Harriot also shared with the Algonquians the desire to determine his relationship to the metaphysical forces responsible for illness, and communicating the invisible-bullets theory provided a meaningful way of formulating the connections between disease and these forces for him, just as it had for the Algonquians. Several medical theories of disease as an entity separate from the body and its humors were already circulating throughout Europe, and Harriot's work for his patrons had brought him into contact with some of them.[68] In particular, the German-Swiss physician Paracelsus had developed medical philosophies that disease originated outside the body; he argued that all diseases "issue from the Entity of Poison."[69] Paracelsian physicians repudiated the Galenic system of the humors, arguing that the seeds, or "fathers," of disease, not the humors, or "mothers" were responsible for illness.[70] Paracelsus rejected the prevailing humoral model of the body, in which physical processes were maintained by the regular circulation of fluids, or humors. Instead, he posited that invisible forces called *archei* or "Alchemists" ruled each organ, distilling pure nutrients from impure or unnecessary matter to maintain the body's normal functions.[71] Disease occurred when these Alchemists failed to separate poisonous from pure elements; the poison became localized in an organ, and sickness proceeded from such "impure Seedes."[72]

Much as the Algonquians attributed illness to a supernatural force, sometimes conceptualized as a Thunder-bird or -being that shot balls of disease into the body, so Paracelsians argued that disease originated in atmospheric explosions that penetrated and diseased bodies. Paracelsus described disease as an "invisible thunderclap in nature shaking the body as long as it passes through it, until it settles and concentrates towards some particular place."[73] According to the "gunpowder theory of thunder and lightning," aerial niter (or salt) and sulphur reacted in the air to explode and create thunder and lightning.[74] An analogous process occurred in the body when these chemicals entered through respiration to "react in certain burning disorders or diseases"[75] that resulted from a "Nitroso-sulphureous upset in the body."[76]

Both Paracelsian philosophies and accompanying chemical medicines were filtering throughout multiple levels of English society by the 1580s, despite attempts by the College of Physicians to maintain the authority of Galenic philosophies. Chemical medicines were widely acknowledged as effective cures, even by members of the College of Physicians, and they were employed by a diverse group of practitioners, from university-educated Galenic physicians to Paracelsian physicians and unlicensed practitioners.[77] In addition, Paracelsian philosophies were transmitted throughout England along with more prevalent alchemical knowledge and occasionally in published recipes for chemical therapies.

Harriot had encountered Paracelsian philosophies in the course of his work for his patrons, Ralegh and, later, Henry Percy, Ninth Earl of Northumberland, and through his interests in alchemy. His patrons' libraries provided access to both Paracelsian therapies and theories: for example, Percy's library included an anti-Paracelsian text by Thomas Erastus and translations of Paracelsian texts by Gerard Dorn, an early Paracelsian, while Ralegh had well-known alchemical interests. Moreover, Harriot conducted his own alchemical experiments in 1599–1600 (and perhaps as late as 1604), a period during which he noted that he relied on the text *Apologia chrysopoeiae et argyropoeiae adversus Thomam Erastum,* a 1590 work by Gasto Claveus called Dulco, which was a defense of Paracelsus and response to Erastus.[78] In Virginia, Harriot seems to have understood the Algonquians' description of disease as caused by bullets shot by invisible spirits through Paracelsian theories that disease was caused by invisible explosions.

Harriot's connections to Paracelsian medical theories and to alchemical practices ensured that he had an epistemological framework different from Lane's through which to approach the Roanokes' medical knowledge. While Lane's narrative subordinated the invisible-bullets theory to a providential explanation, Harriot's list and description of sucking treatments elevated the invisible-bullets theory to a strategy for understanding the metaphysical forces that caused disease. In the context of Paracelsian philosophies, the invisible-bullets theory could have appeared to offer a tool with which to explain and subsequently to influence disease. Harriot's and the Roanokes' shared understanding of disease as an external entity originating in invisible forces made the description of disease as "invisible bullets" a cogent explanation for an otherwise strange illness.

Harriot's presentation of the invisible-bullets theory as a compelling explanation of disease also meant that he faced different consequences for describing the Algonquians' medical knowledge than Lane did. Paracelsian medical philosophies were supported by assumptions that medical practitioners could control illness if they discovered its secret causes, for Paracelsian philosophers incorporated Neoplatonic theories that language could influence the natural world when practitioners discovered the invisible bonds between words and things. They held that the body was part of the microcosm, or terrestrial world, and was linked to the macrocosm, or cosmos, "by innumerable bonds of sympathy," meaning that illness was a manifestation of events in the macrocosm.[79] In order to diagnose and cure disease, the Paracelsian physician sought to "make himself a part of the phenomenon he is investigating"[80] in order to understand the "bonds of sympathy" that united humans and "the firmament," that is, to discover the appropriate linguistic analogy for describing and manipulating the chemical processes at work in the body and in the cosmos.[81] Employing the proper words for natural phenomena allowed physicians to manipulate those phenomena, for "Words are treated as if they are equivalent to things and can be substituted for them. Manipulate the one and you manipulate the other."[82] Such theories would have formed part of the European context in which the *Report* was read; they would consequently have raised questions regarding Harriot's motives for describing the Algonquians' illness as sent by invisible bullets and would have fostered existing suspicions regarding Harriot's unorthodox philosophical practices.

In English as well as Algonquian contexts, then, Harriot appeared to claim or already to possess access to power to control disease through invisible means. As historians of science have already pointed out, Harriot possessed a "reputation for impiety" as a result of his philosophical interests.[83] For some in England, Harriot's alleged impiety was directly connected with his experiences in the New World: for example, he had created an Algonquian alphabet that was said to look "like Devills."[84] This reputation, when considered along with Harriot's description of New World illness, could have facilitated conceptions of "Harriot the impious conjurer."[85] In the context of Paracelsian medical philosophies, the "invisible bullets" would have acted as a secret analogy or key into New World illnesses. With knowledge of this key, Harriot could claim special insight into the sympathies among words, illness, and the cosmos and consequently the ability to manipulate the chemical processes that caused disease. His description of the "invisible bullets" thus threatened to cast his *Report* as the product of investigations into secret natural processes undertaken with the goal of improving his own knowledge and status. Rather than merely describing Virginia's natural resources, Harriot seemed also to seek special knowledge of Virginian medical phenomena in order to increase his own power. Transcribing the Roanokes' medical knowledge was thus simultaneously useful and dangerous for the arguments that he sought to make about the New World: if presenting the Algonquians' medical knowledge allowed Harriot to promote Virginia's environment as healthy, describing the invisible-bullets theory simultaneously raised questions about his motivations for depicting Native knowledge.

Cataloging Encounter

Harriot addressed the controversial nature of his medical knowledge by revising his relationship to Algonquian medical knowledge in the *Report*'s catalog of Virginia's medicinal plants. In particular, his description of tobacco, or *uppówoc,* as the Roanoke and Harriot himself called the herb, clarified his relation to the forces responsible for disease and healing. In both Algonquian and European contexts, *uppówoc* was valued for its spiritual and physiological effects. The herb played a key role in coastal Algonquian rituals intended to influence non-human forces and to secure their power for the Algonquians' interests.[86] *Uppówoc* was also an important part of Algonquians' attempts to understand natural and supernatural phenomena: "tobacco had the power to put one into a spiritually exalted state which was necessary even for secular enterprises. Because of this power, it made a particularly appropriate gift to the spirits and means of addressing them."[87] Thus, if the invisible-bullets theory provided a means by which the Algonquians could explain illness as caused by metaphysical powers, their ceremonies for *uppówoc* provided strategies with which such powers had traditionally been accessed and harnessed.

In Europe, Nicolás Monardes's herbal, *Historia medicinal* or *Joyfull Newes,* introduced tobacco and Native ceremonies for using the herb, which Monardes described as diabolic magic.[88] As I explain below, Harriot also described tobacco in the *Report,* but while Monardes relied on second-hand accounts from soldiers and travelers for information about tobacco and Native practices, Harriot described his own participation in the Roanoke Algonquians' rituals for smoking tobacco. And although Harriot frequently cited Monardes when describing Virginian medicines such as sassafras, he did not refer specifically to Monardes in his description of tobacco. Nonetheless, as I explain below, his report of the Algonquians' medical knowledge evoked *Joyfull Newes* in several ways.[89]

Monardes reported that Natives in Spanish America took tobacco in order to enter trances in which they conversed with the devil. When the Natives had an important matter to discuss, the leading priest or religious practitioner:

> did receive the smoke of them at his mouthe, and at his nose with a Cane, and in takyng of it, he fell doune uppon the grounde, as a dedde manne, and remayning so, according to the quantitie of the smoke that he had taken, and when the hearbe had done this worke, he did revive and awake, and gave them their answeres, according to the visions, and illusions whiche he sawe, whiles he was rapte of the same maner, and he did interprete to them, as to hym seemed beste, or as the Devill had counseled hym, giving them continually doubtfull answers.[90]

Monardes added that the "rest of the Indians for their pastime, doth take the smoke of *Tobaco,* too [*sic*] make them selves drunke withal, and to see the visions and thinges that doe represent to them . . . and other times they take it to knowe their businesse, and successe."[91] Monardes often referred to tobacco's medicinal virtues as marvelous and reported that Europeans and Natives alike successfully employed tobacco for various medicinal purposes. However, he connected only the Natives' "marvelous" uses for the herb to communication with the devil by attributing both the Natives' "delight" when smoking tobacco and their visions to the devil.[92] He aligned Native uses for tobacco with witchcraft and signaled to readers that Natives employed their knowledge of tobacco to obtain information from diabolic forces.

Monardes explained that the Natives turned to diabolic forces because "the Deuill is a deceiuer, & hath the knowledge of the vertue of Herbes, so he did shew the virtue of this Hearbe, that by the meanes thereof, thei might see their imaginations, and visions."[93] Having lived much longer than humans, the devil was believed to possess knowledge of natural or medicinal virtues that were hidden from humans as a result of original sin and of humans' concomitantly incomplete knowledge. As Monardes explained, the devil deceived the Indians into believing that tobacco would allow them to share in his knowledge by offering them insight into the secret parts of their imaginations and, consequently, to knowledge of supernatural realms hidden from the reason. The devil took advantage of tobacco's psychological and physiological effects in order to insert his own ideas into Natives' minds and to make them believe that they had achieved special insight into their futures. Moreover, Monardes's description of the Natives' visions suggested that they possessed strong faculties of the imagination, which made them susceptible to being deceived by the devil and to following his practices. Not only did America produce herbs that could induce trances, but the climate also supported strong imaginations, which inclined people native to the Americas to practice witchcraft.

Considered alongside Monardes's account of Natives' tobacco-induced trances in Spanish America, Harriot's description of the Roanoke Algonquians' sacrifices and ceremonies involving "strange gestures, stamping, somtime dauncing, clapping of hands, holding vp of hands, & staring vp into the heauens, vttering therewithal and chattering strange words & noises" suggested that the Roanoke also employed tobacco to influence events by communicating with diabolic powers (16). Since Monardes had already publicized the virtues and medicinal effects of tobacco, Harriot's description would have signaled that Virginia possessed valuable medicinal commodities. But because the two men had different relationships to Native sources and medicinal herbs, the stakes of reporting on magical practices from the New World were different for Harriot than for Monardes. The connections that Monardes drew among New World medicines and Native medical practices, witchcraft, and faculties of the imagination raised the question of how smoking tobacco would influence the minds of Spanish and English colonists who, like Harriot, had been exposed to the New World's climate and who encountered Native medical knowledge firsthand. Moreover, Harriot explained that he had experimented with *uppówoc* by imitating the Roanokes' practices. He wrote: "We ourselues during the time we were there vsed to suck it after their maner, as also since our returne, & haue found manie rare and wonderful experiments of the vertues thereof" (16). Harriot's engagement with medical practices involving an herb that Native Americans allegedly employed to communicate with the devil and to see into the future would have further implicated him in attempts to obtain secret knowledge of New World medicines and illnesses. Moreover, when considered alongside the interpretation of the invisible-bullets theory as a secret key into the causes of Virginian diseases, Harriot's observation and report of tobacco could have raised suggestions that he had also employed tobacco to harness diabolic forces. Consuming tobacco likewise raised concerns that its medicinal and hallucinogenic virtues would open English smokers' minds to insights similar to those Natives in Spanish American enjoyed by communicating with the devil.[94] Harriot's travel to and experiences in an environment that was perceived as threatening to English bodies and minds would thus have raised questions regarding whether his constitution had been altered and how he would respond to diabolic strategies intended to deceive people into practicing witchcraft.

While Harriot followed Monardes's account of tobacco's marvelous properties, he managed his participation in allegedly diabolic practices and addressed concerns regarding his mental faculties by placing the Roanokes' practices for smoking tobacco in a catalog of Virginian commodities. In the catalog, Harriot described resources from silk grass to sassafras by situating objects in categories that identified them according to their appearance and uses. The catalog foregrounded New World objects over individual experiences and opinions. Indeed, while previous explorers of Virginia had described their emotional responses to unfamiliar scenes, Harriot's catalog focused on New World objects' external attributes and practical uses. For example, Arthur Barlowe wrote that "climing towardes the toppes of the high Cedars, that I thinke in all the world the like aboundance is not to be founde: and my selfe hauing seene those parts of Europe that most abound, find such difference as were incredible to be written."[95] Rather than describing the appearance and number of cedar trees, Barlowe turned inward, to his emotional response and to conventions of medieval travel narratives that expressed sensations of wonder in response to the unfamiliar or fantastic.[96]

Although Harriot observed the same cedars, he cataloged the trees by placing them into a system that identified them by describing their qualities, as well as their commercial and use value. He wrote, for example: "*Cedar,* a very sweet wood & fine timber; wherof if nests of chests be there made, or timber therof fitted for sweet & fine bedsteads, tables, deskes, lutes, virginales & many other things else, (of which there hath beene proofe made already) to make up straite with other principal commodities will yeeld profite" (9). Harriot presented utilitarian information that displayed cedar's use for future colonists, rather than describing his subjective response to the experience of observing cedar trees.

The catalog likewise transformed Harriot's firsthand observations of the

Algonquians' ceremonies and his experiences smoking *uppówoc* into descriptions of an object. The catalog highlighted tobacco's uses as a medicinal herb and a commodity rather than its status as a vehicle with which to access metaphysical powers. As the form of the catalog maintained readers' focus on objects useful for colonization and settlement, it also distanced Harriot from his experiences in Virginia. Rather than constructing his own power as a knower of mysterious non-human powers, Harriot employed the catalog's object-making strategies to create a space from which he could safely observe and even imitate Native medical knowledge. He did not deny that the Roanokes' ceremonies for "delight[ing]" their "gods" with tobacco were effective or that his mental faculties might respond to tobacco in the same way that Natives' did; instead, he described his observations of those ceremonies and noted that tobacco had healthful effects on the colonists who smoked it (16). The catalog established Harriot's ability to obtain information about New World medical knowledge without engaging in inappropriate practices; it positioned him as a "scientific knower" who "discovers through a self-distanced reading of the natural world"[97] even while allowing him to maintain his investigations of knowledge that defined him as an "impious conjuror" in Europe.[98] Harriot's interest in occult philosophies facilitated his investigation of New World medical knowledge, but it did not exclude his use of the disinterested perspective associated with early modern philosophies. Finally, while Harriot did not explicitly describe Native medical knowledge as diabolic, his turn to the classificatory strategies of the catalog to describe practices for smoking *uppówoc* began to posit differences between Native and colonial medical knowledge and practices. The correspondences between Harriot's and Monardes's accounts of Native practices for smoking tobacco suggested that the Algonquians relied on diabolic sources to see into their futures. While Harriot smoked the same herb and employed the same "manner" the Algonquians did, the catalog form allowed him to emphasize tobacco's appearance and utilitarian features and in this way to separate English use of tobacco from practices of witchcraft (16).

The *Report*'s "texture"—its fractured narrative and its turns from narrative to list to catalog forms—confutes the idea that Harriot's *Report* represented only European knowledge and desires for power. When read in intercultural contexts, Natives' and colonists' medical communications, such as Harriot's list of causes for disease and the Algonquians' image of disease as objects sent by non-human forces, are seen to contain elements of both European and indigenous systems. In his study of the Spanish conquest of Mexico, Serge Gruzinski attributes the modes of expression that followed the conquest to "mestizo processes," that is, to "mechanisms that occur on the edge of stable entities labeled cultures or civilizations, . . . a kind of disorder that might suddenly scramble impeccably structured—and allegedly authentic—units."[99] Overlap, interaction, and interpenetration characterized encounters between Native and European ideas and practices. Elements that had originally belonged to one culture "evolved, coexisted, interacted. Fragments of one were combined with fragments of the other, forming varied, shifting configurations," as Natives and colonists alike attempted to explain a devastating illness.[100] As a consequence, the relationship between Native and European practices was not always characterized by opposition or insurmountable difference; rather, such difference had to be created and maintained after colonial encounters.

In Ossomocomuck, the Roanoke Algonquians seem to have interpreted the mysterious illness by piecing together stories of disease that were composed out of pre-existing ideas and some of the elements that circulated in encounters with the English colonists. The Roanokes incorporated Europeans and their technology into theories of disease as caused by witch balls or projectiles. Similarly, Harriot drew on a system of disparate, sometimes conflicting medical philosophies to describe the illness: the Roanokes' descriptions of disease, Paracelsian philosophies, new English words for projectiles, and older environmental theories of disease causation. Rather than projecting or ventriloquizing English knowledge in Native mouths, Harriot transcribed Native medical knowledge by listing the Algonquians' theories of disease. Moreover, he did not apply pre-formulated conceptions of the differences between Native and European medical knowledge to describe the Algonquians' medical practices. Instead, he developed these differences by employing the catalog's rhetorical strategies to distance himself from the Algonquians' uses for tobacco. In Virginia, encounter produced both destruction and creativity: it wreaked havoc on Algonquian bodies while simultaneously inspiring the adaptation of medical theories to explain the appearance of an unfamiliar disease and the apparent connections between the arrival of the English and illness.

The conception of disease as an external entity that was shot into bodies shared by Harriot and the Carolina Algonquians meant that the rhetorical and medical practices with which Harriot and the Roanoke responded to the illness were at least partially intelligible to the other party. The medical knowledge in Harriot's *Report* may thus be seen as the product of communications regarding unfamiliar medical phenomena and their causes. The multiple modes of representation that Harriot employed reflect these communications: the Algonquians' attempts to cure their illness and to represent the consequences of colonization and Harriot's attempts to grapple with the implications of encountering and reporting the invisible-bullets theory. His shift from the narrative form of *historia* to a list of possible causes and his use of the catalog form allowed Harriot to establish different relations to Native knowledge, even within the same text, and in this way to promote Virginian colonization without compromising his reputation. Alternately acting as a participant in and a distanced observer of Native medical practices, Harriot could present firsthand information regarding Virginia's environment and catalog the virtues of tobacco while avoiding suggestions that he participated in practices considered diabolic.

CHAPTER 2

Healing, Medical Authority, and Moral Degeneration in New England

Plague and Providence at Patuxet/Plimouth

ILLNESSES SUCH AS the one Harriot described in his *Briefe and True Report of the New Found Land of Virginia* continued to devastate Native peoples throughout the Americas. In the seventeenth century, some tribes lost up to 95 percent of their members as a result of epidemics that swept the coast of New England. Southern New England was especially hard hit by unfamiliar illnesses between 1616 and 1619, and English explorers reported that New England Algonquians said that the "mortality" was "the greatest that had ever hapned in the memory of man, or been taken notice of by tradition."[1] Thomas Dermer, one of John Smith's associates, reported in 1619, when the epidemics were waning, that such mortality had left "antient Plantations, not long since populous now utterly void."[2] Furthermore, Native peoples in southern New England, like the Roanoke Algonquians, connected the epidemics with the arrival of Europeans: in the 1640s, an Algonquian man informed English missionaries that "about two yeers before the *English* came over into those parts there was a great mortality among the *Indians,* and one night he could not sleep above half the night, after which he fell into a dream . . . [in which a] man all in black, with a thing in his hand which hee now sees was all one *English* mans book . . . told all the *Indians* that God was *moosquantum* or angry with them, and that he would kill them for their sinnes."[3] As the Roanoke Algonquians associated great power but also great danger with the English colonists, so the man connected divine anger and English religious practices with the "great mortality."[4]

The diseases and consequent deaths altered political alliances and rivalries among New England Natives while also transforming the role of *powahs.* They found that their practices and medicinal cures were largely ineffective in curing their peoples' illnesses, thus raising significant questions about their ability to negotiate with the non-human powers who sent disease for their peoples' well-being. Weakened by the epidemics, the Wampanoags, who lived primarily on the east side of what is now Narragansett Bay, agreed to pay tribute to the Narragansetts, who lived on the bay's west side. The Narragansetts had remained relatively healthy throughout the epidemics, and they began to enjoy privileged access to trade routes as a result of their health and greater numbers.[5] When English colonists arrived on the shores of New England, the Wampanoag sachem Massasoit entered into an alliance with them with the goal of strengthening his position in Narragansett Bay.

Meanwhile, the Separatist colonists (later called Pilgrims) who settled at Patuxet—or Plimouth, as they called their settlement—had an experience of the New World environment very different from the one Harriot had promoted by citing his men's health, for half the colonists died of starvation, famine, or disease within a year of their arrival. Moreover, their actions, specifically, their preemptive attack on several Massachusett Indian men in 1623, raised suspicions that exposure to New England's environment had corrupted their morals and degraded their Christian behavior. The medical encounters that took place among the Plimouth colonists and the Wampanoag Indians after such illnesses thus occurred in a context in which both Wampanoag and colonial conceptions of disease and medical authority were unstable. Both colonists and Natives found that communicating medical knowledge could not only restore communities and individuals to health but could also secure positions of power and respect in cross-cultural contexts as well as in transatlantic exchanges.

In this context, colonist Edward Winslow described medical encounters in *Good Newes from New England,* a history of the colonists' experiences in 1622–23, including, as he wrote, "things very remarkable at the Plantation of *Plimouth* in New England" that revealed "the wondrous providence . . . of God" working for the colonists.[6] Winslow recounted the ways in which God's

"All-ordering Prouidence" (15) and "extraordinary meanes" (13) preserved his elect from a variety of hardships, including drought, starvation, illness, frigid winters, poor shelter, inter-colonial strife, and "Saluages" (A2v). Additionally, Winslow related the medical practices that he employed to cure Massasoit from a fatal illness, an act that confirmed an alliance between the Plimouth colonists and Wampanoags.[7] But Winslow also described events less complimentary of the colonists and less promising for settlement in New England, especially the religious community the Separatists sought to establish. The Plimouth leaders, including Winslow and Governor William Bradford, had maneuvered to position the colony as the region's economic and political power, but these efforts had been challenged by the founding of a second colony, called Wessagusset, and by tensions with the Massachusett Indians that developed when the Wessagusset men stole corn and the Massachusett subsequently refused to trade with them. Simmering tensions had finally erupted in 1623, when Miles Standish, Plimouth's military leader, led an attack on the Massachusetts for allegedly plotting to attack Wessagusset; this attack culminated when Standish decapitated the Massachusett leader Wituwamet and killed six other Massachusett men.[8] In *Good Newes,* Winslow addressed criticism of the colonists' violent actions and attempted to justify the apparently preemptive attack.

Although *Good Newes* has until recently received little more than passing mention from literary scholars, historians of cross-cultural encounters in New England have argued that Winslow established conceptions of Natives as savages and devil worshipers that were later employed to justify colonial policy during the Pequot War.[9] Noting that *Good Newes* "contains the first detailed English description of the religious practices of the New England indigenous peoples," Alfred A. Cave argues that Winslow's account nevertheless reflects "Puritan preconceptions" about those practices.[10] As Dana D. Nelson points out in her work on race and early American literature, classical accounts of wild men often shaped colonists' expectations of Native Americans, resulting in descriptions of Natives as uncivilized and barbaric. Writing that "American explorers and colonists refused to see anything but the Indian they had fictively created in advance of contact with him," Nelson argues that colonists' representations of Natives remained unchanged even after they had encountered Natives in the New World.[11] Colonists employed literary strategies from England to incorporate new or unfamiliar experiences into a stable narrative of European cultural authority, and they defended this authority by constructing boundaries between colonial and Native American cultures.

But "fictive" constructs of Natives as barbaric were not consistently used in colonial encounters.[12] Indeed, in *Good Newes,* Winslow altered his previous statement, made in a 1622 account of the colony, *A Relation or Journall of the beginning and proceedings of the English Plantation setled at Plimouth in New England, by certaine English aduenturers both Merchants and others* (also called *Mourt's Relation*), that southern New England Natives had no religion. By contrast, in *Good Newes,* he detailed the Wampanoags' religious ceremonies and the medical practices with which *powahs* communicated with divine beings. Winslow's interest in Natives' religious and medical practices was not limited to documenting his observations as a bystander; he drew on local medicinal herbs and Wampanoag medical knowledge and labor to cure Massasoit. In addition, he rhetorically patterned the medical and spiritual care he provided for Massasoit and other Wampanoags after the actions of Tisquantum, a Patuxet Indian who served as the Plimouth colonists' translator. As Winslow reported, Tisquantum claimed the ability to interpret and control disease by stating that the colonists kept illness in their storehouse for gunpowder, an interpretation that indicated Tisquantum's powerful position as an intercultural mediator as well as his ability to access the powers responsible for disease. Winslow presented himself as a similar vehicle of divine power during his cure of Massasoit, and he temporarily took on *powahs'* responsibility of providing medical and spiritual leadership for the Wampanoags.

By modeling his medical practices after those of Tisquantum, Winslow emphasized the interconnected medical and spiritual roles he possessed in Algonquian contexts, in this way offering evidence of the colonists' Christian behavior and countering criticism of their violent treatment of the Massachusetts. But if Tisquantum's and Winslow's medical practices marked a moment in which both colonists and Natives drew on medical knowledge to communicate their mutual reliance on one another, they later revised these alliances: Winslow added a moral—or cultural—history to *Good Newes* in which he cataloged the Algonquians' "Religion, and sundry other Customs" (52). He positioned Native medical knowledge as an object of analysis in his moral history, thus classifying the Algonquians as heathens in order to construct cultural distance between them and the colonists where geographic distance did not exist. Meanwhile, Massasoit rejected English missionaries' attempts to convert his people and to replace *powahs* with colonial ministers.

"So healthfull and hopefull a country": Illness and Transatlantic Travel

Delivering "good newes from New England" was a more difficult task than Winslow's title might seem to suggest. The colonists and their religious leaders had voiced concerns regarding the physical, cultural, and spiritual degeneration that travel to New England was thought to cause, concerns that were only heightened when the Plimouth colonists attacked the Massachusett Indians. One of the earliest warnings came from the Separatists' deacon Robert Cushman, who had voiced concerns about the degenerative effects of transatlantic travel in a sermon he delivered at Plimouth in 1621. Cushman employed medical rhetoric to draw connections between colonists' behavior—the symptoms either of charity or of "self-love"—and the health of their souls.[13] He urged colonists to examine their actions for signs of self-love just as they would examine their bodies for symptoms of humoral imbalance, and he instructed them to watch especially for sins that might disrupt their spiritual "balance" or "health." He wrote:

> If God see this disease of selfe loue so dangerous in vs, then it standeth vs all in hand to suspect our selues, and so to seeke out the roote of this disease, that it may be cured. If a learned Physitian, shall see by our countenance and eye, that we haue some dangerous disease growing on vs, our hearts will smite vs, and we will bethinke our selues, where the most griefe lieth, and how it should come, whether with cold, heate, surfeit, ouer-flowing of bloud, or thorow griefe, melancholy, or any such way, and euery man will bestirre himselfe to get rid of it, and will preuent all wayes that feed the disease, and cherish all courses that would destroy it.[14]

In Cushman's sermon, the physician diagnosed illness by observing the patient's appearance—the "countenance and eye"—and linking it to a "dangerous disease" caused by invisible, humoral conditions: "cold, heate, surfeit [excess], ouer-flowing of bloud, or thorow griefe, melancholy." The colonists were to apply this same scrutiny to their actions, in order to discover the "roote" of the "disease" of self-love, that is, the selfish, ungodly desires that allowed sin to grow, just as the humors imbalanced the body and caused disease. On the other hand, spiritual health would be manifested by visible signs of charity and unselfishness that would culminate in Native converts, for Cushman wrote that the colonists' ability to keep their communal body free from the disease of self-love would be a "notable president [precedent] to these poore Heathens, whose eyes are vpon you."[15] The colonists' charity would indicate their spiritual health at the same time that it operated as a tool of conversion, for it would "preach louder to them, then if you could crie in their Barbarous language," thus converting the Natives through example.[16] By contrast, the absence of converts or, even worse, intercultural violence provoked by the colonists could signify that the diseases of self-love and dissension had broken out among the colonists.

Cushman drew explicit connections between the disease of self-love and the New World environment. He noted that colonists in Virginia had undergone a moral transformation after arriving in the colony, writing "It is reported, that there are many men gone to that other Plantation in *Virginia,* which, whilest they liued in England, seemed very religious, zealous, and conscionable; and haue now lost euen the sap of grace, and edge to all goodnesse, and are become meere worldlings."[17] Just as the Virginian environment could modify English colonists' humors, so it also degraded the godly behavior they had previously exhibited in England. Moreover, Cushman admitted that New England was filled with so many "hardship[s] and difficulties" that not every person could expect to survive, much less to maintain his or her Christian "humors."[18] He wrote that "men which have a large heart, & looke after great riches, ease, pleasure, dainties, and jollitie in this world (except they will live by other mens sweat, or have great riches) I would not advise them to come there, for as yet the country will afford no such matters."[19] Cushman's sermon offered a warning regarding the dangers of selfish desires in New England, where the extreme climate and the scarcity of food exacerbated actions motivated by self-love. Moreover, his sermon identified the colonists' behavior as a symptom of their spiritual "health" and their ability—or inability—to withstand the degeneration aggravated by environmental influences, from harsh weather to ungodly company.

By the time *Good Newes* was published in 1624, Cushman's sermon was three years old, and, in light of the Plimouth colonists' failure to win any Native converts and their attack on the Massachusetts, the sermon seemed more diagnostic than cautionary. Winslow noted that the natural and cultural environment had altered the colonists' bodies and behavior, despite the fact that *Good Newes* was ostensibly a promotional account. As Winslow explained, the colonists had experienced numerous difficulties during their first years at Plimouth: after half of them had died during the first winter, the remaining settlers struggled for several years to locate dependable sources of food and shelter. Winslow admitted in 1622 that the colonists had not readily adapted to the New World's climate and food, writing that "We found great Mussles, and very fat and full of Sea pearle, but we could not eat them, for they made vs all sicke that did eat, as well saylers as passengers."[20] Moreover, as Winslow explained, the "cold and wett lodging had so taynted our people, for scarce any of vs were free from vehement coughs, as if they should continue long in that estate, it would endanger the lives of many, and breed diseases and infection amongst vs."[21] Although Winslow also complimented New England's environment, his promotional statements were undercut by his admission that the climate "taynted" colonists' bodies.[22]

Furthermore, Winslow acknowledged that the New World threatened to taint colonists' Christian behavior and English identities. He observed that the Wessagusset colonists had suffered through the same starvation and cold that had decreased the Plimouth colonists' numbers so drastically; however, some of the Wessagusset men had sought food and shelter at a nearby Massachusett village. According to Winslow, several of "their company abased themselves by vndirect means, to get victuals from the *Indians*" (34); some of the men were even "turned salvage" (44). These men "liued and suffered [the Natives] to lodge with them, not having sword or gun, or needing the same" (41). As Winslow wrote, the Wessagusset men had become a "*stain to* Old England *that bred them, in respect of their liues and manners among the* Indians: *So, it is to be feared, will be no less to* New-England, *in their vile and clamorous reports, because shee would not foster them in their desired idle courses*" (To the Reader). The Wessagusset colonists' behavior and "*clamorous reports*" reflected poorly on New England's ability to sustain settlers and, just as Cushman warned, on colonists' ability to maintain English customs and civility (To the Reader). Moreover, the Wessagusset colonists' adaptation to Native practices raised the possibility that the Plimouth colonists, whose own stores of food were meager, might also be motivated to modify their English customs in order to survive. Winslow's rhetoric of "tainting" and "staining" to describe the physical and cultural repercussions of settlement suggested that New England's environment provoked devastating, potentially fatal alterations not only in English bodies but also in English customs and behavior.

The Plimouth colonists' attack on the Massachusetts occurred just before Winslow published *Good Newes,* and the violence only heightened anxieties regarding colonial physical, cultural, and moral degeneration. As John Canup has explained, the attack was an attempt "to eradicate incipient savagery in other nearby English settlements that might, through an example of degeneration, encourage the same tendency in Plimouth."[23] Yet the colonists' action against the Massachusett also reflected back on them: the attack suggested that the colonists themselves had failed not only to establish peaceful relations with area Native peoples but also to maintain civilized Christian behavior. In a letter written shortly after the attack, the Separatist colonists' pastor in Leiden, John Robinson, raised questions regarding the colonists' behavior by lamenting that they "had [not] converted some [Natives], before you had killed any."[24] Even more critically, he suggested that their behavior reflected the degenerative effects of the New World by calling the Wessagusset colonists "heathenish Christians" and by suggesting that the Plimouth colonists' actions had made them a "terrour to poore barbarous people."[25] Robinson's comments raised the possibility that travel to New England's environment had tainted and stained the colonists by transforming their English customs and morals into heathenish ones.

Epidemic, Encounter, and Incomplete Narratives

If Winslow was to promote New England as "healthfull and hopefull" in the context of the colonists' attack, he needed to prove that the colonists had maintained their physical, cultural, and religious identities (A2r). *Good Newes* responded to Robinson's critique and concerns that the colonists' actions would be interpreted as evidence of their degeneration: Winslow detailed their dealings with the Massachusett and Wampanoag peoples and the tensions and decisions leading up to the attack on the Massachusett. In particular, his report of Massasoit's cure directly addressed critiques of colonial behavior: he interrupted his depiction of intercultural tensions by embedding a medical narrative of Massasoit's cure within the longer history of Plimouth. This inner narrative, or *historia,* halts the account of the attack for eight pages while Winslow described the medical practices he employed to heal Massasoit and the Wampanoags' response to his healing actions. As Matt Cohen has pointed out, the embedded medical narrative "block[s]" the account of the colonists' uncharitable actions by forcing readers to depart momentarily from the sequence of events that concluded with their "heathenish" actions and to focus instead on Winslow's charitable healing of Massasoit.[26]

Winslow's knowledge of *historia* could have derived from his experience as a printer's apprentice: like Harriot, he had received a formal education in England, after which he was apprenticed to a printer, John Beale, who published several books on natural philosophy, the Americas, and medicine during Winslow's apprenticeship. These publications included Francis Bacon's *Essays; An Itinerary written by Fynes Moryson Gent,* a 1617 travel narrative in which a Spaniard who had syphilis traveled to America to learn from Native Americans how to cure himself; and Gervase Markham's 1615 *The English Huswife, Containing the Inward and Outward Vertues Which Ought to be in a Complete Woman,* which, despite its title, offered advice to both female and lay medical practitioners regarding how to cure a variety of illnesses.[27] In New England, Winslow employed the form of the *historia* to link his medical practices to Massasoit's physical state.

As Winslow explained, he traveled from Plimouth to the Wampanoag village Sowams after the colonists received word that Massasoit was ill and "like to die" (25).[28] Noting that it was a Wampanoag custom to visit friends when ill, Winslow traveled to Sowams because he hoped to confirm the colonists' friendship with Massasoit and, if necessary, with his successor (Figure 3). Winslow was no stranger to the journey to Sowams or, for that matter, to Wampanoag manners and medical practices: he had already traveled to Massasoit's village to relay messages from Governor Bradford. During one of these journeys, in 1621, Winslow noted that many Wampanoag people entertained the travelers (who included Tisquantum, as translator) even before they arrived at their destination, and the men were well fed with bread, fish, and acorns.[29] Furthermore, Winslow smoked tobacco and spent the night with the Wampanoags, an experience that included sleeping in Massasoit's house. Finally, Winslow noted at the end of *Good Newes* that he had observed the Wampanoags' medical practices, "being necessarily called at some times to be with their sicke" (54).

By the time he arrived at Massasoit's bedside in early 1623, then, Winslow had interacted with many of the sachem's advisors and family members, and he would not have been surprised to see either Massasoit's *powahs* in the

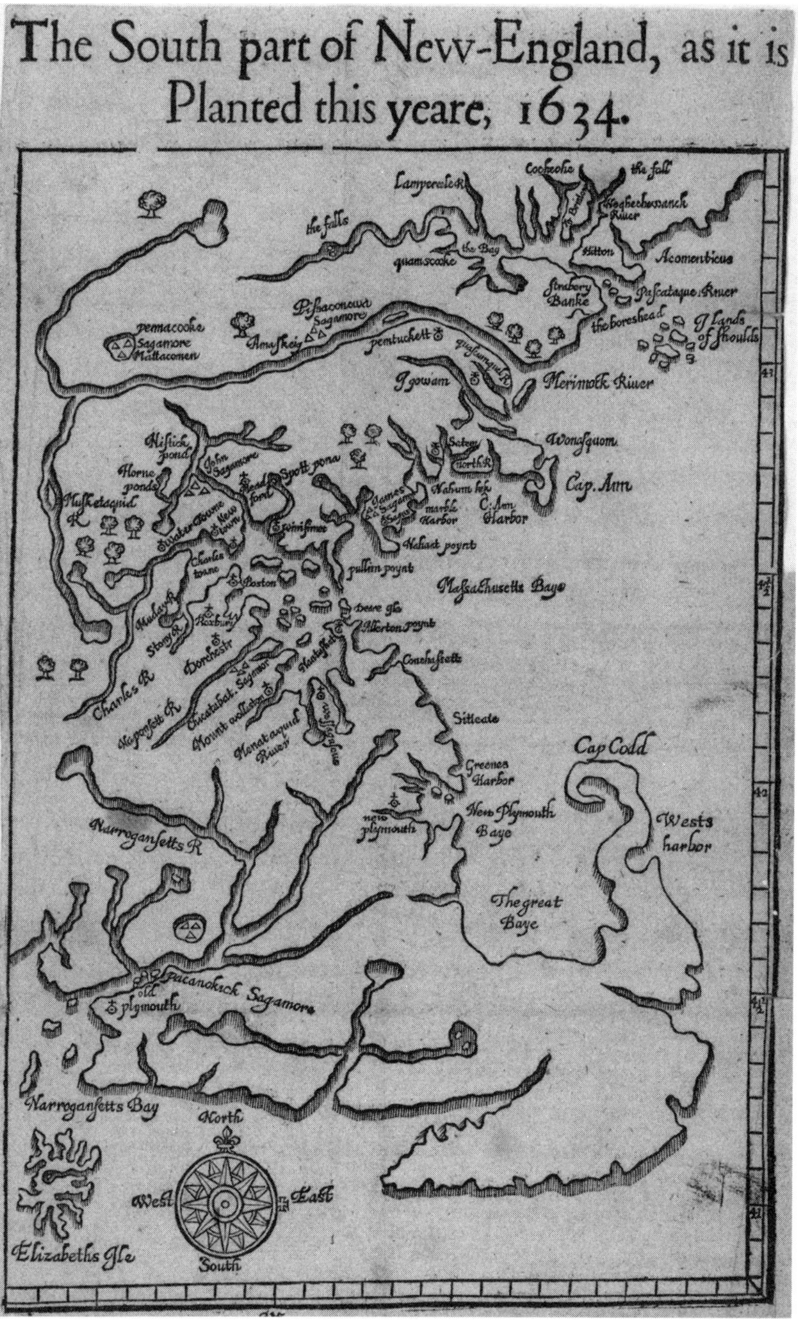

Figure 3. William Wood, *New England's Prospect* (London, 1635). Courtesy of the John Carter Brown Library at Brown University.

midst of a healing ceremony in which they made a “hellish noise” or “six or eight women, who chafed his armes, legs, and thighs, to keepe heat in him” (28). After waiting for the *powahs* to complete their ceremony, Winslow came forward to pay his respects to Massasoit. He offered the sachem conserves, a fruit-based medicinal concoction, that he had brought from Plimouth. As Winslow explained:

> hauing a confection of many comfortable conserues, &c. on the point of my knife I gaue him some, which I could scarce get thorow his teeth. . . . Then I desired to see his mouth, which was exceedingly furred, and his tongue swelled in such a manner, as it was not possible for him to eat such meat as they had, his passage being stoppt vp: then I washed his mouth, and got abundance of corruption out of the same. After which I gaue him more of the confection, which he swallowed with more readinesse; then he desiring to drinke, I dissolued some of it in water, and gave him thereof: within halfe an houre this wrought a great alteration in him, in the eyes of all that beheld him. (28–29)

Winslow placed each development in Massasoit’s cure, from the first dose of conserves “on the point of my knife” to Massasoit’s “great alteration” within a narrative form that linked each of Winslow’s actions to the sachem’s changing symptoms (28–29).

Like the medical practitioners who employed the narrative forms of *historia* to draw connections between their actions and patients’ improvement, Winslow employed temporal markers such as “then,” “after which,” and “within halfe an houre” to describe his successive ministrations in response to Massasoit’s physical condition. Winslow’s account of his healing actions parallels the structure of the entries in Markham’s *English Huswife;* these entries instruct practitioners to apply successive treatments according to the patient’s condition. For example, for the pestilent fever, “you shal cause the party first to be let blood, if his strength will beare it: then you shall give him cool Julyps made of endine . . . if the parties mouth shall through the heate of his stomacke, or liuer inflame and grow sore, you shall wash it with the sirrop of mulbuerries.”[30] The instructions concluded by explaining how to make a suppository that would certainly bring “ease to the party.”[31] In this entry, the practitioner’s actions respond to alterations in the patient’s body, so that if readers adhered to the narrative of the cure by matching healing practices to the pattern of physical changes, they could be assured of success. Winslow’s account of his practices in *Good Newes* mirrored the structure of the *Huswife*’s entries by connecting his actions to Massasoit's symptoms and gradually altered body. First, Winslow's dispensation of "comfortable conserues" set the narrative in motion, after which Massasoit's difficulty swallowing the medicine prompted Winslow to apply further medical care by washing the sachem's mouth (28). Massasoit responded to this treatment by swallowing a small amount of the concoction, and the medicine further opened his mouth, eventually enabling him to take a drink. Winslow's narrative form linked Massasoit's increasingly diminished symptoms and eventual return to health to Winslow's conserves, in this way creating a causal relationship between Winslow's applications of medicine and Massasoit's improvement.

However, Winslow did not complete his administration of medicines from Plimouth or, by extension, his narrative of medical care. As he explained, he had broken the second bottle of "physicke," or medicine, that he had brought to Sowams from Plimouth (29). As a consequence, he sent a messenger to Plimouth to declare "our good success [and] the state of [Massasoit's] body," as well as to request Samuel Fuller, Plimouth's physician, to send "such physicke as [he] durst administer" to Massasoit (29). But Winslow did not wait for the messenger's return to continue his cure, for Massasoit asked Winslow to make "some English pottage," a broth that Massasoit had previously eaten at Plimouth (29). This request halted Winslow's medical narrative, for the sachem's direction, rather than the narrative structure linking physical symptoms and corresponding treatments, began to shape *Good Newes*.[32]

Winslow transformed his narrative of healing into a recipe in which he described the local ingredients he used to concoct the broth that ultimately returned Massasoit to health. He turned from linking Massasoit's symptoms with corresponding treatments to recounting the herbs in the broth. Furthermore, he inserted the Wampanoags' medicinal knowledge into the non-narrative form of the recipe by explaining that he began to make the broth by asking a Wampanoag woman to prepare some corn, or grains, by grinding it into grit. Next, Winslow searched the area for medicinal herbs but reported that he "could not find any but strawberry leaves" and sassafras root, both of which he boiled and strained to make a broth (30). He did not provide an explanation for why he chose strawberry leaves and sassafras for the broth, but it is possible that he drew on Native medical and natural knowledge of the plants when making his decision to include them. As Roger Williams reported, the Narragansett cultivated strawberry fields, and it is possible that Winslow found strawberry leaves because the

Wampanoags had planted them.[33] Far from being a random discovery, Winslow's use of strawberry leaves was dependent on Wampanoag natural knowledge and labor.

Winslow's decision to add sassafras depended on both Native and European knowledge of the root: although sassafras was indigenous to the New World and only became known in Europe as it was transported back by European explorers, by the seventeenth century the root was known throughout Europe as a much-touted cure for syphilis, or, as it was then called in England, the French pox. In addition, sassafras was employed to break up obstructions in the digestive system, much as Winslow seems to have used it. Winslow could certainly have been applying knowledge from European medical recipes when he decided to add sassafras to Massasoit's concoction. However, Natives in New England also used sassafras to cure various ailments: the Mohegan Samson Occom included sassafras in an herbal he wrote in 1754, as a cure for "sore eyes,"[34] and Occom's descendant Gladys Tantaquidgeon described the virtues of a sassafras tonic "which was used as a soothing wash for sore eyes."[35] As Winslow explained, Massasoit had lost his sight as a consequence of his illness, but after drinking the broth, the sachem's "sight mended more and more; also he had three moderate stools, and took some rest," his health being so much improved that those observing him made "no doubt of his recovery" (30). Massasoit's improved eyesight, along with the fact that New England Algonquian medical recipes used sassafras to heal ocular conditions, suggest that Winslow may have relied on Native medicinal knowledge of sassafras and its uses to make his broth.

By writing a recipe for the broth, Winslow departed from the narrative strategies of *historia,* which sometimes contained recipes but which rarely separated the account of ingredients from the case narrative, as Winslow disconnected his account of the broth from his narrative of Massasoit's changing symptoms. Early modern case narratives traditionally included information about the patient and his or her social rank and lifestyle and about the place where the cure took place; these details took prominence over the recipe's list of ingredients.[36] Winslow began his narrative of Massasoit's cure by describing the sachem's sick bed and the respect given to him by his attendants, but unlike conventional *historia* of cures, Winslow's privileged the recipe for the broth with which he cured Massasoit by departing from his earlier focus upon Massasoit's body. His fractured narrative and list of ingredients reflect Massasoit's requests for treatment, the Wampanoag woman's expertise, and the Wampanoags' agricultural labor and medical knowledge of local herbs and their properties.

Plague and Medical Authority

In addition to incorporating Wampanoag herbal knowledge into his account of Massasoit's cure, Winslow drew on Algonquian conceptions of medical authority to describe his actions and their reception at Sowams. Massasoit's requests for treatment as well as Winslow's subsequent actions and his presentation of them in *Good Newes* reflect the Wampanoags' understanding of Winslow as a *powah* who could appeal to spiritual forces for healing and maintain communal health. In order to understand the authority Winslow took on at Sowams, it is necessary to examine his earlier description of Tisquantum's actions, which Winslow also depicted as those of a *powah*. Medical practices allowed both Tisquantum and Winslow to communicate their respective relationships to the divine forces who caused disease, a relationship of interest to Wampanoag and English audiences alike.

Winslow explained that Tisquantum had claimed medical authority on the basis of his relationship to and influence over the colonists, who, he said, kept disease in their storehouse for gunpowder. In 1622, Winslow wrote, Tisquantum circulated an explanation for the contact-era epidemics that had devastated Native communities. Winslow noted that Tisquantum, "to the end he might possesse his Countrymen with the greater feare of vs, and so consequently of himself, told them [the Wampanoag] wee had the plague buried in our store-house; which, at our pleasure, wee could send forth to what place or people wee would, and destroy them therewith, though wee stirred not from home" (10). Tisquantum seems to have drawn connections between the widespread diseases and the settlement of European colonists in places recently depopulated by illness. Indeed, colonist Thomas Morton wrote that Massasoit was concerned when hearing of the English storehouse of plague because of the recent "great mortality" that southern New England tribes had experienced.[37] By locating the plague in the colonists' storehouse for gunpowder, Tisquantum drew on and contributed to descriptions of disease as bullets that Natives throughout the Americas developed after the arrival of colonists and devastating epidemics. Like the Roanoke Algonquians, who, as Thomas Harriot had reported, attributed a mysterious illness to "inuisible bullets" from the colonists' guns and ultimately from non-human forces, so Tisquantum's story explained the devastating plague by connecting the illness to the colonists and their technologies.[38]

In the context of these connections between guns and illness, Tisquantum's attribution of disease to the colonists would have indicated to his Native audience that the colonists were powerful beings with the ability to control and direct disease. Algonquians attributed natural events, including disease, to "many divine powers," spiritual beings called *manitou* whose power was immanent in natural phenomena (52).[39] Although all Native people acknowledged the presence of *manitou, powahs* could acquire *manitou* themselves and, by extension, special knowledge of spiritual realms. By drawing connections between the colonists' presence and the Wampanoags' illness, Tisquantum suggested that the colonists possessed *manitou* who gave them control over disease or, alternatively, that they were themselves beings with special powers enabling them to send and heal disease.

Tisquantum's explanation of disease indicated his ability to mediate between the Wampanoags and the forces responsible for their illnesses. In his capacity as the colonists' translator, Tisquantum already occupied a privileged space from which he could influence political relations and economic exchanges. By defining the colonists as entities who controlled disease and by claiming to influence their decisions to send disease on the Wampanoags, he demonstrated that he possessed spiritual and medical insight as well.[40] As Winslow explained, Tisquantum obtained status as a political and religious leader after circulating his story of disease, for when the Wampanoag people heard Tisquantum's claim to interpret even mysterious plagues, they responded by offering him gifts and holding "him in greater esteeme than many of their *Sachims*" (8). Southern New England Algonquians accorded such gifts and respect to *powahs* as payment for their services; these gifts indicated the community's reliance on *powahs* while simultaneously ensuring that they would remain in the community's service. Tisquantum's power was thus contingent on his success communicating with the colonists and the *manitou* who sent disease. As a *powah,* his cultural status depended not only on his spiritual knowledge but also on his ongoing ability to reciprocate gifts with healing.

Tisquantum was able to achieve status as a powerful medical practitioner because he provided an explanation for illnesses that had frustrated many *powahs'* medical knowledge. The contact-era epidemics had significantly destabilized *powahs'* cultural authority, while also dealing a sharp blow to their spiritual and medical status. Natives' deities were reported to be unable or unwilling to help during the epidemics, and "their *Powwows* themselves were often smitten with deaths stroke," indicating that the *manitou's* anger persisted or that the *powah* was responsible for sorcery.[41] As colonists observed, the *powahs'* "seruice of their God is answerable to their life, being performed with great feare and attention."[42] In such cases, the *powah* was "seen as someone not truly in touch with spiritual forces, whose pretensions to *manitou* were actually rejected by the spiritual world, or worse, who was an outright charlatan."[43] After the epidemics, *powahs* themselves had theorized that the god Kiehtan was angry and had sent an incurable disease against which their cures were useless. They abandoned burial rituals, being "amazed to see their Wigwams or streets lie full of dead bodies, and neither *Squantum* their good, nor *Abbamoch* their bad God could help them."[44] In the physical and cultural devastation that followed, the space of cultural authority *powahs* had occupied was often left vacant, opening space for new leaders to assume positions of power, individuals such as Tisquantum, "whose claim to office were based on personal charisma and the establishment of wide networks of obligation and support."[45]

Tisquantum drew on Native understandings of the causes of disease, but he also adapted these conceptions to include the fact that the colonists' arrival had followed on the heels of the epidemics. His account of disease contained elements that were recognizable to both the colonists and the Wampanoag, as suggested by the Wampanoags' gifts and "esteem" for Tisquantum and Massasoit's anger on discovering that his people were "seek[ing] after *Tisquantum*" for protection (9). When Hobbamock, a Wampanoag translator, questioned whether Tisquantum's claim that the colonists had control over disease was true, one of the colonists (perhaps Winslow) responded by saying that the "God of the English had it in store, and could send it at his pleasure to the destruction of his and our enemies" (11). Neither fully endorsing nor fully repudiating Tisquantum's interpretation of disease, the colonist acknowledged its accuracy while attempting to revise its meaning and to recontextualize Tisquantum's story in a providential context. Communicating his interpretation of the diseases and acting as the Wampanoags' mediator endowed Tisquantum with a position of power in both Wampanoag and colonial eyes. Yet the different responses—from gifts to anger—that Tisquantum's story evoked from the Wampanoag suggest that, although his story had great power and the ability to influence local politics, this position of power was also unstable.

Colonial responses to Tisquantum's story varied as well: most commentators focused on the translator's desire for political and material gain. William Bradford, for example, claimed that "Squanto sought his own ends, and played his own game, by putting the Indians in fear, and drawing gifts from them to enrich him self."[46] As scholars have argued, such comments interpreted Tisquantum's actions through English anxieties regarding their own economic desires.[47] In contrast to Bradford's account, however, Winslow described the translator's story as an act with spiritual elements and implications, with the result that Winslow's account represented Native understandings of disease and medical authority. In addition to obtaining wealth and power, Tisquantum told his story to "possesse his Countrymen with the greater fear of vs, and so consequently of himselfe" (10). For English readers, the word "possess" would have referred to an idea or attitude dominating or controlling a person and to mental and physical possession by a divine or diabolic spirit.[48] As Karen Ordahl Kupperman has pointed out, many colonists "accepted the idea that the Indians worshipped their deities . . . out of fear"; they consequently represented Natives' religious sensibility as founded on fear and wonder of divine powers.[49] Winslow used "possess" throughout *Good Newes* to describe such "fear," or spiritual influence. For example, he wrote that God possessed the "salvages" with "astonishment and fear" of the colonists, in this way saving them from being "swallowed . . . up" (A2v). By describing Tisquantum's story as possessing the Wampanoags with fear and respect, Winslow registered the spiritual insight and concomitant medical knowledge that Tisquantum possessed in a Wampanoag context.

Instruments of Healing

Winslow drew on his observation of Tisquantum's medical and spiritual authority—as well as his own understanding of the connections between medicine and religion—to communicate the significance of his medical practices to Wampanoag and English audiences. In particular, Winslow drew parallels between his and Tisquantum's medical practices: in the space opened up by the broken bottle of medicine from Plimouth and his fractured medical narrative, Winslow presented himself as a medical practitioner who, like Tisquantum, could provide both physical and spiritual comfort. As Winslow pointed out, Tisquantum had acted in the capacity of an "instrument" by mediating between the Wampanoags and colonists in order to facilitate economic and political alliances and by negotiating between divine and human realms to preserve the Wampanoags' health (8). Winslow described his own medical practices in the same terms: after concocting and administering the medicinal broth to Massasoit, he noted that he had "no doubt of his [Massasoit's] recouery, himself and all of them acknowledging vs the instruments of his preseruation" (30). Much as Tisquantum claimed to communicate with *manitou* or their representatives to interpret the plague and protect the Wampanoag, so Winslow presented himself as a mediator between the sachem and the divine power responsible for his illness. In this way, he rhetorically constructed parallels between Tisquantum's claims to control illness and his own medical practices.[50]

Winslow's healing actions communicated the nature of his relationship to the metaphysical powers responsible for disease, a relationship that held crucial consequences for the ways in which both the Wampanoags and the colonists' supporters in England perceived Winslow and the other colonists at Plimouth. Just as Tisquantum received gifts to "worke their peace" and to protect the Wampanoags from disease, so Winslow received "gifts" of information as well as respect after curing Massasoit (8). Perhaps most significantly for Winslow, Massasoit informed him, through the translator Hobbamock, that the Massachusett were plotting to attack Wessagusset. Massasoit's gift displayed his respect for Winslow and his medical knowledge by acknowledging the colonist's ability to communicate with powerful spiritual forces. As he recounted the gifts he received, Winslow indicated that he achieved the status and the respect usually accorded to *powahs,* much as Tisquantum had received gifts and recognition for his special abilities to influence the colonists.

Winslow also assumed the medical and spiritual responsibilities that traditionally accompanied reciprocal relationships between *powahs* and the community. After Massasoit had recovered, he asked Winslow to administer medicine to other Natives stricken with illness, "requesting [him] to wash their mouths also, and giue to each of them some of the same I gaue him, saying, they were good folke" (30). Winslow explained that he acquiesced, virtually accepting the responsibility of serving as a healer for the entire community even though "it were much offensiue to me, not being accustomed to such poysonous sauours" (30). Winslow's reputation as a powerful medical practitioner and healer became known throughout the region. Even Corbitant, a Wampanoag sachem under Massasoit's leadership who, the colonists feared, was planning to align against Plimouth with the Narragansetts, sought to secure Winslow's medical practices for himself, asking "if in case he were thus dangerously sicke, as *Massassowat* had been, and should send word thereof to *Patuxet* for *Maskiet,* that is, Physicke, whether . . . I would come therewith to him" (33).

Accepting the responsibilities of a healer allowed Winslow to present himself as a spiritual leader as well, for as he explained, the Algonquians accepted his religious instruction along with his medicine. Massasoit's cure engendered "much profitable conference [on religious matters] which would be too tedious to relate, yet was no lesse delightfull to them, then comfortable to vs"; these conversations indicate the physical and spiritual healing that Winslow's medical practices brought about (34). Coming just after the contact-era epidemics, Winslow's message of Christianity could have "appeared intellectually and emotionally appealing" to the Wampanoags because it offered the promise of spiritual and physical protection particularly vital in the wake of the shamans' inability to cure the epidemics.[51] By holding "comfortable," that is, medicinal or healing, conversations with the Algonquians regarding spiritual matters, Winslow presented himself as bringing healing not only to Massasoit's body but also to the Algonquians' spiritual "illness" (34).

For both Winslow and Tisquantum, communicating medical knowledge made available new positions of authority in Wampanoag and intercultural contexts. For Tisquantum, drawing connections between the colonists and the contact-era epidemics allowed him to step into the vacuum left by *powahs* who had been unable to cure the Wampanoags' illnesses. Drawing on Native theories regarding *manitou* along with his observations of the colonists' gunpowder, Tisquantum provided a theory of disease that the Wampanoags found familiar and that simultaneously explained the appearance of non-Native people and their technologies. At the same time, Tisquantum's new status among the Wampanoag people made him all the more powerful in the colonists' eyes, for he could employ his new medical authority for or against their goals. For Winslow, providing medical and spiritual healing to the Wampanoags similarly indicated his relationship to the non-human beings responsible for illness and demonstrated his medical, spiritual, and political power. Winslow could assume a position of medical authority at Sowams for many of the same reasons that Tisquantum claimed power over disease: his ability to cure Massasoit indicated that he could restore the Wampanoags' relation with the forces that controlled illness.

Physic and Moral Degeneration

For Winslow, communicating medical knowledge at Sowams had transatlantic repercussions as well as cross-cultural ones. His successful replacement of physic from Plimouth with Wampanoag medicines and medicinal knowledge emphasized for European audiences the priority of local, firsthand knowledge in diagnosing and curing illnesses in New England, including the colonists' disease of self-love. In his narrative, Winslow had attributed the sachem's initial improvement to the "confection" prepared at Plimouth by the physician Samuel Fuller, in advance of Winslow's departure (28). Fuller did not accompany Winslow to Sowams, and neither Fuller nor Winslow seems to have known much about Massasoit's symptoms before Winslow departed, for Winslow wrote only that the colonists heard that Massasoit was "like to die" (25). Therefore, Fuller would have made the confection by relying on his knowledge of the temperaments, or the ideal balance of humors, or fluids, within a body, and New England's environment, rather than on particular experiential knowledge of Massasoit's physical condition.

Winslow's description of the medicine from Plimouth as "physicke" supports this interpretation of Fuller's practices, for physic traditionally included advice or medicine that would restore or maintain patients' humoral balance (29). Practitioners of physic employed their analyses of urine and reports from patients, rather than observation-based diagnoses, in order to treat illnesses.[52] Physic consequently required knowledge of the various temperaments and humors, as well as the causes, signs, and diagnoses of disease, but not of individual bodies and their conditions. By first connecting Massasoit's improvement with "physicke" from Plimouth, Winslow's narrative initially reinforced the authority of European medical philosophies to heal moral and physical illnesses in the Americas without experiential knowledge of the particular illness or its causes. In the context of criticism of the colonists' actions from important figures such as Robinson, the successful use of physic could suggest that it was possible to diagnose New World maladies without possessing firsthand information of conditions in New England.

But Winslow left his narrative of physic incomplete, and this fractured narrative subsequently destabilized the connections between physic and medical authority. He rhetorically replaced physic with medicinal knowledge founded on his experiences at Sowams and on Wampanoag knowledge, for the recipe represented local ingredients, and the broth was so effective that it made the second bottle of physic sent from Plimouth useless and unnecessary. The medicine Winslow concocted out of ingredients from New England had so altered and restored Massasoit's body that by the time Fuller sent additional medicine, Winslow did not dare "giue him any physicke which was then sent, because his body was so much altered since our instructions; neither saw we any need" (31). The physic, prepared by an absent physician, according to a theoretical understanding of Massasoit's body and of humoral principles, now endangered the sachem's newly restored health. Although Winslow's turn to describe Native medical knowledge and practices left his narrative of physic incomplete, his recipe also undermined the causal connections between physic and Massasoit's improvement and, by extension, the authority of physic, or of knowledge at a distance. Instead, experiential medical knowledge successfully cured Massasoit just as, Winslow suggested, firsthand knowledge of intercultural relations would best resolve conflicts in New England. Indeed, Winslow's opportunities to minister to the Wampanoags' spiritual needs offered skeptical readers such as Robinson firsthand evidence of the Plimouth colonists' efforts to convert the Algonquians, their attack on the Massachusett notwithstanding. By disrupting the narrative of physic with the recipe of local ingredients and description of his medical practices at Sowams, Winslow suggested that experiential knowledge from New England could best "cure" diseased bodies and behavior while restoring balance to cross-cultural relations.

A New World of Wonders: Cures and Their Causes

Yet even as Winslow sought to defend the colonists' actions by incorporating local medicinal knowledge into his healing practices, his reliance on Native medicinal knowledge and New England medicines raised questions about the sources of his own medical knowledge. Winslow had stressed his lack of medical expertise by writing that that he was "vnaccustomed and vnacquainted in such business, especially hauing nothing to make it comfortable [medicinal], my Consort being as ignorant as my selfe" (29).[53] After Massasoit recovered, Winslow "blessed God for giuing his blessing to such raw and ignorant meanes" (30). His language of absence—his frequent references to his "ignorance," to "raw and ignorant meanes," and to being "vnaccustomed and vnacquainted" with medical philosophies—suggested that his cure depended on other than human forces, not his own acumen (29–30). Despite the fact that Winslow attributed the cure to God's blessing, his alleged ignorance of medical knowledge also opened up the possibility that his cure depended on diabolic, rather than divine, forces.

Furthermore, the experiential and medicinal knowledge that Winslow privileged in his recipe was sometimes considered to lie outside the realm of knowledge approved for humans. In particular, sassafras was believed to possess mysterious curative properties that extended beyond the scope of orthodox philosophical investigation (Figure 4). Early modern descriptions of sassafras reflect uncertainty regarding how to explain the root's virtues: practitioners named sassafras after one of the diseases it cured, departing from the accepted method of describing medicines by referencing the humors they counteracted or qualities they exhibited.[54] Moreover, both explorers and physicians remarked that sassafras had surprising qualities, which they attributed to preternatural causes. In one of the first European descriptions of the root, the French traveler Jacques Cartier described the effects of a sassafras broth on his men, who were suffering from a mysterious illness (probably scurvy). Cartier wrote: "As soon as they had drunk it they felt better, which must clearly be ascribed to miraculous causes; for after drinking it two or three times they recovered health and strength and were cured of all the diseases they had ever had."[55] Similarly, the Spanish physician Nicolás Monardes wrote that Spanish colonists who took sassafras "were healed of many euills, which surely it doeth bryng admiration, that one onely remedy should do so variable and so merueilous effectes."[56] Monardes and Cartier explained sassafras's ability to heal many different diseases not by pointing to the root's qualities or temperament, usually expressed in terms of the Aristotelian elements of hot, cold, moist, and dry, but by suggesting that sassafras worked by invisible, "miraculous" powers.[57]

Medicines that lacked apparent causes for their curative properties were believed to possess occult, or hidden, virtues, which were unintelligible (their causes could not be known) and insensible (they were incapable of being known through manifest qualities). As a consequence, as Keith Hutchison explains, "Occult qualities could . . . be detected experimentally, but could not be studied scientifically, since *scientia* in the Aristotelian tradition was, above all, a knowledge of causes."[58] One might be able to detect the *effects*

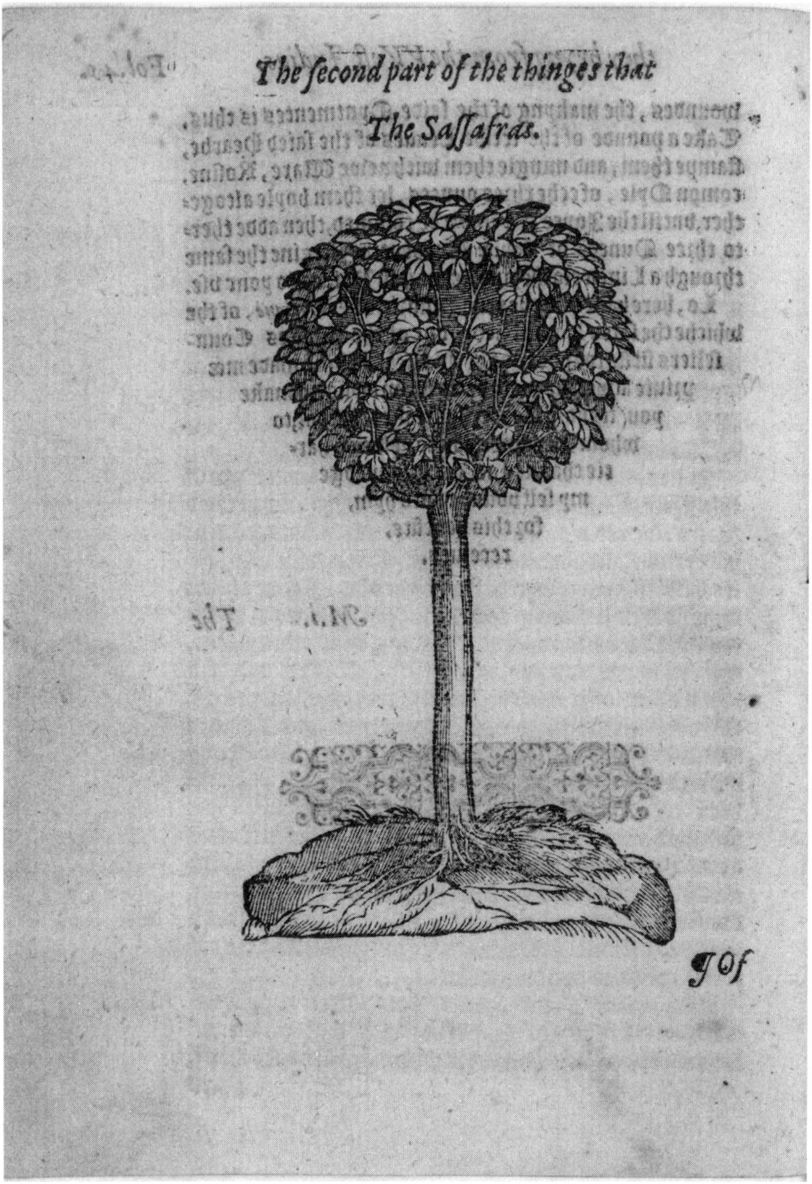
The second part of the thinges that

The Sassafras.

Of

Figure 4. Nicolás Monardus, *Joyfull Newes Out of the Newe Founde Worlde* (London, 1577). Courtesy of the John Carter Brown Library at Brown University.

of medicines with occult virtues, but the qualities ultimately responsible for those effects were hidden from the senses. Such medicines were excluded from philosophical investigation, although special insight obtained through witchcraft or diabolic communications could provide knowledge of occult virtues, for the devil's knowledge of natural causes exceeded that of humans. Consequently, investigation of occult virtues was considered un-philosophical and unchristian, commonly connected with supernatural revelation, and "closely associated with mysticism and demonism."[59]

Winslow's ability to cure Massasoit with medicines known to possess miraculous virtues, along with his claimed ignorance of medical philosophy, left him open to suggestions that the medicinal broth worked on the basis of hidden, or occult, medicinal qualities and that Winslow's cure was indebted to his investigation of hidden, potentially diabolic knowledge.[60] In the context of Cushman's warning about the New World's degenerative effects, Winslow's cure could suggest that New England's environment had strengthened his faculties of the imagination and had inclined him to accept knowledge obtained through illicit means, as Harriot's presentation of the invisible-bullets theory suggested that he sought invisible means of controlling natural phenomena. Moreover, in his travels to Sowams and his participation in Wampanoag medical systems, Winslow, like Harriot when he smoked tobacco with the Roanoke Algonquians, left no question as to his exposure to medical and religious practices that the colonists and their ministers considered dangerous for Christians to encounter. Roger Williams later acknowledged these dangers, particularly the possibility that proximity to heathen practices would result in participation in them. Williams commented that he reported *powahs'* actions by drawing on the Narragansetts' "owne Relation, for after once being in their Houses and beholding what their Worship was, I durst never bee an eye witnesse, Spectatour, or looker on, least I should have been partaker of Sathans Inventions and Worships."[61] Although the parallels between Winslow's cure and *powahs'* practices allowed Winslow to represent the medical and religious significance of his medical practices for the Wampanoags, these similarities also suggested to English audiences that he might have displayed too much "curiositie" regarding New World medicines and practices with hidden causes.[62] Winslow's practices invoked the possibility that, like the colonists in Virginia who had lost "the sap of grace . . . and are become meere worldings" after experiencing the degenerative effects of the New World, he had lost an understanding of the difference between diabolic and divine medical knowledge and had investigated practices that would be considered diabolic in England.[63]

Diabolism and Difference

Winslow protected himself from accusations that the New World had altered his knowledge and behavior by adding religion to the distanced perspective that colonists like Harriot claimed in classificatory forms in order to identify Native medical practices as heathen. In the last section of *Good Newes,* he attached a moral history of the Algonquians' religious, medical, political, and domestic practices. Winslow's history was preceded by moral histories written by Spanish travelers and priests; for example, José de Acosta's *Naturall and Morall Historie* gave a "*proper historie of the Indians,*"[64] an account of the Indians' "*mores*—of customs"; it was a "true history"[65] of the Indians based on "*much conference and travaille among the Indians themselves.*"[66] In his account of indigenous religious practices in Spanish America, Acosta detailed sacrifices of both humans and animals in order to illuminate the differences between Catholicism and Native religions, which otherwise seemed to share similar ceremonies. Acosta's descriptions established not only the paganism of the Indians in New Spain but also their idolatry and barbarism.[67]

Similarly, Winslow's moral history provided a descriptive account of New England Algonquians, including their religious and medical customs, as well as their political structures and domestic traditions. Winslow focused in particular on Native medical philosophies, which he observed when he traveled to Sowams "to be with their sicke" (54). He described the gods that the Wampanoags worshipped, *powahs'* charms and reliance on a power they called Hobbamock and whom Winslow speculated was the devil, and the sacrifices that the Wampanoags and Narragansetts had made to appease Kiehtan during the recent epidemics. He also explained that the Wampanoags "told me I should see the Diuell at those times come to the [ill] party," but Winslow "assured myself and them of the contrary" and, as he writes, "so [it] prooved" (54).

Winslow's moral history classified the Algonquians' medical practices as heathen by connecting them with ceremonies he deemed pagan. Winslow wrote that the Wampanoags sometimes sacrificed children to obtain divine blessing, although he also reported that they "grow more and more cold in their worship to *Kiehtan*" (55). By contrast, the Narragansetts "exceed in their blinde devotion" to Kiehtan, offering him many sacrifices; indeed, the Wampanoags attributed the Narragansetts' ability to withstand the contact-era epidemics to such oblations (55).[68] By connecting Native medical practices with sacrificial rituals, Winslow classified them as barbaric behaviors, for, as Anthony Pagden points out, "Cruelty and ferocity, the marks of unrestraint, were from the beginning the distinguishing features of a 'barbarous' nature."[69] Winslow's moral history marked *powahs'* magical practices as diabolic and heathen by defining the Algonquians' religious beliefs as actions that were the "mark of the savage regardless of time or place."[70]

Winslow contrasted *powahs'* medical knowledge and practices with his own healing strategies, in this way legitimizing empirical medical knowledge, even if connected with medicines possessing mysterious virtues, for colonists' use. Unlike the Algonquians' sacrifices, Winslow's firsthand exploration of mysterious medicinal virtues resulted in opportunities to convert the Wampanoags.[71] When placed against *powahs'* heathen ceremonies, Winslow's medical practices showed that colonists' exploration of the medicinal powers of unfamiliar herbs could improve practitioners' understanding of medicinal virtues and provide opportunities to display Christian charity. Winslow's classification of Native medical knowledge as heathen made religious beliefs, rather than environmental influences, the primary context through which to understand cultural difference and degeneration.

For early modern Europeans, religion was a repercussion of civilization, so that cultures lacking civilization and order were thought to be incapable of developing religion until they had been civilized. By contrast, cultures that had some form of spiritual beliefs, even if adjudged misguided or unchristian, possessed a foundation of civility and social order, however meager, on which Christian beliefs could be established.[72] Winslow's report in the 1622 *Mourt's Relation* that the Wampanoags had no religion had suggested that the New England Algonquians were barbaric and uncivilized; their absence of religion made them apt to engage in the same violent actions that, according to colonists, characterized the allied Virginia Algonquians who attacked Jamestown and killed about three hundred fifty English colonists.[73] However, by 1624, the fact that colonists in New England had also behaved violently suggested that particularly New World influences, rather than a lack of religion, was responsible for the recent violence. Like Harriot, then, Winslow had to assure readers that the New World's environment had not changed

English colonists' bodies, health, or, in his own case, behavior. In contrast to his comments in *Mourt's Relation,* Winslow offered a new conception of indigenous heathenism in *Good Newes* by suggesting that, although they did not completely lack religious beliefs, Natives practiced a primitive form of religion that included devil worship and sacrificial ceremonies. The moral history defined the Algonquians as heathens on the basis of their medical and religious practices, in this way classifying them as undeveloped and uncivilized and locating them on the outskirts of civilization.

Good Newes's classification of Native medical knowledge offered new strategies for recognizing and demarcating cultural otherness, for Winslow's moral history began to separate environment and behavior to argue that the colonists had maintained their religious and cultural identity, their location in New England and attack on the Massachusett notwithstanding. The differences that Winslow constructed between the colonists' and Algonquians' medical practices aligned the colonists' religious and cultural practices with those of their supporters in Europe, thereby allowing Winslow to disprove accusations that the New World environment had a degenerative effect on the colonists' behavior and beliefs. Describing the Algonquians' medical practices as heathen established categories that exemplified Natives' difference from English Protestants—both colonists in New England and Europeans in the Old World. When placed against the Algonquians' medical practices, the colonists' religious beliefs indicated not only their cultural difference from the Natives but also their similarity to Christians across the Atlantic. The moral history thus discounted the relations among the environment, behavior, and spiritual health on which Cushman based his analysis of the colonists' actions. Winslow's classification of Native medical knowledge redrew the geographic separation between the Old and New Worlds that the Atlantic created by emphasizing instead the cultural divisions between the colonists and the Algonquians. He constructed differences between colonial and Native medical practices (and by extension, between colonists and Natives) by observing, imitating, and then classifying as heathen Native medical practices. Rather than originating only in the Old World, these differences were also constructed in the New World, in response to encounters with Native medical knowledge and to accusations of colonial degeneration.

Religion, Identity, and Cross-Cultural Encounters

Like Harriot, Winslow employed classificatory forms in order to distance himself from his encounters with Native medical knowledge. However, although Harriot noted that the Algonquians were amazed at the colonists' technologies and could be brought to "feare and loue" English settlers, he did not mark the Roanoke Algonquians as savage nor did he dwell on the status of Native medical knowledge as witchcraft.[74] Instead, he focused on a plant that, when smoked, had the potential to open one's mind to communications with the devil and thus to illicit knowledge. Winslow developed conceptions of Natives' difference by making explicit the status of Native medical knowledge as diabolic and by connecting Native witchcraft with savagery and pagan religious beliefs. Although Harriot created rhetorical distance between colonial and Algonquian uses of tobacco with the catalog of commodities, Winslow's moral history highlighted the fact that the Wampanoags and the colonists appealed to different divine powers. In this way, Winslow began to separate colonists' religious beliefs and intellectual faculties, as well as their medical knowledge, from environmental influences. Winslow did not deny that climate influenced behavior and bodies, but he did raise the possibility that colonists' beliefs and behavior could be maintained even in the New World, the unfamiliar climate notwithstanding.

Colonists did not construct descriptions of New England Natives as heathens and as barbaric only by projecting pre-existing conceptions of witchcraft in New World encounters, as some scholars have argued.[75] Instead, as Winslow's fractured narrative and classificatory strategies make clear, colonists tested a range of responses to Natives and their medical knowledge. They sometimes found Native medical knowledge and conceptions of medical authority to be guides for communicating in intercultural encounters, but they also aligned Native medical knowledge with witchcraft to defend themselves against the possibility that they appeared to have degenerated intellectually and culturally. Natives likewise employed medical knowledge to respond to the unfamiliar diseases that circulated as a result of colonization and that sometimes altered pre-existing structures of power. Some Algonquians interpreted colonial medical knowledge as powerful means with which to cure physical and spiritual diseases and as epistemological resources that aligned with their conceptions of illness and of bodies, while other

Natives maintained their reliance on traditional medical practitioners and ceremonies for preventing disease.

Colonists' and Natives' shared understanding of medical and religious knowledge as interconnected continued to influence colonial encounters. For example, when New England Natives experienced several more devastating epidemics in the 1630s and 1640s, many of them turned to colonial missionaries and religious beliefs in hopes of locating spiritual guidance and restoring their communities to health, just as the Wampanoags had relied on Winslow as their religious and medical healer after their *powahs* proved unable to cure the 1616–1619 epidemics.[76] But if Algonquians in New England began to investigate Christianity after the epidemics, they did not entirely replace their traditional beliefs and practices with European ones. Instead, they recognized parallels between Christianity and their beliefs; they drew on Christianity as a means of living with colonists while maintaining their land claims (although a series of wars would make this goal difficult to attain); and they employed Christianity as a "diplomatic cloak under which to maintain traditional beliefs and customs."[77] Algonquians thus responded to and embraced Christianity on their own terms; for example, we might see their acknowledgment of Christianity's power as part of the practice of rejecting *powahs* if they failed to cure disease.[78] Similarly, Natives continued to draw on their understanding of the *powah's* responsibilities and powers in order to incorporate colonists into their religious and medical practices; for example, the minister Thomas Mayhew "played the role of Christian *powwow* the Indians cast for him" by attending ill Natives on their deathbeds, a role he then employed to attempt to convince the Natives to embrace Christianity.[79]

Just as southern New England Natives incorporated Christianity into their religious and medical systems without repudiating those pre-existing systems, so colonists drew on Native medical knowledge and conceptions of medical authority as they attempted to convince New England Natives to accept Christianity. Colonial ministers did not reject the connections between medical and religious knowledge embodied by *powahs*' abilities to communicate with non-human powers in order to heal disease. Instead, ministers presented themselves as alternatives to *powahs,* and they made medicine part of their spiritual message to Native peoples. In a tract published to promote New England missions in the Old World, the minister Thomas Shepard suggested that medical and religious education could occur simultaneously, and he proposed to "traine up these poore *Indians* in that skill [of finding plants] which would confound and root out their *Powwaws,* and then would they be farre more easily inclined to leave those wayes and pray unto God, whose gift Physick is, and whose blessing must make it effectuall."[80] Ironically, Shepard suggested that ministers could educate Natives about local botanical resources—resources with which many Natives would have been quite familiar already—as an alternative to *powahs'* practices.[81] But Shepard's plan also positioned Natives not as "curiosit[ies] within the New England landscape" but rather as important agents of medical knowledge.[82] Finally, as Shepard reported, potential converts asked "*If they leave off* Powwawing, *and pray to God, what shall they do when they are sick,*"[83] and he sought to fill this absence with medicinal knowledge and Christianity, or the divine "gift [of] Physick."[84] Natives' act of forsaking *powahs* was seen as a visible manifestation of an inner transformation, evidence of the "sanctified living that had to follow regeneration as part of the salvation process."[85]

In this context, it is significant that Massasoit and his successors specifically rejected Christianity. In a tract that Winslow published in 1649, the minister John Eliot noted that "Young *Ousamequin* [Massasoit's son Wamsutta or Alexander] is an enemy to praying to God, and the old man too wise to look after it."[86] Massasoit and his sons, Wamsutta and Metacom (also called Philip), made the decision not to "look after" Christianity, despite their ongoing political alliance with Plimouth.[87] Furthermore, Massasoit actively discouraged Wampanoag peoples under his leadership from accepting Christianity. In a 1653 tract, *Tears of Repentance,* Eliot and Mayhew, who eventually established a church on Martha's Vineyard, reported that the "great *Sachem* on the *Mayn* . . . is a great Enemy to our Reformation on the Island."[88] The ministers noted that this sachem "and those Indians about him" expressed their "discontentment" when a Martha's Vineyard Wampanoag showed interest in Christianity.[89] Additionally, the missionaries discovered that the Gay Head Indians were "obstinately resolved not to admit the *Glad-Tydings* of the Gospel among them (being animated by the *Sachims* of the Continent)."[90] Massasoit's opposition to Christianity and his continuing influence over Wampanoag people in southern New England show that while Winslow obtained temporary medical and religious authority among the Wampanoag, this authority was limited. Powerful Natives in southern New England remained unconvinced of the power and authority of colonists and their deity.

As Serge Gruzinski points out of the Spanish conquest of Mexico, both

European colonists and Native Americans experienced a "shock of conquest," a jarring realization that they now existed in unprecedented social and epistemological contexts made new by epidemics, invasion, sociopolitical upheaval, and dispossession.[91] As a result, Gruzinski argues, both colonists and Native Americans sought to rebuild their familiar practices with the goals of restoring stability and of adapting to the new world created by colonization. Although Gruzinski argues that New Spain was unique in facilitating intercultural forms of knowledge and communication after conquest, Winslow's and Harriot's accounts show that colonists and Native Americans in British America likewise responded to the shock of conquest by incorporating unfamiliar medical knowledge and practices.[92] Both colonists and Natives such as Tisquantum and Massasoit drew on available ideas and practices as they attempted to regain stability, with the result that they incorporated new medical knowledge into existing traditions, consequently creating new modes of communicating and healing that were not quite reproductions of pre-contact cultural practices.

Although Winslow's classification of Native medical and religious practices as witchcraft began to construct differences between colonial and Native medicine, Eliot and Shepard's reliance on medical knowledge as a path to conversion shows that colonists and Natives continued to share conceptions of disease and healing, especially beliefs that illness had a divine cause. Indeed, colonists continued to recognize the value of non-European medical knowledge in the eighteenth century, especially as European diseases such as smallpox began to affect not just Native Americans but also colonists born in the New World, who no longer possessed the same immunity to the disease that their counterparts in Europe did. In the context of repeated deadly smallpox epidemics, enslaved Africans' testimony regarding their preventive treatments for smallpox offered a compelling method of maintaining colonists' health. Colonial ministers encountered and drew on African medical knowledge even while attempting to convert its sources. Cotton Mather promoted African medical knowledge as a useful, providential gift to his chosen people, even as other colonists countered that such knowledge was untrustworthy.

CHAPTER 3

African Testimony, Dangerous Communications, and Colonial Medical Knowledge in the 1721 Boston Inoculation Controversy

Communicating Disease: Smallpox and the Circulation of Information

In 1721, Reverend Ebenezer Parkman, of Westborough, Massachusetts, received "two instance [letters] from friends who had just been innoculated [*sic*] for smallpox, [and] immediately burnt them both for fear of catching the disease from them."[1] The letters arrived during a smallpox epidemic that struck Boston after several enslaved Africans on board a ship from the West Indies contracted the disease in June 1721. Although city officials quarantined the Africans who first exhibited symptoms, smallpox spread throughout Boston, becoming an epidemic that would kill over eight hundred citizens before ending a year later. Parkman's decision to burn the letters indicated not only colonists' fear of contracting smallpox but also their concerns regarding inoculation, a preventive treatment for smallpox, and, by extension, concerns regarding how to recognize safe, or "healthy" forms with which to communicate disease. It is significant that Parkman's fears were not allayed by his knowledge that the letter writers had been inoculated; instead, he worried that the writers might have transmitted smallpox virus in their written communications.

Such concerns that inoculated patients would transmit smallpox were articulated most publicly and forcefully during the epidemic by the physician William Douglass, who argued that inoculation was an unsafe method of preventing smallpox because the "*Communication of Constitutional Distempers, is a difficulty which will require some series of Years to obviate.*"[2] Douglass expressed concerns that inoculation could communicate, or transmit, undesirable elements, including fatal doses of the smallpox virus and other illnesses present in the donor's blood. He worried that inoculation, like Parkman's letters, would invisibly communicate diseases that would be fatal to their recipients.

Parkman's concerns regarding the parallel repercussions of inoculation and of letter writing point as well to the ways in which, during the 1721 epidemic, anxiety about inadvertent, fatal transmissions of disease was not limited to medical practices but extended as well to acts of communicating medical knowledge. Indeed, Douglass's reference to inoculation as the "*Communication of Constitutional Distempers*" posited an equivalence between medical and literary communications that connected the safety of inoculation with the "health" or trustworthiness of information about inoculation and of the source of that information.[3] In fact, Douglass's arguments against inoculation frequently manifested concerns about appropriate forms of transmitting both smallpox viruses and medical knowledge. Douglass objected to inoculation not only because it was an untested practice that might transmit diseases already in the patients' blood but also because pro-inoculators based their arguments on communications from sources who, Douglass alleged, were unreliable.

Douglass's rival, Cotton Mather, shared his understanding of the connections between medical and literary communications, but Mather disagreed about how to interpret inoculation and knowledge of the practice. Mather, who presented inoculation to Bostonians as an effective prevention for smallpox, argued that the procedure transmitted only a small dose of smallpox that would not harm patients. Moreover, he explained that he had first learned of inoculation when his African slave Onesimus informed him of firsthand experiences with inoculation in Africa. Drawing on the rhetorical strategies of the plain style, which posited a close relation between words and the truths they represented, Mather offered Onesimus's testimony as trustworthy, unbiased evidence that inoculation worked to prevent smallpox. By contrast, Douglass insisted that only multiple tests and careful evaluation could prove that inoculation would not cause a full-blown case of smallpox and further spread the disease. Moreover, he argued that Africans' testimony contained irrational ideas that threatened to compromise colonial medical knowledge. For Douglass, both forms of medical communication hid dangerous elements under an appearance of efficacy. In a dispute that raged alongside the epidemic, Mather and Douglass debated the nature of medical communications: both inoculation and African testimony.

Historical and literary studies of the inoculation controversy, as it is now called, have explained Mather's and Douglass's respective responses to inoculation and to African testimony by describing the two men as opposing figures who occupied contrasting cultural and epistemological positions. Mather, who originally studied medicine at Harvard when he thought a stammer would prevent him from preaching, was not a licensed physician, but he did own the most extensive medical library in the colonies.[4] Moreover, he argued that he was uniquely authorized to attend to his congregants' bodies and souls, since his status as a minister gave him insight into the ultimate, spiritual causes of disease. Mather's numerous sermons on medical topics, such as *Seasonable Thoughts Upon Mortality: A Sermon Occasioned by the Raging of a Mortal Sickness in the Colony of Connecticut, and the Many Deaths of Our Brethren There* (published in Boston in 1711), illuminate his view of the body and soul as interconnected and the concomitant need for remedies that addressed both the physical and spiritual causes of disease. Historians and literary scholars have suggested that Mather promoted inoculation because he "hoped to improve his own position as a figure of importance in New England society" and to defend ministers' influence in both religious and political affairs.[5] Much to Mather's dismay, however, many colonists refused to accept inoculation, giving what historians suggest was one of the last fatal blows to ministerial authority.[6]

By contrast, Douglass, who had received an official medical degree in Europe before immigrating to Boston, has been seen as representing an emerging skepticism that was directed both at the "knowledge-claims" of "sectarian 'enthusiasts'" in England and at ministers "who claimed individual and unmediated inspiration from God, or whose solitary 'treading of the Book of Nature' produced unverifiable observational testimony."[7] Douglass's insistence that inoculation undergo careful testing countered Mather's belief that inoculation could be trusted to transmit a safe dose of smallpox. Moreover, Douglass argued that ministers lacked authority to produce medical philosophies, claims that "represented the earliest calls for medical professionalism heard in the colonies."[8] Indeed, during the controversy, Douglass organized the first colonial medical society and contributed to a new newspaper, *The New-England Courant,* both of which offered venues from which colonists could critique the ministers without fear of retribution. Literary historians have consequently seen Douglass as fostering a new, genteel colonial culture founded on rationality and print that sought to "create a sphere that was liberated from the pulpit."[9] Although Douglass's point of view accorded with perspectives that have come to be recognized as modern—such as theories that spiritual entities did not intervene in natural realms and that repeated experiments were necessary to prove a theory—his opposition to inoculation has paradoxically been seen as a barrier "in the path of scientific progress," especially since inoculation eventually became the preferred method of preventing smallpox until Edward Jenner introduced vaccination in 1796.[10]

Despite their differences, however, Mather and Douglass had more in common than studies of the controversy have heretofore acknowledged. In particular, the two men shared a position of geographic and cultural distance from metropolitan centers of knowledge production: Mather because his colonial birth marked him as a Creole whose humors were believed to differ from those possessed by his counterparts in Europe, and Douglass because, as a Scotsman who had immigrated to the colonies, he experienced "overlapping provincialisms."[11] Although Mather and Douglass held opposing views of African medical knowledge, for both men, interpreting African knowledge—and, in Mather's case, exchanging medical knowledge with Africans—allowed them to signal their conceptions of authoritative medical knowledge and thereby to counter biases from Europe regarding their own medical practices. Meanwhile, by communicating knowledge of inoculation in the early eighteenth century, Africans took on authority—at least momentarily—as firsthand witnesses and practitioners of a medical practice that powerful colonists such as Mather perceived as valuable.

Africans and their medical knowledge played a crucial role in the inoculation controversy and in Mather's and Douglass's formulations of their respective arguments. For Mather, representing Africans' testimony about inoculation during the controversy allowed him to position himself as an authoritative collector and evaluator of medical knowledge useful in the Americas and in Europe. Mather presented Africans' words as a transparent reflection of inoculation, in this way suggesting that these two medical communications could be trusted to transmit information straightforwardly, without fear of side effects or unreliable evidence. To counter Mather's promotion of inoculation, Douglass wrote a history of inoculation in which he charted the circulation of knowledge about the practice in order to expose the dangerous nature of both inoculation and African testimony. Unlike Mather, Douglass designated African medical knowledge as witchcraft and described Africans' minds as irrational. But rather than being motivated by biological views of Africans' bodies as possessing unique characteristics, Douglass drew on new Lockean conceptions of the relation between words and things to trace Africans' medical knowledge to ideas in their minds rather than to phenomena in the world. Although Mather died a few years after the controversy, Douglass returned to the topic of inoculation and African knowledge in his *Summary, Historical and Political of the First Planting, Progressive Improvements, and Present State of the British Settlements in North America,* in which he finally admitted that inoculation was effective, even while writing African knowledge out of inoculation's history.[12] He used classificatory forms to identify African medicine as skill using poisons, in this way adapting the categories in which colonists had previously placed Native American medical knowledge in order to mark the medical practices of enslaved Africans as dangerous.

William Douglass's History of Inoculation

Although many physicians in the eighteenth century responded to epidemics by using the rhetorical strategies of *historia* to write case studies of the illness, Douglass wrote a case study not of patients' symptoms but of pro-inoculators' arguments.[13] He sought to expose the weaknesses in the pro-inoculators' position by diagnosing the dangers both in their communications and in the practice of inoculation. In a history of inoculation's origins and entrance into Boston, Douglass employed narrative forms to connect the unsanctioned circulation of knowledge about inoculation with the dangerous circulation of disease that inoculation allegedly facilitated. His history of inoculation was published serially, with its first part appearing in the *Boston News-Letter* on July 17, 1721, and the sequel in the first issue of James Franklin's newspaper, the *New-England Courant,* published almost a month later. The articles traced Europeans' earliest encounters with inoculation, and they chronicled the transmission of information about the practice throughout the Mediterranean and the Atlantic worlds, from Greece to Constantinople to England to Boston.[14]

Douglass's "History" of inoculation assembled details regarding each "discovery" and use of the procedure, and he presented these details in a narrative that provided evidence that the practice was unsafe. In the *Boston News-Letter*, Douglass began the narrative by justifying his reasons for writing:

> it may be agreeable to some of your Readers to know the History of this affair from its Origine; how it came to be divulged here, The Success of the first Essay to put it in Practice, with the Character of the Operator; some loose hints from the accounts our Turkey Royal Society Communicators give of it, tending to discourage this Wicked and Criminal Practice, concluding with a disswasive from the same.[15]

In Douglass's version of inoculation's origin story, two medical practitioners, Jacobus Pylarinus and Emmanuel Timonius, observed practices of inoculation in Turkey and transmitted this information to the Royal Society, after which it was published in the Royal Society's *Philosophical Transactions* in England. A copy of the *Transactions* made its way to Douglass in Boston and, eventually, to Mather, when Douglass loaned the publication to the minister. As Douglass argued, Mather's first promotion of inoculation rested on a few "loose hints" that the minister gleaned from the *Transactions* and rushed into use, rather than on extensive testing of inoculation.[16]

Douglass added to the "History" in the first issue of the *New-England Courant*, in which he provided "A Continuation of the History of Inoculation in *Boston*, by a Society of the Practitioners in Physick."[17] He described in detail the local debates about inoculation, and he emphasized what he saw as the ministers' rash support for the procedure. He highlighted the clergy's disregard for colonists' concerns by placing Mather's actions to promote inoculation in a temporal sequence in which the people's objections opposed each of the minister's acts. In each case, the powerful leaders overturned the citizens' opposition. For example, Douglass explained that, after the ministers had encouraged Boylston to practice inoculation, the selectmen, "in duty bound to take Cognizance of the Matter," called a meeting and agreed that the practice of inoculation was untrustworthy.[18] Nonetheless, Douglass explained, the ministers continued to promote inoculation solely on the "Merits of their Characters," thereby overruling the selectmen's decision.[19] In the "History," the people's and city officials' objections to inoculation were countered at every turn by the ministers, a sequence that made the ministers' move to "set themselves up for Judges of a Man's Qualifications in the Practice of Physick" all the more egregious.[20] As *historia* described a patient's symptoms in order to support a physician's diagnosis, so the "History" exposed Mather's misuse of information in order to point readers toward Douglass's final "disswasive": the conclusion that inoculation should be rejected until the city officials and physicians agreed that it was an effective practice.[21]

But Douglass's "History" of inoculation did not conclude with the promised "disswasive" to Mather's arguments for inoculation, for Douglass interrupted the "History" with an alternate account of inoculation's origin and uses.[22] He interjected a satire into the fragmented narrative of inoculation's discovery; in the satire, Douglass farcically suggested some potential uses for inoculation. He also acknowledged Africans' role in the controversy as sources of information about inoculation, thus including a source of knowledge about inoculation that he had heretofore omitted from the "History." The satire took the form of a framed tale: in the opening frame, an anonymous writer informed the *Courant*'s editor that his brain had concocted a "Project."[23] He explained that he had read Douglass's "History" of inoculation as well as a story about the colonists' plans for an expedition against the Abenaki Indians in Maine, both of which had been printed in the previous issue of the *Courant*.[24] The writer found that these stories "lodged together in the same Apartment of my Brain, and by next Morning formed themselves into the following Project, . . . for reducing the Eastern Indians by *Inoculation*."[25] He presented his account as the result of his unconscious, the consequence of the two stories accidentally lodging in the same part of his brain. No carefully constructed linear narrative or a "History" organized by chronology or cause and effect, the "Project" was created by the seemingly random mixing of several histories.

The ideas and anxieties expressed in the "Project" disrupted Douglass's "History" by shifting his narrative of inoculation's origins in the circulation of documents among European men of science to a different story, which lacked the "History's" clear temporal sequence. This competing account replaced the "History's" European physicians and fellows of the Royal Society with enslaved Africans who employed inoculation throughout the Americas, in order to cure a number of diseases. The anonymous writer suggested outfitting inoculators with a mixture of "Negro yaws and confluent smallpox," two diseases for which Africans employed inoculation as a preventative.[26]

According to this satirical logic, the colonists would inoculate the Abenaki Indians, a move that would end the war by infecting the Native warriors with contagious doses of smallpox that the inoculated men would carry back to their villages and spread to others. The fragmented "History" and the satire registered anxieties regarding political tensions with the Abenakis as well as concerns regarding colonists' encounters with Africans and their medical knowledge in the context of the smallpox epidemic. In the fragmented non-narrative space of the satire, Douglass acknowledged the role that African medical knowledge played in the 1721 controversy, and he nodded as well to contexts in which colonists valued African medical knowledge. Douglass's attempt to interpret the significance of African medical knowledge was manifested by his rhetorical shift from the narrative "History" to the satire, which alluded to alternate understandings of inoculation even as it acknowledged perceived threats to the colonial political and physical body.

Douglass's satire certainly should not be read straightforwardly, as an indication of his approval of inoculation, for, as I explain below, he expressed concerns regarding the validity of African medical knowledge by critiquing Africans' testimony as a communication that appeared trustworthy but that hid dangerous elements. However, it is worth pausing, as Douglass did when shifting from his "History" to the satire, to consider how these rhetorical moves mark his encounters with African medical knowledge and to ask how African medical communications influenced the controversy and Douglass's medical writing. As I show in the following sections, Douglass's mention of both yaws and smallpox in the satire referenced medical practices employed by Africans in the Caribbean, where they were often accorded space in which they could employ inoculation to cure illnesses, especially yaws. Moreover, Africans' practices of and communications about inoculation accorded them medical authority that colonists throughout the Americas acknowledged as useful. During the controversy, for example, Mather emphasized the efficacy of African medical knowledge, in this way proposing an alternate conception of medical communications, one that challenged Douglass's history of the controversy.

Inoculation in the Atlantic World

Douglass's inclusion of both yaws and smallpox in his "Project" invoked contexts in which Euro-colonial medical practitioners not only perceived African medical knowledge as beneficial but also acknowledged that Africans' remedies superseded their own. African medical practices, including inoculation, were well known throughout the British West Indies for their efficacy treating and preventing both smallpox and yaws. As Richard B. Sheridan points out, Douglass had traveled to Barbados in 1717, where he could certainly have observed slaves infected with yaws as well as the medical treatments that Africans employed to treat this illness in the Caribbean.[27] Both yaws and smallpox were a scourge on slave ships and plantations: yaws, in particular, was endemic on the coast of Africa but grew to epidemic proportions on slave ships. The disease spread rapidly throughout African and African Creole communities in the West Indies, subsequently disabling large portions of planters' enslaved workforce. Yaws was extremely contagious and communicated by physical contact, with the result that, as the physician John Williamson pointed out, "white people naturally feel a horror in exposing themselves to the risk of infection."[28] Indeed, European medical practitioners were so fearful of being infected with yaws that they frequently allowed enslaved Africans to employ their own cures for the disease. Slaves with yaws were usually quarantined and sometimes placed under the care of an African who had already had the disease; such immune healers were usually left unsupervised to apply traditional African medicines or remedies developed in the Caribbean.[29]

European and colonial plantation physicians frequently admitted that African treatments for yaws were more effective than their own procedures, which sometimes involved doses of mercury. Inoculation was among these African remedies: children were inoculated against yaws in Africa, and some slaves relied on inoculation to prevent yaws in the West Indies as well.[30] In the early eighteenth century, colonial physicians and natural historians commented that enslaved Africans possessed knowledge of a range of treatments for yaws, which Douglass would likely have observed or heard about while traveling in the West Indies. Henry Barham, whose *Hortus Americanus* circulated in manuscript in the early eighteenth century before it was published in 1794 and who advised Hans Sloane, a physician and a Fellow of the Royal Society, on his natural history of Jamaica, identified several roots that Africans used in "venereal cases," a category in which European and colonial physicians included yaws.[31] Moreover, Barham described "an old negro woman so called, who, with a simple decoction, did wonderful cures in the most stubborn diseases, as the yaws, and in venereal cases, when the person has been given over as incurable by skillful physicians, because their Herculean medicines failed them; viz. preparations of mercury and antimony."[32] Sloane had less success discovering the remedies that Africans employed to treat yaws; as he reported, he had heard of Africans possessing knowledge of "some specific Herbs to root [yaws] out," but he admitted that he was unable to discover the identity of the plants.[33]

Knowledge of Africans' use of inoculation to treat yaws must have circulated orally among enslaved peoples and sometimes among planters for many years before European physicians began to publish accounts of these treatments. When the medical practitioner John Quier contributed to a collection of medical reports from the West Indies, he acknowledged that inoculation had already been in use in the Caribbean for some time. Quier noted that he used inoculation to prevent both yaws and smallpox in an epidemic of 1768 because "Inoculation had been frequently practised with success in this country, according to the methods formerly in use."[34] As William Hillary pointed out, enslaved Africans were accustomed to treating yaws in order to prevent successive infections: "*Yaws* seldom fail to attack the Negroes in Africa, at one time or other in their Life-time, but most frequently the Children and young People; and that they very rarely or never have it a second time, if they have been perfectly cured the first time, either in their own native Country by their Negro Doctors, or after they arrived here."[35] Hillary further explained that "yaws" is an African word, a statement that would have suggested to European readers that the illness and its treatments originated in Africa.[36]

By the end of the eighteenth century, descriptions of Africans' knowledge of inoculation as a preventive treatment for yaws were common in printed accounts of the West Indies. Bryan Edwards explained that one of his slaves informed him that the "Natives of the Gold Coast give their children the *yaws* (a frightful disorder) *by inoculation;* and she described the manner of performing the operation to be making an incision in the thigh, and putting in some of the infectious matter."[37] Although Africans had initially employed inoculation without much supervision by colonial physicians, plantation owners and medical practitioners eventually appropriated inoculation as a treatment for yaws, so that the physician Benjamin Moseley could claim inoculation as a colonial practice, writing that "The cure of the *yaws* is now understood by skilful practitioners. Inoculation is performed with success."[38] Douglass's travels to the Caribbean and his proximity to Africans' treatments for yaws show that his satirical account of African knowledge during the controversy was not the random thoughts of an unconscious mind but rather was based on his encounters with African medicine.

Douglass would also have learned of African medical knowledge of inoculation from local sources in New England, for Mather made African testimony about inoculation a primary element of his argument during the controversy. Knowledge of inoculation could have been transmitted from Africa to Boston as early as 1706, when Mather's congregation purchased an African slave as a gift for their minister. Although it is not clear when this African, whom Mather renamed Onesimus, told Mather about inoculation, Mather knew of the procedure at least by 1716, as he indicated in a letter to John Woodward, one of the fellows of the Royal Society. Mather wrote:

> I do assure you, that many months before I mett with any Intimations of treating y^e^ *Small-Pox,* with ye Method of Inoculation, any where in *Europe;* I had from a Servant of my own, an Account of its being practised in *Africa.* Enquiring of my Negroman *Onesimus,* who is a pretty Intelligent Fellow, Whether he ever had y^e^ *Small-Pox;* he answered, both, *Yes,* and, *No;* and then told me, that he had undergone an Operation, which had given him something of y^e^ *Small-Pox,* & would forever praeserve him from it; adding, That it was often used among y^e^ *Guramantese,* & whoever had ye Courage to use it, was forever free from ye fear of the Contagion. He described ye Operation to me, and shew'd me in his Arm ye Scar, which it had left upon him; and his Description of it, made it the same, that afterwards I found related unto you by your *Timonius.*[39]

Mather's description of Onesimus as a "*Guramantese*" is difficult to translate exactly, but it probably places Onesimus's country of origin in West or central Africa.[40] Smallpox had existed in West Africa for centuries by the eighteenth century, and it is quite probable that inoculation had long been used there as well, as indicated by Yoruba smallpox gods dating to pre-Christian history and by accounts of inoculation being used "from time immemorial" reported to European travelers.[41] Knowledge of inoculation seems to have been widespread throughout the continent: Donald R. Hopkins concludes that by the mid-eighteenth century, "African tribes further south along the eastern coast had apparently learned, or relearned, inoculation . . . perhaps from the Arabs or the Portuguese."[42]

Throughout Africa, inoculation and other medical practices had been employed to bring about both physical and spiritual healing for individuals and the community for centuries before Onesimus and Mather discussed inoculation.[43] Smallpox epidemics were seen as manifestations of divine judgments, sent by a wrathful god. As Philip D. Curtin has pointed out, smallpox gods were honored throughout West Africa and had special status: "For the Yoruba, Sopona was one of the four divinities invested with special status by Olodumare, the creator god. He was both feared and important, and he was the only deity associated with a particular affliction."[44] Smallpox was often considered the worst of these divine judgments, and medical practitioners treated the disease by petitioning divine powers for healing while simultaneously prescribing treatments such as inoculation.[45]

Several methods of inoculation seem to have been in use in Africa: as the physician James Kirkpatrick reported by relating information from the "Ambassador from *Tripoli* [who] affirmed that in *Africa* the Disease was imparted by passing a Needle and Thread, that had been conducted thro' a well maturated Pustule, through the Teguments between the Thumb and Forefinger, where they may be pierced without wounding the subjacent Muscle."[46] The Scottish physician James Bruce reported in his travel narrative that in eastern Africa, women were responsible for the practice of inoculation. When hearing of an outbreak of smallpox, they:

> go to the infected place, and wrapping a fillet of cotton cloth about the arm of the person infected, they let it remain there till they bargain with the mother how many she is to sell them. . . . This being concluded, they go home, and tie the fillet about their own child's arm; certain, as they say, from long experience, that the child infected is to do well, and not having more than the number of pustules that were agreed and paid for. There is no example, as far as I could learn, either here or in Abyssinia, of this disease returning, that is, attacking any one person more than once.[47]

Medicine men or women also employed healing practices that combined "magical and *supernatural* elements, on the one hand, with medicinal practices and *natural* processes on the other."[48] Such prayers and healing ceremonies cured disease by appealing to the world of non-human spirits to restore relationships between human and non-human realms. Finally, healing practices sought to restore not only physical and spiritual but also social, political, and economic health to communities.[49]

The communication of information about inoculation in the New World probably occurred in a similarly religious context, and Mather's and Onesimus's conversations about inoculation would have been informed by both Puritan and West African medical and religious practices. By the time Onesimus entered Mather's household, he would have observed a variety of medical practices and systems in the course of his travels throughout the Atlantic World. Slaves from various locations in Africa usually arrived in New England after a journey of multiple passages. The Atlantic slave trade fed mostly West Indian markets, but unsold or unwanted slaves might be sent to northern cities, where they formed communities characterized by a diverse mixture of languages, cultures, and nationalities, rather than a unified African culture.[50] Although Africans shared many similar religious and cultural beliefs, their religious systems frequently differed in their specific practices. Despite these differences, however, enslaved peoples in the Americas held knowledge of inoculation in common or employed the practice after learning of it from other Africans.

Although Boston's Africans probably came into contact with the medical and religious beliefs of their masters and other slaves from a perspective of cultural disorientation, they seem to have responded to such pressures by adopting some of their masters' beliefs while maintaining elements of their own medical and religious practices. Onesimus underwent lessons in Protestant and textual literacy, but he also seems to have resisted these teachings. In 1706, the same year he received Onesimus from his congregation, Mather wrote *The Negro Christianized,* a pamphlet in support of converting slaves. Onesimus was one of the "Negroes" Mather sought to "Christianize," and this education included spiritual tenets as well as the skills necessary to read the Bible.[51] As Mather noted in his diary, he planned for Onesimus to "be sure to read every Day" and from there to "go on to Writing."[52] Moreover, Mather determined that Onesimus would also be "frequently catechized."[53] It is thus likely that Onesimus learned to read the Bible—or Mather's simplified catechism in *The Negro Christianized*—and he must have become familiar with Protestant interpretations of illness and healing as signs of divine judgment or approval. These lessons, as well as Onesimus's pre-existing understanding of disease and healing as having metaphysical origins, would have allowed him to explain Africans' practice of inoculation in terms both familiar and appealing to colonists such as Mather.

Yet Onesimus apparently did not wholly embrace Christian religious beliefs, for Mather reported in 1716 that Onesimus "proves wicked, grows useless, Froward, Immorigerous [or uncivil]."[54] It was in this same year that Mather first wrote about learning of inoculation from Onesimus, and, interestingly, it was also the year that Onesimus obtained a degree of official independence from his owner. Mather wrote that, having considered how best to "Dispos[e]" of Onesimus,[55] he agreed to "Release" Onesimus to "Enjoy and Employ his whole Time for his own purposes, and as he pleases," in exchange for Onesimus's continued help when the Mather family was in need and for five pounds, which Onesimus was to pay within six months.[56] Kathryn S. Koo speculates that Mather's dissatisfaction with Onesimus's behavior may have stemmed from the fact that Onesimus had already gained some autonomy by 1716, for he had been already allowed to earn his own wages, to marry, and to maintain a separate household in Boston.[57] He seems to have employed his knowledge of colonial religious and textual practices to separate himself from Mather and to claim the authority to determine his own actions and beliefs. At the same time, Onesimus seems to have resisted a complete conversion both to Christianity and to Mather's authority. Although we cannot be certain that communicating his knowledge of inoculation influenced Mather's decision to agree to manumission, Onesimus did obtain medical authority as a firsthand observer of a medical practice unfamiliar to colonists around the same time that he obtained his manumission. As with the slaves who used inoculation to treat yaws in the Caribbean, Onesimus's knowledge of a treatment for a deadly disease endowed him with status as an expert on a medical practice that prevented diseases feared by colonists. We should consequently be wary of treating Onesimus as a rhetorical figure that either Mather or Douglass created in order to advance their arguments for or against inoculation, for Onesimus clearly maintained some control over his labor and his medical and spiritual knowledge.[58]

Onesimus's relative autonomy, his actions to resist Christianity, and his medical knowledge disrupted the narratives that both Mather and Douglass attempted to construct regarding the conversion or Christianizing of "Negroes" and the origins of inoculation. Although Onesimus's testimony regarding inoculation was compelling and useful to Mather, his refusal to submit entirely to Christian beliefs and discipline motivated Mather to alter his plans for his slave and to allow Onesimus more independence, even as Mather continued to rely on his former slave's testimony. Similarly, the connections among practices of inoculation employed in Boston and in the

Caribbean disrupted Douglass's "History" of inoculation by providing examples of effective uses of inoculation and of powerful medical knowledge held by enslaved Africans. The texture of Douglass's writing—his shift from the historical narrative to the satire of inoculation—manifested his attempt to explain how inoculation—and, by extension, African medical knowledge—could appear effective in some contexts and endanger colonists in others. Meanwhile, Onesimus, like Africans throughout the Americas, employed his knowledge of inoculation as a form of medical authority that colonists both recognized and sought to control, though not always successfully.

African Witnesses and the Plain Style

Douglass and Mather disagreed about how to interpret Africans' knowledge of inoculation because they held different views on the nature both of oral testimony and of inoculation, specifically, what these two communications transmitted. Mather accorded Onesimus's testimony authority by representing his slave's words, and, by extension, inoculation, as trustworthy medical communications; to do so, he drew on the tradition of the simple, unbiased witness and the rhetorical strategies of the plain style. Mather argued that one could read African testimony straight-forwardly, as a guide to an unfamiliar medical practice, and he held that one could likewise "read" inoculation as a preventative practice that would perform its intended function without side effects. To support these arguments, Mather offered a transcription of Onesimus's statements about inoculation:

> There is at this Time a considerable Number of *Africans* in this Town, who can have no Conspiracy or Combination to cheat us. No body has instructed them to tell their Story. The more plainly, brokenly, and blunderingly, and like Ideots, they tell their Story, it will be with reasonable Men, but the much more credible. For *that these* all agree in *one Story;* 'That abundance of poor Negro's die of the *Small Pox,* till they learn this *Way;* that People take the Juice of the *Small Pox,* and *Cut the Skin,* and put in a drop; then by'nd by a little *Sick,* then few *Small Pox;* and no body dye of it; no body have *Small Pox* any more.' Here we have a clear Evidence, that in Africa, where the Poor Creatures dye of the *Small Pox* in the common way like Rotten Sheep, a Merciful God has taught them a *wonderful Preservative.*[59]

Mather's description of Africans' speech as broken and blundering and of slaves as "Ideots" did not mean that they were insane or witless but rather indicated their status as unlearned, or nonprofessionals. As Stephen Shapin has pointed out, in "routine medieval and early modern English usage, an 'idiot' was simply a lay, uneducated, or common person, and that was the major basis on which 'tales told by idiots' might signify nothing."[60] Michel de Certeau observes that the idiot traditionally acted in European discourse as an "'illiterate' who lends his word the support of what his body has experienced and adds to it no 'interpretation.'"[61] European travelers to the Americas who hoped to authorize their reports of seemingly marvelous sights and experiences often replaced the idiot with Native Americans, whose simplicity and savagery were presumed to make them incapable of misrepresentation or deceit. As de Certeau writes, the "cannibal came to rest in the place occupied by the *Idiotus,* which for two centuries had been the only place that could authorize 'new language.'"[62]

Mather's description of slaves' simple speech and "clear Evidence" substituted the African witness for the idiot and the Native, thus defining Onesimus as a figure whose simplicity and unlearnedness made him an ideal instrument through whom God could communicate his will.[63] Indeed, despite the fact that Mather himself had attempted to teach Onesimus to read and write, the historical meanings of the "idiot" as one who was unlearned or common meant that Mather could still present Onesimus as an "idiot" in order to signal that his testimony was unbiased and trustworthy. Moreover, Mather had described Africans' intellectual capacity in *The Negro Christianized,* saying that "their *Stupidity* is a *Discouragement.* It may seem, unto as little purpose, to *Teach,* as to *wash an AEthopian.*"[64] This comment suggests that Mather believed that Africans retained their simple minds even after they had been educated; rather paradoxically, this simplicity also made them ideal witnesses. Finally, although slaves' speech did point to their position of servitude, an inferior position to be sure, it also defined their testimony as uncorrupted by artifice or bias.

In this context, Onesimus's broken and blundering testimony reflected his simple, honest character and his ability to speak about "the true, the given, nature of things."[65] Mather could rely on Onesimus to offer "clear evidence" of inoculation's success because he believed his slave's words reflected only his experience, unmediated by text-bound philosophies and uncorrupted by personal motives.[66] Mather's transcription of his conversation with Onesimus positioned the slave as an unlearned witness whose simple wisdom surprised allegedly more sophisticated readers. Onesimus took on the role of the uneducated, yet wise African slave whose innocent perspective and unfamiliar dialect produced "a speech which is unaware of what it expresses before decipherment can provide it with meaning and practical usage"; such speech discovers great truths to so-called civilized peoples.[67]

Africans often appeared in this role in intercultural dialogues and in conversations printed in anti-slavery tracts. For example, Thomas Tryon presented a dialogue between a "Christian, That was his *Master* in *America*"[68] and a slave who is "identified in the text as an indigenous voice of wisdom."[69] The slave's straightforward honesty and unsophisticated perspective exposed the hypocrisy and greed of Europeans who claimed to be enlightened Christians but who mistreated their slaves. The slave's understanding surpassed that of his Christian master because it came from the natural wisdom of experience, that is, from "so much understanding, as not to content our selves to *see with other mens Eyes.*"[70] In much the same way that colonists described Natives' speech to pit "primitive babble against 'civilized' readers' 'reasonable' expectations, thereby conveying a distinctly Protestant feeling of cosmic rupture between man's reason and objective cosmic truth," so authors such as Mather and Tryon described dialogues with slaves to expose the shortcomings of "civilized" behavior and knowledge.[71] Given these traditions of Africans as simple, yet wise, witnesses, we should not see Mather's representation of Onesimus's and other Africans' patois as a suggestion that they had "as little mastery over the procedure as they [had] over language" but rather as linguistic markers familiar to Europeans throughout the Atlantic world as signs of trustworthy testimony.[72]

Mather's interpretation of Onesimus's words as a truthful account of inoculation suggested that communications of words and of disease could be trusted to transmit their objects straightforwardly. His view of medical communications during the controversy was indebted to his sense that signs—whether words from an African slave or symptoms on a body—could be trusted not to hide falsehoods or dangerous elements. Like many ministers in New England, Mather employed the plain style to mediate between his audience and divine truths, whether expressed in scripture or in natural phenomena such as Africans' words and bodies. The plain style brought "words and things" into "closer relationship"; its rhetorical authority was founded on the belief that words could be arranged to reflect things as they appeared in the world.[73] According to this nominalist conception of language, developed by natural philosophers and linguists in Europe, "words represent reality to our understanding."[74] This emphasis on connecting words and things to produce knowledge inspired literary styles and forms that made "language reflect the rudimentary composition and order of nature."[75] Ministers acted as authoritative mediators for divine truth: they made it seem as though the "medium by which the Spirit moved has become transparent: . . . the person, and the human instrumentalities of writing and speech, vanish, leaving communication to occur between pure Spirit (the living Word) and the hearts of those who believe."[76]

As a minister who regularly employed the plain style to offer his congregation access to divine truths, Mather sought to transfer this authority to his acts of recording African testimony, in order to present useful evidence from his sources and to assure his audience that they would not be infected by the "manners of the Heathen," as some anti-inoculators argued.[77] Just as ministers employed their "privileged discernment" to determine whether their parishioners' testimonies of faith contained evidence of grace, so Mather analyzed Onesimus's testimony to ascertain whether it was a trustworthy account, and he employed his "ministerial expertise" and the plain style to present the testimony as trustworthy.[78] Mather's transcription of Africans' testimony suggested that their simple words suited the "nature and order" of inoculation—its status as a safe prevention for smallpox.[79] Furthermore, Mather's description of Africans' "Story" as "clear Evidence" posited a direct correspondence between inoculation and Africans' words and bodies, such that slaves' simple speech and scarred but healthy bodies were clear signs that inoculation was both effective and safe.[80] In the same way, Mather's promotion of inoculation as a safe, effective prevention rested on his interpretation of the pustules and pocks that appeared on inoculated patients as the direct and only repercussions of the practice. As Mather pointed out, "*The Operation has been performed on a Hundred & more, in the Town of Boston: And not one of them has miscarried.*"[81] Thus whereas anti-inoculators argued that inoculation could invisibly transmit diseases that would remain hidden in patients for years, only to surface after they had survived smallpox, Mather argued that inoculation could be trusted to transmit only a small dose of smallpox.

Similar to the "skilful Physician well-prepared," who "well and wisely managed" the inoculation and transmitted an appropriate dose of smallpox virus, enough to induce a brief case of the disease but not so large as to endanger the patient, so Mather's transcription ensured that Africans' communications about inoculation had their desired effect on his audience.[82] In particular, Mather, like colonial ministers who interpreted natural phenomena as the work of divine approval or judgment, presented African testimony and inoculation as signs of providence. Onesimus's testimony had special significance as a revelation of God's will for the colonists, for, as Mather wrote, as a medical "*Preservative,*" inoculation could save the lives of many Bostonians; as "*wonderful*" knowledge, inoculation would motivate patients to acknowledge God's providence.[83] Slaves' testimony and firsthand experience offered empirical evidence of invisible spiritual truths, specifically of God's providential intervention into the course of the epidemic to heal mercifully his chosen people.

At the same time that Mather positioned himself as a spiritual authority capable of interpreting the work of God in nature by transmitting Africans' testimony, so he also used his transcriptions of African medical knowledge to define his place as a valuable producer of medical knowledge in a transatlantic context. Mather did not only "authenticate [and make] distinctive his source" when quoting Africans' speech; he also sought to authenticate his own status as a colonist capable of locating and applying trustworthy medical knowledge.[84] As Ralph Bauer has argued, in a system of "epistemic mercantilism," colonists were positioned as collectors of knowledge they sent to the metropole, where men of science transformed it into facts.[85] However, Mather attempted to revise this system with his transcriptions of Onesimus's knowledge: Mather directed the safe interpretation and use of Africans' testimony in order to establish his ability not only to collect but also to evaluate medical knowledge and practices, his colonial birthplace notwithstanding. Mather's promotion of African knowledge and of inoculation stood as evidence of his ability to analyze medical communications and to make decisions about which communications offered evidence of divine, providential truths rather than diabolic or heathen communications.

Speaking "Negroishly": Infectious Evidence, Words, and Minds

Although Douglass, like Mather, acknowledged both that African knowledge could be useful and the African origins of inoculation, he ultimately disputed the safety both of inoculation and of African testimony.

He revised Mather's interpretation of slaves' "blunderingly" speech as an indication of Africans' characters as trustworthy witnesses by shifting the criteria with which Mather judged modes of communication.[86] Douglass's comment in his satire that the *"Ammunition"* with which colonists would face the Abenakis would be *"of the best Proof"* suggested that inoculating the Abenakis with yaws and smallpox would certainly kill them, but it is also possible to read this *"Proof"* as epistemological ammunition.[87] The "proof" or quality of the ammunition would thus refer also to the status with which African medical knowledge was endowed during the controversy as "proof" or evidence of inoculation's success. Just as he connected communications about inoculation with the procedure itself, so Douglass conflated Africans' testimony regarding inoculation—their words and pockmarks that Mather interpreted as "proof"—with inoculation, or the practices that would make one "proof" against, or immune to, smallpox. African testimony thus possessed medical significance not only because it transmitted information about a medical practice but also because, as Douglass alleged, it communicated medical knowledge that endangered Natives' (and by extension colonists') health.

The multiple meanings of "proof" connected Douglass's questions about the safety of inoculation with his interpretation of Africans' transmissions of medical knowledge. Douglass admitted that his concern regarding the hidden maladies transmitted by inoculation might seem a "*Chimerical* or conjectural fear: but as all constitutional Distempers have some *Idea* or *Seminium* in every drop of our juices, the *acute Distemper* according to its nature soon shows itself, the *Chronical* ails act slowly & imperceptibly on our Bodies."[88] Like the inoculated Abenaki warriors, who would discover the adverse effects of inoculation only after returning home, so inoculated colonists might escape the smallpox epidemic only to be stricken later with an illness passed along during inoculation. Whether it transmitted full cases of smallpox itself or other diseases, inoculation deceptively carried secret "*Constitutional Distempers*" that were revealed when patients believed themselves safe.[89] Eventually, Douglass suggested, the "*Idea* or *Seminium*" transmitted with the smallpox virus would "show itself" in the form of a new and deadly illness.[90] Douglass's "Project" thus defined inoculation as an apparently safe but eventually fatal procedure by exposing a gap between its appearance and its dangerous reality.

Douglass's comments manifested anxieties that African communications—both inoculation and slaves' testimony—likewise hid dangerous epistemological elements. Although Douglass, like Mather, made the oral medium and plain style of slaves' medical testimony a key factor in determining its veracity, he offered a competing, critical evaluation of slaves' speech and status. He wrote:

> Their second Voucher is an Army of half a Dozen or half a score *Africans,* by others call'd Negro Slaves, who tell us now (tho' never before) that it is practised in their own Country. The more blundering and Negroish they tell their Story, it is the more credible says *C.M.; a paradox in Nature;* for all they say true or false is after the same manner. There is not a Race of Men on Earth more *False Lyars,* &c. Their Accounts of what was done in their Country was never depended upon till now for Arguments sake.[91]

Douglass pointed to the same plain, or simple, stylistic attributes that Mather had emphasized in Onesimus's speech, but he did not construe slaves' "blundering and Negroish" style as an indication of honesty. Rather, Douglass classified slaves as an entire "Race of Men [of] *False Lyars*" by connecting their "blundering" speech with their "Negroish," or African, backgrounds and reading both as an indication of their intellectual capacities.[92] Consequently, he suggested, Africans' "Story" reflected neither the truth about inoculation nor their virtuous characters but rather indicated slaves' inability to speak in more than one manner, that is, to learn to think and speak rationally. Their particular sounds or styles of speech did not reflect personal attributes of honesty or education; instead, everything the "Army" of Africans said revealed their status as uneducated and thus untrustworthy witnesses.[93]

The connections Douglass drew between Africans' speech and cultural background suggested that slaves possessed undeveloped intellectual faculties, which allegedly predisposed them to mistake dangerous medical practices for trustworthy knowledge, similar to Harriot and Winslow's suggestion that Native Americans possessed strong faculties of the imagination that inclined them to accept knowledge obtained in communications with the devil. Douglass developed these conceptions of Natives' and Africans' mental faculties by suggesting that Africans' words did not reflect things in the world, such as diseases and cures, as Mather had argued, but rather that they corresponded to sense impressions or ideas in Africans' minds. This argument reflected emerging conceptions of the mind presented in John Locke's

An Essay Concerning Human Understanding, which suggested that, far from mirroring things themselves, words were "external sensible Signs, whereby those invisible *Ideas,* which possess his Mind in so great variety, might be made known to others."[94] Words corresponded to the impressions that things made in the mind, rather than to the real essences of things.[95] Language was thus "based not on the reality of words but on the rationality of speakers"; consequently, words could conceal human fallibility and their mental failures.[96] As Locke wrote, "*Words in their primary or immediate Signification, stand for nothing, but the* Ideas *in the Mind of him that uses them,* how imperfectly soever, or carelesly those *Ideas* are collected from the Things, which they are supposed to represent."[97] Such rationalist conceptions of language raised the possibility that descriptions of natural phenomena were subjective and fallible, regardless how plain the style with which they were presented. In this context, firsthand reports, based as they were on potentially fallible sense impressions, required careful evaluation to ensure their accuracy, thus making rationality and learning crucial to determining a witness's credibility.

Douglass's criticism of African speech suggested that, in the case both of inoculation and of conversations about the practice, the source of communication—whether a donor's blood or witnesses of medical practices—determined the safety of the malady or medical knowledge transmitted. Just as inoculation could potentially transfer unknown "*Chronical ails*" and fatal doses of smallpox, so medical communication could transmit poisonous or untrustworthy evidence that compromised the authority of the knowledge being transmitted.[98] In the case of African testimony, Douglass argued that slaves' minds transmitted deceitful or inaccurate information, the product of their irrational thoughts. He developed this interpretation of African speech in a pamphlet published a few months after his "History" appeared, likening African medical knowledge to the "*successful Wickedness*" practiced by "Pharaoh's *Magicians,*" who imitated God's "*own Judgments.*"[99] In this way, Douglass compared slaves to the Egyptian magicians who successfully performed the same wonders as Moses and whose acts led the pharaoh to conclude that Moses' god was no more powerful than his magicians. The connection between inoculation and witchcraft that masqueraded as legitimate knowledge supported Douglass's interpretation of Africans' "blundering and Negroish" words as a sign of their irrational minds, which, he suggested, had inclined them to mistake dangerous, untested procedures for trustworthy medical knowledge.[100] Douglass thus reinterpreted Africans' speech as reflecting not the nature of inoculation but rather slaves' irrational thoughts.

As colonists' words and actions were read by European audiences as signs of the status of mental faculties influenced by the American climate, so Douglass interpreted Africans' testimony as a sign of their wits. In this context, Africans' "Negroish" style of speech exposed not only the dangerous status of Africans' medical knowledge but also the nature of their temperaments.[101] Douglass's attention to Africans' modes of communication and their intellectual faculties complicate analyses of his opposition to inoculation as driven by biological conceptions of difference that drew connections between slaves' skin color and their testimony. Instead, Douglass opposed Africans' knowledge on the basis of the argument that their minds could not be trusted to produce rational thoughts.[102] Moreover, Douglass developed previous colonial accounts of Native medical knowledge as witchcraft to suggest that, like Natives, Africans credited diabolic practices and knowledge.

Classifying African Knowledge

Douglass ultimately had the last word in the inoculation controversy, for he returned to his history of inoculation thirty years after the controversy and the epidemic had ended. Mather had died in 1728, but he no doubt would have been pleased to find that Douglass eventually admitted that inoculation was effective. Far from crediting Mather with his new conclusions, however, Douglass insisted that only time had proven inoculation's success, and he acknowledged neither Mather's nor Onesimus's role in inoculation's history.

Douglass also revised his prior accounts of African knowledge: he classified African medicine as dangerous not because it was irrational knowledge or witchcraft that masqueraded as trustworthy information but because Africans' medical practices were founded on skilled knowledge of poisons. In his *Summary, Historical and Political of the First Planting, Progressive Improvements, and Present State of the British Settlements in North America,* Douglass wrote: "The American Indians are noted for their traditional knowledge of poisonous herbs and antedotes; but I do not find that our Indian venefici are so expert in the veneficium art, as the negroes of Africa, who give poisons, which in various, but certain periods, produce their mortal effects, some suddenly, some after a number of months or years."[103] The description of African poisons fatally sickening their recipients years after they were administered replicated Douglass's critique of inoculation and African medical knowledge during the controversy. Just as inoculation initially appeared to make patients immune to smallpox only to infect them with other "*Constitutional Distempers,*" so African poisons turned out to have fatal effects years after they were applied.[104]

But Douglass did not compare such hidden dangers to witchcraft masquerading as reliable knowledge, as he had during the controversy. In the *Summary,* he classified African medicine as the "veneficium art," or knowledge of poisons, rather than of magical ceremonies and practices.[105] African knowledge remained untrustworthy but not because of Africans' trust in diabolic knowledge. Instead, Africans' medical knowledge was threatening because they possessed knowledge of natural poisons whose effects, although initially hidden, would fatally affect patients. Douglass supported this new conception of witchcraft as practices that appeared supernatural but merely had hidden natural causes by drawing linguistic connections between witchcraft and herbal poisons in a footnote. As he wrote: "Originally *veneficium,* or witchcraft, did not signify an explicit covenant with the devil; but the study of the poisonous qualities of herbs, and these herb-women were called *veneficae,* or witches. The witchcraft of our times is a pavid superstition and ignorance, therefore it prevails in Lapland; and other obscure ignorant parts of the world."[106] Categorizing African medical knowledge as "veneficium" supported Douglass's argument that Africans possessed not diabolically inspired knowledge but a "veneficium art,"[107] or skill with the "poisonous qualities of herbs," which only appeared to be preternatural because they had delayed effects.[108] By drawing attention to an "original" signification for witchcraft that involved experiential knowledge of herbs, rather than diabolic insight, Douglass identified a natural cause for Africans' mysteriously fatal medical practices. In this way, he separated himself from beliefs that witchcraft originated in a secret alliance with diabolic powers that allowed humans to perform preternatural acts.

Douglass's classification of African knowledge as poison separated his own medical practices from those of Mather and African slaves (and from colonists such as Thomas Harriot and Edward Winslow), who each credited the ability of non-human, supernatural forces to influence the material world. At the same time, Douglass signaled to readers in England that he had maintained his ability to differentiate authoritative forms of knowledge from untrustworthy ones, his long stay in the New World notwithstanding. During the controversy, he had compared Mather's certainty that inoculation was an effective medical practice to the "*Infatuation*" of "*hanging those suspected of Witchcraft*" that had plagued New England when Mather had infamously supported prosecuting witches at Salem on the basis of empirical evidence such as witnesses' testimony.[109] Similarly, Douglass argued, Mather's eagerness to promote inoculation led him to mistake Egyptian witchcraft for God's "*own Judgments,*" or providential medical knowledge;[110] Mather had subsequently infected the colonists' minds with the infatuation of "*Self-procuring the Smallpox.*"[111] As Douglass pointed out, New England often fell victim to such "Infatuations," which "seemed to return to us after a Period of about Thirty Years, *viz.* from the *Massachusetts-Bay* being colonized *Anno* 1628, to the Persecution of the Quakers, Thirty Years; and so from Infatuation to Infatuation."[112] The periodic return of mental infatuations, like the return of smallpox epidemics after several decades, suggested that accepting irrational ideas and crediting witchcraft were as endemic to New England as smallpox was. In the context of beliefs that British American colonists' bodies and minds degenerated as a result of exposure to the American climate, the recurrent infatuations suggested that the American environment had altered colonists' minds, with the result that they were easily transfixed by one infatuation after another.

As an immigrant to New England, Douglass shared the same natural and cultural environments as the colonists who participated in various infatuations and who interpreted Africans' allegedly diabolic knowledge as a providential answer to smallpox. Indeed, if in Boston Douglass could claim the authority of professional medical knowledge that colonial practitioners such as Mather and the inoculator Zabdiel Boylston lacked, he did not possess the same medical authority in transatlantic contexts. His colonial location distanced him from institutions such as the Royal Society and the Royal College of Physicians, and his immersion in the New World climate meant that his humors and intellectual faculties could have been compromised by that environment. Although Scottish emigrants did employ their transatlantic travel as an opportunity to improve their social standing and to compete with their counterparts in England, they also experienced many of the same accusations of degeneration leveled against British Americans as well as English views of Scotland as provincial.[113] Even some creole, or American-born, colonists made Douglass's Scottish dialect an object of ridicule during the controversy, by calling it a "coarse Dialect" and insisting that he "speak English."[114] Interestingly, Douglass's speech underwent the same scrutiny and accusations to which he had subjected African testimony. Douglass's Scottish identity, reflected in this case in his style of speech, marked him as provincial in transatlantic contexts and as an outsider in Boston and suggested that his medical knowledge, like his speech, might be incomprehensible or untrustworthy. In this context, Douglass had to address the question of whether his mental faculties had been affected by the colonial environment and, by extension, whether he could found medical knowledge on "*Observations* made, and *Experiments* taken."[115] He had to provide proof that his own mind had not become susceptible to crediting the latest infatuation.

Douglass's new classification of African medical knowledge in his *Summary* reflected back on his own medical practices and vindicated his intellectual capacity. His discovery of the natural sources of Africans' medical knowledge illuminated Douglass's ability to employ observation to arrive at natural explanations for seemingly preternatural events. Instead of attributing Africans' mysterious medical knowledge to communications with the devil, Douglass reported that a natural, albeit hidden, cause was responsible for Africans' cures and poisonings. Only misguided, credulous beliefs in the powers of supernatural forces to influence disease might mistake Africans' medical practices for witchcraft. In this way, Douglass separated himself both from Mather—whose part in the Salem witch trials exemplified his belief that witchcraft was a real, present threat—and from African slaves—whose preventative and curative medical practices were indebted to influences from metaphysical beings. Years after the controversy had ended, Douglass defended his capacity to found colonial medical knowledge on experimentation by showing that his medical practices had resulted in increased knowledge of natural poisons rather than of the invisible world.

Douglass's description of African testimony marks a key moment in the history of colonial medical writing, for it demonstrates a shift in colonists' methods for classifying Native and African medical knowledge as witchcraft. Rather than attributing Natives' and Africans' medicine to actual communications with the devil, colonists began to suggest that these peoples mistakenly credited illness and healing to diabolic communications because they possessed inferior mental faculties. This move reflects colonists' growing hesitancy to claim that they had investigated and discovered a diabolic cause for Native and African medical knowledge. Yet Natives, Africans, and colonists continued to share the belief that medical knowledge included an empirical element—such as herbal knowledge or experimentation—and a final, metaphysical cause of disease. For Native, African, and colonial practitioners alike, then, treating the visible symptoms of disease was still not equivalent to exploring or understanding the final cause of disease; such medical practices merely intervened in the visible or surface manifestation of an entity with a deeper, hidden logic and cause. However, colonial medical practitioners such as Douglass began to stop short of speculating about the nature and identity of this final cause and to focus instead on the illness's visible effects. Colonists began to argue that if witches or magicians had power over people, it was because their credulous minds and strong imaginations deceived them into believing that fanciful forces had real effects on the natural world. Less a faculty that the devil influenced to achieve his will, the imagination was increasingly defined as a faculty that led people away from reason, inclining them to believe mistakenly in the influence of supernatural powers in the material world.

Douglass's classification of Africans' knowledge throughout the *Summary* also worked to counter perspectives that his medical writing was supported by degenerate humors, shaped by the American environment. Douglass began the natural history by explaining that he had employed strategies of classification, quantification, and categorization for clarity and exactness. However, he categorized African medical knowledge under the same "heads," as Native American medical and religious practices.[116] Douglass himself admitted this inconsistency in his classifications by writing that the "barbarous" state of Native culture made it impossible to provide a "clear, exact, and full account."[117] Similarly, he described Native and African medical knowledge throughout the *Summary* in "*loose particulars,*" footnotes, digressions, and repetitive comments.[118]

In a similar fashion, Douglass wrote that it was impossible to create a complete account of New World illnesses, explaining that the idea of producing a "history of epidemic yearly constitutions, in Sydenham's manner would be writing of a novel."[119] The physician Thomas Sydenham was famous for his "manner" of writing a history of all diseases present in a particular season and locale, and many physicians began to follow his example by keeping accounts of diseases and their daily or seasonal manifestations.[120] However, employing this method could have highlighted Douglass's provincial position by defining him as a collector of particulars regarding New World diseases and medicines but not as a practitioner who possessed rational wits that made him capable of explaining their causes. Moreover, a complete history of all colonial diseases would communicate to European medical practitioners exactly how many diseases Americans faced, potentially suggesting that the colonists lived in an unhealthy environment.

Douglass frustrated derogatory views of colonists and of New England's climate by playfully connecting his classificatory form to his humors. He wrote: "This history was not composed into a regular, full body, before it began to be published: and its being published only at various times of leisure, and humour of the writer, it seems to become too much of a miscellany, but without neglecting the principal view or design."[121] Douglass's description of his "humour" played on the word's references both to the fancy and to the temperament, and it raised the possibility that the *Summary*'s apparent irregularities could be attributed to his physical and mental state, which had determined how he arranged the work.[122] As Douglass knew, the fact that the *Summary* had become a miscellany might have been read by medical practitioners in the metropolis as literally determined by his humors, which by 1755 would have been thought to bear the marks of the colonial environment. In this context, the *Summary*'s swelling, erratic style might be interpreted as a sign that Douglass's wits had altered in the colonies, making it difficult for him to transform experiential particulars into a coherent theory or catalog of colonial diseases and medical knowledge.

But Douglass stated clearly that it was this "humour" for random organization and publication that kept the natural history from overwhelming and boring readers with too much information.[123] As he wrote, "Notwithstanding of the designed brevity, conciseness, or summary (which spoils the fluidity or fluency of stile), it swells too much; therefore at present to ease some of our readers, we lay aside or defer the designed short description or natural history of these things, which are used by the Indians as food, medicines, or traffic."[124] Douglass's footnotes, various "heads" for classification, and "*loose particulars*" reflected the complexity and great quantity of colonial medical knowledge, as well as the fact that it would not fit into categories established in the metropole.[125] Colonial natural historians regularly noted that American nature frustrated received categories, often in order to explain that Europeans' expectations of America did not match the reality and to demonstrate the value of firsthand knowledge of the Americas over expectations originating in the metropole.[126] Similarly, Douglass redefined what might appear as disorderly classification by stating that his decision to write a miscellany was inspired not only by the difficulty of categorizing New World knowledges and diseases but also by his sense that readers would appreciate reading a miscellany rather than an extensive list of American medical phenomena. He thus framed his particular form of classification as a sign of his mental ability to organize medical knowledge from the colonies without losing his "principal view of design."[127]

Inoculation and African Networks of Medical Communication

Although Douglass did include African medical knowledge in the *Summary,* he did not mention inoculation or the role Africans had played in the inoculation controversy. Instead, he returned to his claim, made in the "History," that knowledge of inoculation entered the colonies via the *Philosophical Transactions* of the Royal Society that he had lent to Mather in 1721. Thus, although Douglass finally admitted in the *Summary* that the "novel practice of procuring the small-pox by inoculation, is a very considerable and most beneficial improvement in that article of medical practice," he occluded the role that African testimony played in the controversy and in promoting inoculation, not even mentioning African knowledge in order to dismiss it.[128] In the *Summary,* Africans appeared to contribute nothing to colonial medical philosophy; they were incapable of offering any information of value to colonial knowledge. Instead, their medical practices revolved around the discovery and application of poisons. Douglass's classification of African medical knowledge as the study of poisonous herbs ultimately sought to erase Africans' knowledge of useful remedies and to occlude Africans' testimony regarding inoculation from colonial medicine. Colonists continued to employ strategies of attributing witchcraft to misguided mental faculties, and, as chapter 4 shows, they began to link Africans' mental faculties to their Old World African climates in order to separate colonial and African intellects further.

Yet if African medical knowledge of inoculation was erased from Douglass's *Summary,* it did not disappear among African communities. New World Africans continued to practice inoculation in their own communities, often unbeknownst to colonists. Indeed, enslaved Africans seem to have transmitted their knowledge of inoculation secretly, rather than sharing it with colonists as Onesimus had. In New York, Cadwallader Colden wrote with surprise that his slaves employed a "common practice in their country" to prevent smallpox and had known of inoculation for years before colonists did.[129] Moreover, the South Carolina physician James Kirkpatrick noted in his *Essay on Inoculation* that he had "inoculated a Negro Boy of Major *Pinckney's* who did not take. He had no manner of Complaint from it, was purg'd, and the Incision healed. He continued as healthy as ever after it."[130] The fact that the young boy neither manifested the effects of inoculation nor contracted smallpox suggests that he had been inoculated somewhere else, whether in Africa or somewhere in South Carolina, and that knowledge of inoculation continued to circulate along pathways hidden to colonists.

CHAPTER 4

Obeah, Slave Revolt, and Plantation Medicine in the British West Indies

Secret Knowledge, Rebellion, and James Grainger's West-India Georgic

JUST AS AFRICANS throughout North America continued to use knowledge of inoculation to maintain the health of their communities, so enslaved Africans in the British West Indies also employed their medical knowledge to strengthen communal bonds. In several locations, they drew on obeah—a "medicinal complex" of interconnected herbal and spiritual practices—to maintain the health of slaves on plantations as well as to signal their relationship to other New World Africans and to colonists throughout the Americas.[1] Africans in the Caribbean often employed these medical practices in secret, to accomplish purposes that were perceived as beneficial by the participants. In Jamaica in 1760, rebelling slaves were inspired by an obeah man, who offered them medicines said to make them invincible to planters' bullets. Led by a slave named Tacky, the rebels attacked several plantations and a fort in Saint Mary Parish; they escaped to the hills for nearly a year before colonial authorities re-enslaved and punished them.[2]

One of the first colonial texts to describe obeah after Tacky's Rebellion, as the 1760 uprising was called, was the physician James Grainger's 1764 georgic poem *The Sugar-Cane,* which, as its title suggests, celebrated sugar and its commercial importance to the British Empire by offering practical instructions regarding sugar production and cultivation in neoclassical poetic language imitative of Virgil's *Georgics.*[3] But Grainger's "West-India georgic" poeticized many more subjects than sugar cane, including tropical flora and fauna, hurricanes, tragic love stories, and, in its final book, African and colonial medical knowledge.[4] In particular, Grainger described obeah, explaining that it was composed of "magic spells" (4.381) that both healed and produced disease and therefore did "mischief" as well as "good" on plantations (144). Scholars have cited colonial histories from the 1770s and 1790s as the most influential representations of obeah, while in the nineteenth century sensational novels such as William Earle's *Obi; or the History of Three-Fingered Jack* (1800) contributed to making obeah a popular literary and dramatic subject.[5] However, *The Sugar-Cane* described obeah at a particularly crucial moment, just after Tacky's Rebellion began to make clear to colonists that obeah could pose a major threat to plantation hierarchies.

Grainger's poem also participated in an English "georgic revolution," in which poets imitated the structure and themes of Virgil's *Georgics* by writing four-book, didactic poems that suggested agriculture would usher in the Roman Empire's Golden Age of peace and prosperity. As Anthony Low has argued, the georgic revolution responded to a literary taste for classical poetry and to sociopolitical transformations brought about by England's emergence as a nation-state and empire. Georgics accorded new significance to labor, with the goal of increasing enthusiasm for agricultural innovation.[6] While the hard work of farming had rarely been considered an appropriate subject for poetry, eighteenth-century georgics such as James Thomson's *The Seasons,* John Dyer's *The Fleece,* and Christopher Smart's *The Hop-Garden* elevated the work of farmers and field hands while also celebrating the superiority of British commodities. Describing otherwise prosaic, utilitarian practices with the "address of a Poet"[7] neoclassical georgics followed Virgil's classical example by transforming hard work and skilled labor "from [their] shameful place at the bottom of the social ladder to a new pioneering role as the shaper of history and the benefactor of humanity."[8] Patriotically linking agriculture to the expansion of the British Empire and providing pleasing descriptions of English country life as well as didactic advice regarding agricultural innovations, georgics presented farming as a civilizing, progressive activity crucial to Britain's imperial glory.[9] Similarly, in the British Americas, poets imitated classical georgics by employing their themes and conventions to celebrate colonial staples, from indigo to sugar cane, and to depict the cultivation and civilization of wild lands.[10]

Yet Grainger departed from the georgic's conventional form in a number of ways, with the result that, scholars have argued, the poem fails to achieve the georgic's formal and thematic conventions. Georgics were narrative poems whose structure mirrored the linear process of producing a crop; they opened with images of uncultivated wilderness and moved on to describe acts of planting, cultivating, and harvesting, before concluding with visions of productive, settled estates. For example, Book 4 of Virgil's *Georgics* opens with instructions for bee-keeping that emphasize scenes of "quiet Station"[11] and "rest."[12] However, in the case of *The Sugar-Cane,* the "design begins coherently, [but it] soon shows signs of distraction."[13] *The Sugar-Cane*'s first three books follow the georgic narrative by discussing when and how to plant sugar cane; how to cultivate the plants; how to protect the cane from the insects, diseases, and weather specific to the West Indies; and how, finally, to harvest the plants. Yet, as David S. Shields has observed, "In the culminating book, where the vision of accomplished estate should be, Grainger provided an extended discourse on the most problematic aspect of planting—slave management."[14] Scholars have identified this turn to topics related to slavery and the poem's concomitant formal irregularities as the cause of the "lukewarm reception" that *The Sugar-Cane* received in England.[15] As Shaun Irlam has pointed out, "The poem failed to capture the imagination of literary London on two counts: moral and aesthetic."[16] Irlam argues that Grainger's poem failed because it "did not successfully realize the transformation of the plantation into the highly exacting codes of eighteenth-century poetic decorum" but instead instructed planters how to keep their slaves fit for work.[17]

This chapter reconsiders the question of why *The Sugar-Cane*'s georgic narrative falters in the final book by examining the poem in the context of Tacky's Rebellion and the African medical knowledge that inspired the rebellion. I reread *The Sugar-Cane*'s "moral and aesthetic" failures as evidence of Grainger's encounters with obeah and his attempts to interpret that knowledge and its implication for colonists in the West Indies.[18] Before Tacky's Rebellion made obeah the focus of colonists' anxiety regarding slave rebellions, planters subjected Africans' medical practices to relatively little surveillance or control, in this way making it possible for medical practitioners such as Grainger to observe obeah men and women at work and the uses of obeah in African communities. As I show by placing *The Sugar-Cane* in the contexts of colonists' mounting fears of obeah and of Africans' various uses for it, the poem's formal anomalies manifest multiple, sometimes conflicting conceptions of African medical knowledge. Grainger's account of obeah disrupts his georgic narrative on two levels: the poetic description of obeah departs from the conventional georgic narrative, and it acknowledges the recent danger obeah posed to colonists. Meanwhile, prose footnotes provide another perspective on obeah's meaning and uses by reflecting Africans' views of obeah as socially beneficial.[19]

Grainger ultimately rewrote his poetic description of African medical knowledge in a prose medical treatise, entitled *An Essay on the More Common West India Diseases.* In the *Essay,* he addressed the significance of his fractured georgic narrative, particularly the possibility that *The Sugar-Cane*—and his failure to reproduce European literary forms in the colonies—would signal that his mental faculties had degenerated. In the treatise, Grainger enacted his ability to classify, identify, and, consequently, to heal tropical illnesses, and he united practical and sympathetic medical knowledge to allay metropolitan concerns regarding planters' allegedly inhumane treatment of slaves as well as to calm colonial anxieties about future slave rebellions. Finally, Grainger substituted colonial knowledge of slaves' diseases for obeah men's expertise, in this way effacing African medical knowledge from the *Essay.* His medical writing ultimately inspired a genre of prose treatises on plantation medicine, while also giving rise to subsequent analyses of obeah as deceitful practices that slaves mistakenly viewed as witchcraft and to representations of slaves' minds as inferior.

Medical Encounters in the Caribbean

Obeah received relatively little attention from planters or physicians before it emerged as a threat to colonists and to social order on plantations during Tacky's Rebellion. Grainger seems to have constituted an exception to planters' indifference to it, for he noted his interest in Africans' medical knowledge throughout *The Sugar-Cane,* and this interest could have brought him into contact with obeah. As chapter 3's discussion of African cures for yaws showed, colonists commented that Africans possessed herbal knowledge and medical treatments that were extremely effective against tropical maladies. Similarly, Grainger documented his investigation of Africans' knowledge of tropical illnesses and remedies, writing in *The Sugar-Cane*'s preface that "the mention of many indigenous remedies, as well as diseases, was unavoidable. The truth is, I have rather courted opportunities of this nature, than avoided them" (vii). The botanical notes glossing plants and medicines referenced in *The Sugar-Cane's* verses contained such "indigenous remedies," making it likely that Grainger's poetic descriptions of herbs and medical cures also depended on his observations of and conversations with St. Christopher's African and Indian inhabitants (vii). Indeed, Grainger included African and Indian names for plants that, being specific to the West Indies, were unfamiliar to him and to European and colonial audiences. For example, he wrote that wild liquorice was a "scandent plant, from which the Negroes gather what they call *Jumbee Beeds.* These are about the size of pigeon-peas, almost round, of a red colour, with a black speck on one extremity. They act as an emetic, but, being violent in their operation, great caution should be observed in using them. The leaves make a good pectoral drink in disorders of the breast" (38). Grainger described the medicines obtained from wild liquorice by integrating both slaves' medical terminology and their practices, from their name for the plant to their cautious use of "*Jumbee Beeds*" as an emetic.

Grainger's interest in healing tropical diseases and in Africans' medical knowledge could have provided motivation to "court . . . opportunities" to observe obeah (vii). Although it is difficult to know with certainty what aspects of it Grainger would have observed, the informal nature of plantation medicine in the early 1760s and his medical practice—much of which would have been devoted to curing ill slaves—would certainly have offered occasions to encounter obeah. With few previously published plantation medical guides to consult, Grainger would have had to rely on his own observations and medical training to diagnose and cure Africans' maladies and to build a successful practice. Colonial medical practitioners, whose livelihoods in the Caribbean depended on maintaining the health of slaves, faced diseases specific to contexts of plantation slavery, including maladies that Africans had contracted as a result of transatlantic migration and hard labor in cane fields. Grainger was unique among the European doctors who practiced in the Caribbean, for he was the first of a group of medical practitioners who published treatises that focused specifically on slaves' diseases and medicines.[20] Moreover, Grainger's frequent inclusions of slaves' medical knowledge in *The Sugar-Cane* suggest that he was familiar with a range of African medical practices and might have conversed with obeah practitioners or observed their practices. Finally, even with the increased anxiety regarding obeah following Tacky's Rebellion, planters were still in the process of institutionalizing ways for restricting slaves' medical practices, leaving slaves some autonomy to employ traditional remedies.

Traces of possible encounters with obeah appear in Grainger's 1764 medical treatise, *An Essay on the More Common West-India Diseases.* William Wright, a well-regarded physician and a Fellow of the Royal Society, provided footnotes for the second edition of Grainger's *Essay,* in which he commented that Grainger offered a unique perspective on yaws. While colonial practitioners had been writing about yaws for several decades, Wright claimed that Grainger was the first author to have "viewed [yaws] in its proper light."[21] Unlike "Dr. Cullen, and other nosologists" who classified the disease "amongst the *Cachexiae,*" Wright noted, Grainger wrote that yaws "attacks the Negro but once," and he categorized it among other skin diseases to which patients were immune after one infection.[22] Grainger placed his description of yaws "immediately after small-pox," and, according to Wright, was the first European medical practitioner to suggest that inoculation might effectively prevent the illness, despite the fact that, of course, William Douglass and other medical practitioners had discussed inoculation and other African treatments for yaws much earlier.[23]

Wright's overstated claims regarding Grainger's knowledge of yaws notwithstanding, Grainger's classification of the illness among other skin diseases and his interest in inoculation suggest that he had made extensive observations of the disease and of Africans' treatments. As explained in chapter 3, yaws was an extremely contagious disease, and many European physicians hoped to avoid infection by permitting African practitioners, themselves often infected with yaws, to treat patients. Significantly, slaves who practiced obeah were often infected with yaws, and were thus outsiders—often of African, rather than Caribbean, birth, and frequently knowledgeable regarding Old World medical and religious practices. As the narrator of William Earle's novel *Obi; or the History of Three-Fingered Jack* explained, slaves with yaws "are the beings, who, in their seclusion, most frequently practice Obi. The more they are deformed, the more they are venerated, and their charm credited as the strongest."[24] Yaws-stricken patients seem to have become—or perhaps already to have been—obeah practitioners, possibly exploiting the relative freedom their quarantine afforded not only to heal other slaves infected with yaws but also to practice obeah.[25]

Grainger's knowledge of yaws suggests that he had sought opportunities to study the disease, and the correspondences between yaws and obeah practitioners suggests that he could have conversed with obeah men or heard stories of slaves whose illness afforded them a measure of autonomy and freedom to practice obeah. Grainger could thus also have encountered the range of uses to which Africans put obeah, from healing to discovering thieves to obtaining protection from evil. Indeed, Charles Spooner, the colonial agent for St. Christopher's and Grainger's brother-in-law, testified regarding obeah before Parliament, noting that: "From their [obeah practitioners'] Skill in Simples, and the Virtues of Plants, they sometimes operate extraordinary Cures in Diseases which have baffled the Skill of regular Practitioners, and more especially in foul Sores and Ulcers. I have myself made use of their Skill for the Last with great Success. There are no Laws in St. Christopher's or Grenada, nor do I believe in any of the Leeward or Ceded Islands, which take cognizance of Obeah, or its Professors."[26] Grainger's familial relation to Spooner, as well as the fact that he stayed with Spooner when he visited England in 1763, shows that Grainger had access to first-hand information about obeah, its potential dangers, and its uses.[27] Grainger's representation of obeah may thus be seen as one aspect of his more extensive practice of investigating and integrating African medical knowledge.

"Wonder-working charms" and the Georgic Form

Throughout most of *The Sugar-Cane,* Grainger employed the georgic structure to present his observations of West Indian maladies, flora, fauna, and insects as information useful for planters who wanted to understand the various stages of sugar cane planting and production. However, in Book 4, he departed from the georgic's teleological drive toward settled estates. Rather than providing expected images of plenty and peace, Grainger made Africans' health the primary subject of Book 4, by offering advice to planters regarding how to choose, maintain, and control their slaves. He provided descriptions of the illnesses to which enslaved Africans were susceptible, while also instructing planters how to season, or accustom, their slaves to the tropical environment. The images of African bodies suffering from various tropical maladies not only contrasted with the georgic's conventional images but also made it difficult even to imagine the possibility of a peaceful plantation.

Instead of completing the georgic's traditional narrative, Grainger described African medical knowledge, in particular, the signs that slaves exhibited under obeah's spell and the practices with which obeah men allegedly influenced slaves. Slaves infected with obeah:

> . . . mope, love silence, every friend avoid;
> They inly pine; all aliment reject;
> Or insufficient for nutrition take:
> Their features droop; a sickly yellowish hue
> Their skin deforms; their strength and beauty fly.
> Then comes the feverish fiend, with firy eyes,
> Whom drowth, convulsions, and whom death surround,
> Fatal attendants! (4.371–78)

Grainger listed the transformative effects that obeah had on slaves' behavior and bodies: "bewitch'd" (4.369) slaves exhibited unusual conduct, by isolating themselves from their "friend[s]," withdrawing from their communities, and refusing to eat. In addition to making slaves "inly pine" obeah altered their bodies, turning their skin "yellowish" and sapping their "strength and beauty." Eventually, "fatal attendants," symptoms of a slow yet certain death, descended on the body: "drowth"—the "drought" or thirst that often accompanied "the feverish fiend"—and convulsions took over slaves' bodies before finally causing death. Grainger's account of obeah acknowledged the existence of a powerful obstacle to colonial physicians' attempts to maintain slaves' health and tranquil plantations. Obeah made slaves ill and rebellious, as Grainger explained: "Luckless he who owns, / The slave, who thinks himself bewitch'd; and whom, / In wrath, a conjurer's snake-mark'd staff hath struck!" (4.368–70). Obeah—as the cause of slaves' illnesses—thwarted planters hoping to season their slaves efficiently to the West Indian climatological and cultural environment, for slaves who believed themselves "bewitch'd" not only maintained their belief in elements of Old World African medical and religious practices but also refused or were too ill to work (4.369).

In addition to describing diseased and disobedient slaves, Grainger listed the specific ingredients that composed obeah men's potions and "charms" (4.386):

> Fern root cut small, and tied with many a knot;
> Old teeth extracted from a white man's skull;
> A lizard's skeleton; a serpent's head:
> These mix'd with salt, and water from the spring,
> Are in a phial pour'd; o'er these the leach
> Mutters strange jargon, and wild circles forms. (4.387–92)

The descriptions of fields of sugar cane in the previous three books give way in the fourth to images of diseased African bodies and of obeah men gathering colonists' teeth in order to make deadly potions. The account of obeah thus indefinitely delays the poem's concluding representation of production and prosperity, for Grainger's departure from the georgic's conventional narrative form registered the danger that obeah posed to colonists' lives and livelihoods after Tacky's Rebellion, leaving no room for images of peaceful estates. Indeed, Grainger's reference to the "Old teeth extracted from a white man's skull" in the obeah man's phial manifested the direct threat to colonists that obeah had recently posed, while the images of ill slaves represented the ways in which obeah disrupted orderly production on sugar plantations. Yet Grainger did not complete his description of obeah's connections to slave rebellion, especially the recent uprising in Jamaica and the punishments that obeah practitioners had received. Instead, he shifted his description of obeah to footnotes in which he provided an alternative view of obeah as a powerful, potentially useful system of knowledge.

Grainger employed footnotes throughout *The Sugar-Cane* in order to support the poem by elucidating poetic descriptions that readers in Europe might otherwise have found confusing. As he explained, "some notes have been added, which, it is presumed, will not be disagreeable to those who have never been in the West-Indies" (vii).[28] Some notes provide a classical history for objects in the poem; for example, they support the reverence accorded to plants such as sugar by charting its long history and documenting its appearance in literary works. The notes also maintain the poem's formal integrity by removing utilitarian information and prosaic content from the body of the text. Many notes explicate unusual words or references to Caribbean flora and fauna—from mosquitoes to cockroaches—with which European readers might be unfamiliar; others provide the botanical names for plants that Grainger identified by their popular or common names in the poem. The notes often take over the page, thus requiring the reader to stop reading the poem in order to examine the footnotes, some of which extend for several pages. For example, as figure 5 shows, Grainger's note on sugar cane took up several pages, in which he quoted ancient references to sugar and described the various places sugar had been cultivated, even as his verses instructed planters how to choose a location for cane fields. The footnotes thus made *The Sugar-Cane* all the more unusual as a georgic poem, for the combination of poetic verses and scientific notes created a hybrid text composed of multiple forms and a mixture of elevated language and straightforward botanical descriptions. Yet the notes' function is ultimately to complement the poem's

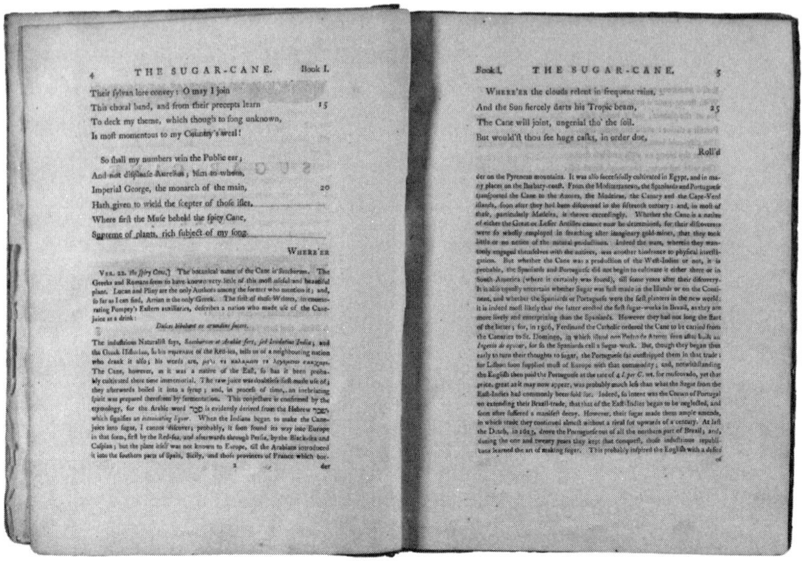

4 THE SUGAR-CANE. Book I.

Their sylvan lore convey: O may I join
This choral band, and from their precepts learn
To deck my theme, which though to song unknown,
Is most momentous to my Country's weal!

So shall my numbers win the Public ear;
And not displease Aurelius; him to whom,
Imperial George, the monarch of the main,
Hath given to wield the scepter of those isles,
Where first the Muse beheld the spicy Cane,
Supreme of plants, rich subject of my song.

Book I. THE SUGAR-CANE. 5

Where'er the clouds relent in frequent rains,
And the Sun fiercely darts his Tropic beam,
The Cane will joint, ungenial tho' the soil.
But would'st thou see huge casks, in order due,

Figure 5. James Grainger, *The Sugar-Cane* (London, 1764). Courtesy of the John Carter Brown Library at Brown University.

narrative, so that the poem maintains its authority even when the footnotes and verses appear to struggle for priority on the page.[29]

However, Grainger's footnotes on obeah departed from the complementary function that the botanical, historical, and explanatory notes served, for they contrasted the poetic description of obeah as a potion composed of white men's teeth, and they departed from the "world's" "laugh[ter]" at obeah (4.385). In the notes, Grainger acknowledged that just as obeah men "can do mischief, so they can also do good on a plantation, provided they are kept by the white people in proper subordination" (144). Rather than supporting Grainger's representation of obeah in the poem, the notes on obeah contradict the poem by admitting that obeah men could serve useful, positive ends on plantations. Furthermore, the footnote on obeah suspends the georgic narrative by forcing readers to turn from the poem to the footnote, subsequently leaving the poetic account of obeah's dangers in abeyance and requiring reflection on the frightening consequences of obeah men's practices. By removing readers' attention from the poem, the footnote makes the possibility of a traditional georgic conclusion all the more remote. Furthermore, the footnote undercuts the authority of the poetic description of obeah: as it acknowledges that obeah men might "do good" on plantations, the footnote manifested the conceptions of and uses for obeah held by both Africans and colonists throughout the Americas prior to and shortly after Tacky's Rebellion (144). Far from solidifying conceptions of obeah as purely dangerous, diabolic, or laughable, as later texts would certainly do, *The Sugar-Cane*'s fractured georgic and footnotes communicate a range of opinions about obeah.[30]

The tension between Grainger's footnotes and poem corresponds to the work of "representation" and "criticism" that footnotes began to perform in the eighteenth century.[31] As Frank Palmeri has argued, the shift from marginal notes to footnotes signaled a corresponding shift from models of resemblance—in which both text and marginalia functioned as glosses on the "world as text" and ultimately on divine truth—to models of difference—in which footnotes existed in ironic, critical relation to the text.[32] As Palmeri argues, this "antagonistic" relation between text and footnote created instances of heteroglossia and supplementarity that opened space for the articulation of multiple voices and perspectives and that subsequently undercut the text's authority.[33] In cases when authority is shared by text and footnotes, "meaning emerges indirectly from the patterns of interference between conflicting voices and languages, each of which carries its own presuppositions, interests, and view of the world."[34]

In the case of *The Sugar-Cane,* Grainger's departure from the georgic narrative and the "antagonistic" relationship between the poetic text and footnote reflect his attempts to respond to obeah.[35] In addition, the poem's fragmented narrative, or texture, reflects Africans' reliance on obeah to respond to their encounters with colonists in the context of slavery. As a consequence, Grainger's rhetorical shifts manifest the encounter and adaptation of multiple perspectives regarding obeah: including colonial and African conceptions of obeah as a socially beneficial practice as well as Africans' use of obeah as a mode of resistance to slavery, in the form of armed rebellion and refusals to work. Book 4's texture reflects as well the ways in which colonists began to revise their largely positive views of obeah after Tacky's Rebellion. Finally, as the footnote on obeah supplemented the poetic representation of obeah men's practices, it exposed the fact that the georgic narrative lacked authority in the West Indies. Rather than shoring up the poem's meaning, the footnote extended the problem of authority, in this way making clear Grainger's failure to create an authoritative, complete narrative about obeah. In the section that follows, I first discuss the ways Africans in North America and the British

West Indies employed obeah as a set of strategies with which to "do good" by resisting enslavement and strengthening social bonds (144). Then I examine how Grainger acknowledged various uses for obeah throughout the Americas, even while distancing himself from African medical practices.

Obeah and Afro-Caribbean Medical Knowledge

Grainger's footnoted acknowledgment of the good that obeah men could do on plantations pointed to some of the meanings obeah possessed within African communities throughout the Americas. Africans did not always employ obeah as black magic, with the intent to harm other Africans or European colonists, nor did colonists always perceive obeah as dangerous witchcraft to be controlled. Before the rebellion in Jamaica made obeah an object of colonial anxiety, slaves often enjoyed "wide scope" to employ African and Afro-Caribbean medical knowledge to treat their illnesses and to maintain elements of their traditional religious and medical practices.[36] Moreover, for much of the eighteenth century, the absence of organized medical care for slaves and large numbers of absentee planters meant that slaves could practice obeah without colonial oversight.[37] Obeah men were "almost entirely independent of white control and contributed enormously to the physical and psychological well-being of the slave population and therefore to the health of the society as a whole."[38] Only a few Europeans published descriptions of obeah before *The Sugar-Cane,* and the natural histories that do briefly mention obeah describe it as a secret but not necessarily dangerous practice. Indeed, mid-century natural histories relating encounters between obeah men and colonists report that obeah had socially positive uses.

One of the first European depictions of obeah in the West Indies appears in a natural history of Barbados by Griffith Hughes, a Fellow of the Royal Society who described "*Obeah* Negroes" as "a sort of Physicians and Conjurers, who can, as they believe not only fascinate [slaves], but cure them when they are bewitched by others."[39] Hughes described a case in which an "*Obeah* Negro" healed a woman of her rheumatism with a "Magical Apparatus" composed of various natural objects: "Earthen Basons, a Handful of different Kinds of Leaves, and a Piece of Soap."[40] African healers often used such a medico-religious apparatus to appeal to and influence the entities responsible for the patient's illness and thus to "control or contain the supernatural force that is believed to actually perform the desired cure."[41] In the

Caribbean, obeah offered slaves a method by which they could not only seek healing from diseases but could also access and pacify the supernatural and natural forces to which they attributed their maladies and misfortunes. Obeah practitioners were employed as diviners and healers, and slaves relied on them to avenge wrongs, find stolen property, and heal diseases.[42] Hughes's description suggests not only that obeah men combined religious and herbal knowledge but also that European travelers perceived obeah as a medical practice with magical elements employed for practical purposes.

As Hughes's account suggested, obeah was an inherently neutral practice composed of a mixture of African religious practices and Afro-Caribbean herbal knowledge. As Edward Kamau Brathwaite insists,

> this 'magic' was (is) based on a scientific knowledge and use of herbs, drugs, foods and symbolic/associational procedures (pejoratively termed *fetishistic*) as well as on a homeopathic understanding of the material and divine nature of Man (*nam*) and the ways in which this could be affected. The principle of *obeah* is, therefore, like medical principles everywhere the process of healing/protection through seeking out the source or explanation of the cause (*obi*/evil) of the disease or fear.[43]

Africans in the Americas did not perceive obeah as an intrinsically evil or harmful practice; rather, obeah was used "for protection against sorcerers (*tapu*)" or against slaves whose actions made them outsiders to the Afro-Caribbean community.[44] In contrast to what Europeans designated as black magic (also called witchcraft or sorcery), which was "practiced by genuine sorcerers (*wisiman*), who call up the spirits of the dead, render them slaves to their malevolent will, and force them to work for evil purposes," obeah men used their access to *won,* that is, neutral spirits, for either good or evil purposes.[45]

As Brathwaite has described, obeah was only one component of Afro-Caribbean medical culture, in which "religion [was] the form or kernel or core."[46] Because African medical practice was not characterized by a "specialization of disciplines [or a] dissociation of sensibilities," obeah was part of a network composed of worship, rites of passage, divination, healing, and protection.[47] African medical practitioners possessed herbal therapeutic knowledge as well as several techniques for accessing natural, spiritual, and ancestral deities, whose anger was believed to be the ultimate cause of disease. Different categories of medical practitioners addressed various levels of disease: an herbalist used plant medicines to focus on relieving the visible symptoms of disease, perhaps also drawing on "magicoreligious techniques."[48] While an herbalist could provide protective magic, diviners would diagnose the cause of illness and apply herbal medicines with spiritual powers to heal the patient. Finally, a sorcerer-healer, similar to an obeah man, could both heal and cause disease by using herbal medicines and spiritual knowledge.[49]

While, as Hughes's natural history shows, enslaved Africans used obeah for healing, they also turned to it to seek revenge on or to harm other Africans for reasons they perceived to be socially useful. Writing of his encounters with slaves in Pennsylvania, the Swedish botanist Peter Kalm reported: "Negroes commonly employ it [obeah] on such of their brethren as behave well, are beloved by their masters, and separate as it were from their countrymen, or do not like to converse with them. They have likewise often other reasons for their enmity; but there are few examples of their having poisoned their masters."[50] Noting that obeah was a secret art, Kalm did not describe its ingredients, writing only that "It is full of ******. I purposely omit what he mentioned, for it seems undoubtedly to have been the name of the poison with which malicious Negroes do so much harm, and which is to be met with almost every where."[51] Kalm's description suggests that Africans in Pennsylvania, like their Caribbean counterparts, turned to obeah to maintain their social "health" and solidarity by reproving slaves who embraced Euro-colonial lifestyles and beliefs.[52]

As Kalm's description suggests, obeah offered a set of practices by which Africans throughout the Americas maintained cultural traditions and reinforced belief in the power of *won,* or the spiritual forces inherent in medicines, by appealing to such forces to heal diseases and to punish aberrant or dangerous behavior. After poisoning a Europeanized slave who "behave[d] well,"[53] Kalm reported, "The other Negroes and Negro-women fell a laughing at the complaints of their hated countryman, and danced and sung as if they had done an excellent action, and had at last obtained the point so much wished for."[54] As anthropologists of African cultures in the New World have noted, slaves' dances and songs often transmitted, sustained, and remade Old World beliefs and practices. Like the holidays that provided slaves with an "institutional context" through which they preserved "chants, dances and various other manifestations of African art," obeah offered a framework with which slaves preserved their medical beliefs and their accompanying spiritual significance.[55] By concluding their practice of obeah with a dance, the Pennsylvania Africans likely employed obeah to affirm their cultural solidarity. Just as slaves' dances mixed African religious or medical beliefs with European traditions such as Christian holidays, so the obeah dance fused African religious and medical beliefs with slaves' knowledge of American herbs, thus ensuring the survival of traditional beliefs by attaching them to New World elements. In the context of West Indian plantation slavery, obeah offered an Afro-Caribbean form of "*cultural* resistance, a symptom of Negro protest against compulsory Christianisation, the imposition of European customs and values."[56] Obeah allowed Africans to continue the use of various Old World practices and beliefs, even while adapting these practices to the resources and exigencies of the New World.

Far from remaining stable as it was transferred to the New World, Africans' medical knowledge provided a powerful way of communicating one's medical and sociopolitical status to other Africans and to colonists. As Kalm's account of Africans' use of obeah to poison one of their fellow slaves suggests, Africans employed obeah to communicate a variety of messages about their bodies and about their relation to colonists' power. To Africans who seemed to adopt too many of their masters' viewpoints and ideas, obeah constituted a potentially fatal directive to return to the African community and to maintain resistance to colonists' values and beliefs. For the African men and women who employed obeah, the medical practices signaled their special knowledge of secrets, herbs, remedies, and charms, as well as their relationship with divine forces; obeah marked them as powerful medical practitioners with the ability to influence human and non-human entities. For some Africans, such as the woman Hughes mentioned, obeah offered a solution to illness or, if diseased by obeah, a strategy for temporarily avoiding enforced labor.

For Africans in Jamaica, obeah provided a direct way to resist their enslavement. In 1760, they expanded obeah's uses to inspire violent rebellion against European colonists, but they also continued the practice of using obeah for socially positive ends. As Edward Long reported years later, an obeah man gave the rebels "a powder, which, being rubbed on their bodies, was to make them invulnerable: they persuaded them into a belief, that Tacky, their generalissimo in the woods, could not possibly be hurt by the white men, for that he caught all the bullets fired at him in his hand, and hurled them back with destruction to his foes."[57] The rebel slaves, who numbered over one thousand, killed sixty colonists and devastated several plantations before colonists captured them. The rebellion had surprised the colonists, and the slaves were suppressed only after martial law was declared and military reinforcements arrived. The obeah man was eventually caught by a colonial militia and executed.[58] The revolt cost planters about ten thousand pounds, or one thousand slaves, who were executed or exiled or who committed suicide rather than surrender.[59] Moreover, the rebellion struck fear into planters throughout the Caribbean: colonists expressed consternation that their slaves had surreptitiously organized the rebellion over a period of several years, while maintaining the utmost secrecy, and they focused on obeah's role in stimulating the confidence and bravery that led to the rebels' initial success.[60] Obeah communicated Africans' resistance to their place at the bottom of plantation hierarchies, and it manifested slaves' abilities to rationally plan and execute a coordinated attack.

Degeneration and the Tropics

Grainger shared with Africans the desire to discover how to employ Caribbean herbs in socially and physically healthful ways as well as the motivation to define his relation to various peoples in the Caribbean and in the metropolis. As a result of his experiences in the West Indies, however, he faced questions about the state of his mental faculties, for tropical climates were infamous for degenerating English colonists' minds and morals. Furthermore, Grainger's descriptions of Africans' illnesses and medical knowledge in Book 4 raised questions regarding just how peaceful Caribbean plantations actually were and, by extension, whether it was possible to write a conventional "West-India georgic" that concluded with scenes of peace and prosperity (vii).

The difficulty of maintaining English physical and cultural identities in tropical climates was well known, for travel to the Caribbean posed the danger of physical, cultural, and intellectual transformation for colonists. Both African slaves and British colonists underwent a period of seasoning during which their bodies adapted to the tropical climate and the diseases, especially fevers, specific to the West Indies. The effects of transatlantic travel were visible on English bodies: as James Lind pointed out in his *Essay on Diseases Incidental to Europeans in Hot Climates,* "The whites in general become yellow [in the West Indies]; their stomach could not receive much food, without loathing and reachings [retching]."[61] Lind explained further that the "constitution of Europeans, by length of time, becomes seasoned to the East and West Indian climates, if it is not injured by the repeated attacks of sickness, upon their first arrival. Europeans therefore, when thus habituated, are generally subject to as few diseases abroad, as those who reside at home."[62] Surviving the seasoning period ensured that Europeans could maintain their health even in the unfamiliar disease environment of the Caribbean, but this physical alteration also meant that returning home to England posed a new threat to colonists' bodies, now adapted to the tropical environment. As Lind pointed out, some colonists, "dreading what they may be again exposed to suffer from a change of climate, choose rather to spend the remainder of their lives abroad, than to return to their native country."[63]

Successful adaptation to the tropics rendered colonists' cultural practices, as well as their bodies, out of place in Europe. As with the yellow-tinted skin that marked the effects of the Caribbean climate on colonial bodies, so colonists' behavior was believed to bear the marks of cultural degeneration. For example, Edward Long noted that colonists in the West Indies lost the habits of speech and manners that distinguished them as British. As he wrote, "We may see, in some of these places, a very fine young woman aukwardly [*sic*] dangling her arms with the air of a Negro-servant, lolling almost the whole day upon beds or settees. . . . Her ideas are narrowed to the ordinary subjects that pass before her, the business of the plantation, the tittle-tattle of the parish; the tricks, superstitions, diversions, and profligate discourses, of black servants, equally illiterate and unpolished."[64] The young woman adopted not only the lazy "air" of her "Negro-servant" but also the ideas and belief in "superstitions" that, as Long argued, characterized the minds of "black servants."[65] Indeed, the tropical climate was described as disordering British colonists' minds, for, as William Falconer commented, "The mind is here [in hot climates] open to every impulse; but as these succeed rapidly one to another, they none of them make any very permanent impression, but efface one another in order."[66] The result, Falconer suggested, was a "general depravity in manners" that required a "despotic" government.[67]

As Grainger pointed out, Europeans in the metropolis might possess "antidotes" of reason "to guard" (62) against "Dire spells," but in the Caribbean, colonists' rational faculties were susceptible to environmental influences that could weaken the reason and open the mind to believing in the "spells" it could resist in Europe (2.135). As one colonial writer reported, "witchcraft or sorcery produced the same kinds of 'symptoms' on slaves as on those Europeans . . . 'with weak and superstitious minds . . . when sudden but vast painful afflictions of the mind are brought on.' "[68] The tropical environment made colonists' bodies and minds more like those of their African slaves than like those of Europeans in the metropolis, thereby making it possible that colonists would not only experience diseases similar to those that Africans contracted but also that colonists would adopt similar modes of speaking and thinking.

In this context, *The Sugar-Cane*'s formal anomalies functioned not only as signs of the disorder and degeneration of colonial society but also as indicators of Grainger's own cultural and mental health. *The Sugar-Cane*'s formal failures reflected back on Grainger's literary and intellectual abilities, raising questions about the degree to which the tropical climate had altered his mental faculties. *The Sugar-Cane*'s incomplete narrative had medical significance as a potential sign of colonial degeneration, for georgics were "inscriptive" poems that brought about the things of which they spoke.[69] Georgic poets drew connections between writing and planting by claiming parallels between the poet and the farmer and thereby treating writing as an "artisanal" or "inscriptive" process that enacted, even as it mirrored, the agricultural labor of planting and harvesting a crop.[70] The poet, like the farmer, gathered and ordered the seeds, or subject matter, of his poem to transform raw materials into a pleasing harvest of poetic description. The poetic labor of transforming traditionally mundane topics into pleasing images rhetorically mirrored the farmer's act of civilizing uncultivated fields, so that, as georgics reproduced agricultural processes in didactic narratives, the poems produced the very civilizing effects that they represented. But the georgic's inscriptive qualities also meant that *The Sugar-Cane*'s formal inconsistencies could be attributed to colonists' agricultural and literary practices; the absence of images of harvest in the poem suggested that Grainger had failed to reproduce the georgic's civilizing narrative in the British West Indies. If Grainger could not achieve the georgic's conventional conclusion, in which wilderness was converted into ordered, productive fields, it followed that the tropical climate had altered his civilized, English constitution, leaving him unable to reproduce English cultural practices in the West Indies. Grainger's departure from visions of harvest and peace in Book 4 thus reflected a mind disordered by the tropical climate and a colonial society characterized by upheaval and violence.

The response to *The Sugar-Cane* in England pointed to the difficulties involved in adapting the georgic form to the West Indies. James Boswell explained in his *Life of Johnson* that, when Grainger read a draft of the poem in London, "all the assembled wits burst into a laugh, when, after much blank-verse pomp, the poet began a new paragraph thus:—'Now, Muse, let's sing of *rats*.'"[71] Boswell further commented that Samuel Johnson himself did not care for the poem, writing, "The Sugar-Cane, a poem, did not please him; for, he exclaimed, 'What could he make of a sugar-cane?' "[72] Moreover, critics such as Johnson noted that *The Sugar-Cane* was a "new creation . . . of which an European has scarce any conception," and Grainger himself explained that he introduced "new and picturesque images" into the georgic.[73] While Grainger appeared to have hoped that these new elements would invigorate the georgic form, they seem only to have raised suspicions about his own ability to transfer a classical form to the Caribbean.

While Grainger explained in his preface that he sought to include information in the poem that was the "result of Experience, not the productions of Fancy," his failed georgic raised the possibility that his "Fancy," or imagination, had indeed compromised his writing (v). More specifically, the fractured narrative suggested that travel to the West Indies had altered Grainger's mind and made the construction of the georgic's narrative difficult or even impossible. Moreover, Grainger's account of obeah risked putting him at odds with strategies that medical practitioners in Europe employed to describe the causes of mysterious diseases and cures. As Douglass's classificatory practices in his *Summary* showed, practitioners did not deny that diseases could have final preternatural causes, but they did restrict medical knowledge to discovering the observable environmental causes responsible for disease. Seeking to avoid hypothesizing about occult, or hidden, causes, medical philosophers identified the causes of disease by collecting and correlating observations of visible factors, such as weather, environmental conditions, and patients' physical or constitutional characteristics. "Environmental" medical philosophies postulated that disease was the product of disorder caused by measurable environmental forces, usually "miasma," "vaporous exhalations . . . and particles suspending in the atmosphere."[74] For instance, climatic or environmental variations in the air or new dietary or exercise patterns allegedly relaxed the blood vessels, disrupting the regular circulation of the blood and producing corrosive or corrupted blood that infected the entire body.[75] Physicians theorized, as John Arbuthnot did, that the air "operates sensibly in forming the Constitutions of Mankind, the Specialties of Features, Complexion, Temper, and consequently the Manners of Mankind, which are found to vary much in different Countries and Climates."[76]

But Grainger's representation of obeah's "wondrous power" (4.399) to make "diseases fly" (4.398) did not attribute obeah's capacity to cause and to cure disease to environmental factors. His account of obeah could thus act as evidence that the tropical climate had altered his mind and motivated him to venture too far into the "hidden arcanums or concealed medicines" against which environmental medical philosophies cautioned.[77] In this light, the medical knowledge recorded in *The Sugar-Cane* would appear to be founded not on experience but on hypotheses regarding phenomena about whose causes humans could only speculate. Given the alleged propensity of the West Indian environment to incite the passions of the mind, *The Sugar-Cane*'s fractured narrative and the supplementary account of obeah in the footnotes could appear to represent the work of an excited imagination rather acts of observation and reason. Grainger thus also needed to provide evidence to his English readers that, despite *The Sugar-Cane*'s formal irregularities, he had not experienced physical or intellectual degeneration.

"Imaginary Ills," Obeah, and "Illiterate Africans"

Grainger counteracted questions regarding the effects of the climate on his mind by making learning, rather than the environment, the foundation of intellectual abilities and cultural identities. As Edward Winslow made religion a mark of difference between Natives and colonists and a sign of sameness that connected colonists with Europeans in the Old World, so Grainger contrasted his learning with that of Africans in order to suggest that his knowledge had more in common with that of Europeans in the metropole. He relocated the source of obeah's power from medical potions and practices to Africans' mental faculties by redefining earlier conceptions of obeah as a combination of natural remedies and ceremonies. In his footnote, Grainger explained: the "blacks imagine that its [obeah men's staff] blow, if not mortal, will at least occasion long and troublesome disorders. A belief in magic is inseparable from human nature, but those nations are most addicted thereto, among whom learning, and of course, philosophy, have least obtained" (144). Grainger's attribution of obeah's power to Africans' imaginations linked their medical practices with their Old World, African culture and "learning" rather than with the Caribbean environment that colonists shared with slaves (144). In this way, he extended modes of evaluating slaves' value as workers to categorize their intellectual traits as well. Throughout *The Sugar-Cane,* Grainger explained variations in slaves' abilities on the basis of the African environments from which they hailed. For example, he evaluated slaves' illnesses, even those contracted in the tropics, by identifying their various African origins. He wrote, for example, that "*The Mundingos, in particular,* [are] *subject to worms; and the Congos, to dropsical disorders*" (124). In addition, Grainger connected slaves' physical characteristics to their African climates, writing that planters seeking strong workers for hard labor should "chuse the slave, / Who sails from barren climes; where want alone, / Offspring of rude necessity, compells / The sturdy native" to hard agricultural labor (4.57–60). Similarly, Africans from "many a sylvan realm," (4.89) were "hardy" and purportedly made good laborers in the cane fields (4.96). Grainger interpreted slaves' physical traits by mapping geographical information about Africa onto their bodies. His understanding of Africans' behavior and health suggested that uniquely African environmental features shaped slaves' constitutions even after they had traveled to the Caribbean.

Grainger developed these connections between slaves' physical attributes and Africa's environment by tracing Africans' belief in obeah to their intellectual faculties. His comment that Africans "imagine[d]" that the obeah man's staff would mortally wound them positioned slaves' African cultural origins as the cause not only of the particular diseases they contracted in the tropics but also as the reason for their confidence in "wicked" obeah men, their fear at the "imagine[d]" power of the obeah man's staff (144), and, therefore, their "imaginary" ills (4.367). This description was consistent with earlier characterizations of Africa's hot climate as endowing its inhabitants with a "difference [or kind] of imagination" that made them "great enchaunters" who excelled at "obtaining things, and finding remedies to their necessities."[78] In this context, slaves believed in obeah because their imaginations, strengthened by Africa's heat, left them vulnerable to magical beliefs and to conjurers' deceptive practices. Obeah had power because Africans were willing to believe in and to fear its effects, not because obeah men actually possessed "wondrous power" and medical knowledge (4.399). Africa's hot climate and undeveloped civilization made slaves' minds ripe breeding grounds for both material and epistemological poisons, specifically, obeah.

Grainger suggested that slaves lacked the "antidote[s]" (62) of reason with which Europeans defended themselves from such irrational "poison[s]" as obeah and thus could not protect themselves from their own delusions and the depredations of obeah men (4.394). In this context, slaves believed in obeah because their imaginations left them vulnerable to magical beliefs and to conjurers' deceptive practices. By attributing slaves' "deluded" minds and illnesses to their African constitutions and national origins, Grainger redefined obeah as an Old World, African practice involving witchcraft and deception that slaves had transferred to the West Indies (144). The geography of medical knowledge that Grainger constructed in *The Sugar-Cane* allowed him to attribute Africans' medical practices and mental faculties to their places of origin and learning, rather than to the tropical environment they shared with colonists. Grainger could thus locate Africans at the bottom of a "theoretical hierarchy" based on "proximity to Europe and to temperate climates."[79] His account of obeah as an effect of Africans' mental faculties contributed to emerging understandings of Natives' and Africans' alleged participation in witchcraft as the effects of their mental faculties: Grainger, like Douglass, attributed obeah's mysterious powers to Africans' credulous minds rather than suggesting that obeah practitioners communicated directly with the devil. But Grainger also developed Douglass's account of enslaved Africans' minds by focusing on the African environmental factors shaping slaves' behavior and health; in this way, Grainger raised the possibility that Africans' mental faculties remained stable across time and space. In this way, his explanation of obeah foreshadowed racial explanations of difference, for it suggested that uniquely African features shaped slaves' intellectual and physical natures.

Obeah and Natural History

While Grainger's footnote allowed him to identify obeah with African environments and medical practices, he still had to assure English readers that he continued to enjoy the rational faculties that civilized European nations possessed. Grainger distanced himself from the tropical environment and from encounters with African medical knowledge by rewriting Book 4's medical advice in *An Essay on the More Common West-India Diseases,* a natural history of disease that included descriptions of the maladies that commonly infected slaves and instructions for their cures. Grainger shifted *The Sugar-Cane*'s poetic language into classificatory forms by substituting descriptions of diseases in discrete categories for the georgic's narrative of cultivation. In this way, the medical treatise took up the same question of Africans' medical care that *The Sugar-Cane*'s Book 4 had attempted to address. And like the footnote on obeah, Grainger's medical treatise acted as a supplement that exposed the poem's failure to complete the georgic narrative: while the *Essay* claimed to offer authoritative strategies for healing slaves' illnesses and managing their behavior, it attested to the fact that Grainger had been unable to establish that authority in *The Sugar-Cane.*

In the *Essay,* Grainger classified illnesses in categories that reflected their relationships, the manner in which they might appear in nature, and the symptoms that made them visible. Each disease's character and behavior determined the category in which Grainger classified it, so that, for example, he discussed fevers and skin diseases in separate books, while placing fevers and fluxes in adjacent categories and noting that fluxes "naturally follow" fevers.[80] These rhetorical strategies made disease, rather than the body, the primary object of study: bodies were surfaces on which diseases appeared and on which they could be observed for a time. However, the illness, rather than individual bodies, was of primary importance. Finally, the arrangement of diseases within each book mirrored the progression of ailments slaves might actually be expected to experience over the course of their lives: Grainger began the *Essay* with instructions for seasoning slaves newly arrived in the West Indies and proceeded to discuss care for infant Creoles—Africans born in the West Indies—before concluding with an account of how to ensure that slaves maintained their health and ability to work.

Grainger's account of slaves' diseases in the *Essay* revised his poetic description and explanation of slaves' belief in obeah in *The Sugar-Cane,* for the natural history abstracted diseases from slaves' bodies and minds and from obeah men's charms. He presented diseases as entities for scrutiny rather than as phenomena encountered in a specific place or time, in this way attempting to erase the contexts of slave rebellion and of African medical practices that he had acknowledged in *The Sugar-Cane.* By representing Africans solely as bodies to be healed and controlled, Grainger left unacknowledged the possibility that Africans could act as medical practitioners capable of providing useful medical care on plantations. Moreover, while Douglass had categorized African knowledge as poison in his *Summary,* Grainger effaced Africans' knowledge altogether from his *Essay.* The erasure of Africans as medical practitioners and as individuals with their own interpretations of disease also effaced Grainger's admission in *The Sugar-Cane* that obeah men could, in certain circumstances, be beneficial on plantations. In the *Essay,* Grainger did not acknowledge the medical practices that had recently posed a threat to the slave system and to the hierarchies that ordered plantation society in the West Indies, thus leaving obeah to function as a silenced but productive and "seditious" knowledge.[81] As Homi Bhabha has explained, colonial discourse does not simply construct binary, master-slave relationships, nor do colonizers alone always possess and produce colonial discourse. Instead, dominated or marginalized subjects may be placed within discourse, to increase the "visibility of the subject as an object of surveillance, tabulation, enumeration, and indeed, paranoia and fantasy."[82] By providing instructions regarding slaves' medical care, Grainger quelled fears of obeah-inspired slave rebellion even as he positioned African bodies as "object[s] of surveillance" that, thanks to the *Essay*, could be observed and policed by planters and physicians attuned to the various symptoms that could appear on slaves' bodies and their meanings.[83]

Finally, adopting the form of the natural history allowed Grainger to position himself as an observer of diseases whose primary role was to arrange and order his observations and in this way to replicate in prose the appearance of illnesses in nature. Grainger followed rhetorical strategies for describing and classifying diseases established by the physician Thomas Sydenham, who applied rhetorical strategies already associated with natural histories to identify illnesses by listing the features that distinguished various maladies from one another. While Douglass had departed from Sydenham's ideal of completeness in his *Summary* in order to avoid listing the illnesses present in the colonies and thus to avoid the suggestion that New England's climate was unhealthy, Grainger adopted Sydenham's strategies to position himself as an observer of enslaved Africans' illnesses. By presenting himself as observer, commentator, and physician, Grainger located himself outside the natural history and, by extension, outside the contexts that caused both slaves' and colonists' illnesses.

Grainger did explain that colonists experienced some of the tropical maladies that commonly infected slaves and that, in certain cases, they were more likely to contract some illnesses than Africans. Yet the diseases colonists were likely to share with their slaves included tooth-ache, costiveness, and heart-burn, conditions brought on by diet, relaxation, or "lying with their heads, &c. too slightly covered."[84] The causes for these shared maladies proceeded from physical reactions to the environment, and these reactions suggested colonists' bodies had not adjusted to the Caribbean's dietary and climatological environment but maintained their English attributes. In these cases, the tropical environment continued to endanger colonists, but it did so because their bodies still possessed English attributes or behaviors that signified their ongoing connections with their counterparts in Europe. In this way, Grainger implicitly suggested that colonists and Africans did not share the same diseases or the same relationship to the Caribbean environment.

Sympathy and the Slave Trade

Grainger's *Essay* further addressed colonists' relation to enslaved Africans by marking colonists as benevolent and rational, despite their immersion in the tropical climate. Grainger introduced the *Essay's* "plain and popular style"[85] as a correction to and improvement of prior literary styles for conveying tropical medical philosophies, and he claimed that his "scientifical" and perspicuous manner rejected the "parade of learning" that metropolitan practitioners such as Thomas Sydenham repudiated as based on hypothetical conjectures, rather than observation.[86] Yet Grainger also employed these plain rhetorical strategies to support an argument for colonists' ability to care for their slaves without metropolitan oversight. By employing a prose style characteristic of scientific or medical treatises to recommend the benevolent treatment of slaves, Grainger made the West Indies the source of sympathy for enslaved Africans, in this way uniting planters' pragmatic concerns with "humane and sensible" attributes.[87] He expressed confidence in the "power of medical science to diminish, and greatly too, the number of those who must otherwise be sacrificed to the pursuit of riches."[88] Kinder treatment would make slaves more willing workers, as Grainger wrote: "How shocking to philanthropy it is, to think there are human beings who are made to act from motives of fear only! Surely, were Negroes instructed in the practical principles of Christianity, they would be rendered much better servants, and would prevent much severity whereto they are now unavoidably exposed."[89] At once defending slavery's "unavoidabl[e]" "severity" and chastising planters who forced their slaves to work out of "motives of fear," Grainger suggested that slavery and the slave trade could be humanely and productively maintained if planters modified the most oppressive forms of management with "sensible" medical care.[90]

Grainger's call for planters to treat their slaves with sympathy and benevolence addressed metropolitan biases against allowing planters to determine how and when to end the slave trade. David S. Shields has pointed out that Grainger was "prophetic in seeing that the remedy to the problem of slavery would be found in the metropolis and not in the islands."[91] Yet although Grainger called for metropolitan intervention to end slavery, he also expressed concern about the repercussions of such action. His muse laments that it, and colonists by extension, lacked the power "Which monarchs have, and monarchs oft abuse" to outlaw slavery (4.233). Imperial rulers, Grainger suggested, might:

> quell tyrannic sway; knock off the chains
> Of heart-debasing slavery; give to man,
> Of every colour and of every clime,
> Freedom, which stamps him image of his God. (4.235–39)

By replacing oppression with freedom, Grainger wrote, imperial legislation would "knit the whole in well-accorded strife" (4.241) to make slaves servants "of choice" (4.242). These verses suggested that English legislation to end slavery would transform oppressive relationships between masters and slaves into harmonious, "well-accorded strife" that would, in classic georgic form, civilize the wilderness (4.241). Grainger suggested that laws prohibiting slavery and the slave trade would modify planters' oppressive power to produce a kinder, gentler coercion, thus improving slaves' conditions. In this vision, slaves would become servants with whom planters would struggle against the wilderness to produce fruitful harvests.

Yet as Grainger wrote, monarchs could prohibit slavery, but they "oft abuse[d]" this prerogative (4.233). This characterization of monarchical power as potentially abusive suggested that any laws moderating slavery's oppressive system or the slave trade had to be carefully formulated to account for planters' economic welfare.[92] Grainger's concern regarding laws unfriendly to planters reflected West Indians' complicated relationship with metropolitan commercial legislation: planters sought to secure European markets for their merchandise even while defending their "West India interest."[93] In 1763, the British government, seeking to increase outlets for English and North American manufactures, established a system of free ports in the British West Indies that required the colonies there to compete with North American and French colonial markets, thus raising the possibility that planters might not find outlets for their sugar or that they might have to lower prices to compete with other markets.[94] At the same time, English authors were increasingly expressing sympathetic and humanitarian attitudes toward enslaved Africans, such as those articulated in georgic poems by Grainger's contemporaries James Thomson and John Dyer, while perceptions of colonists as culturally and morally degenerate also circulated in England.[95] Planters increasingly feared that they would lose unrestricted access to the African slave trade, which, they argued, was crucial to maintaining and expanding sugar production. British West Indian merchants and planters therefore insisted that colonial, not English, legislatures should establish guidelines for treating and managing slaves, and they argued that with better treatment, slaves would reproduce naturally and would eventually render the transatlantic slave trade obsolete.[96] Planters soon began to standardize practices for trading and caring for enslaved Africans in order to convince metropolitan audiences that they provided slaves with humane treatment.

The *Essay* reconciled planters' desire to maintain order on plantations with the pressure to treat slaves with compassion. Grainger recommended punishing slaves "for their own as well as their masters' sakes" by arguing that "as Negroes are ignorant, they must be vicious" and therefore required discipline.[97] At the same time, he insisted that slaves should be treated with "humanity," carefully seasoned to the tropical climate and to labor in the cane fields, and should receive prompt and regular medical care when ill.[98] He urged planters to provide slaves with appropriate clothing and to distribute warm blankets when they were ill.[99] With such instructions, Grainger justified his "performance" of practical medical knowledge by simultaneously displaying a sympathetic acknowledgment of slaves' humanity.[100] As a result, his prose treatise represented plantation medical knowledge as simultaneously practical and progressive, sympathetic to slaves yet supportive of planters' economic interests. Moreover, he disproved conceptions that colonial planters were characterized by "tyrannical behaviour to [their] Negroes," while simultaneously supporting arguments that planters could provide care for their slaves' well-being and health.[101]

The *Essay* located the source of humanitarian attitudes in the Caribbean by rewriting *The Sugar-Cane*'s invocation of metropolitan sentiment. In *The Sugar-Cane,* the muse authorized its sympathetic expressions by calling on the patronage of Robert Melville, a "classical scholar," Scottish military officer, and governor of the ceded islands when Grainger wrote the poem.[102] The muse asked Melville to hear and facilitate its description of slavery: "Yet, thou wilt deign to hear; a man thou art / Who deem'st nought foreign that belongs to man" (4.36–37).[103] While *The Sugar-Cane*'s poetic descriptions of slaves depended on Melville's official authority for inspiration and efficacy, in the *Essay* Grainger revised the muse's appeal to metropolitan legislation and official patronage, for the colonial physician expressed Melville's sentiments.

Grainger wrote of his treatise, "if this performance shall produce the salutary effects for which only it was written, I shall think my leisure well employed; for though diseases of Blacks are its primary object, *Homo sum et humani nihil a me alienum puto.*"[104] Quoting in Latin the same line, "I am a man: and Think nothing that is foreign to me" with which the muse had invoked Melville, Grainger appropriated the muse's appeal to official authority by claiming progressive attitudes for the colonial physician.[105]

By uniting pragmatic and practical concerns in the prose style of the colonial physician, the *Essay* rhetorically accomplished the shift from slave to "servant" that *The Sugar-Cane*'s appeal to the power of monarchs to end slavery had only imagined.[106] Plantation medical science answered the poem's call for kings to lift the oppressive bonds of slavery and to transform Africans into "Servants, not slaves; of choice" (4.242). Ultimately, colonial medical practices, rather than imperial oversight or a monarch's "laws" (4.239), would transform oppression and mistreatment into humane relationships between masters and "Servants" (4.232). Grainger's representation of the colonial physician as progressive, humane, *and* practical resolved the conflicts between metropolitan sympathy and West Indians' utilitarian commercial concerns. Importantly, the treatise located the source of such pragmatic humanity in the colonies, where the plantation physician both treated slaves' illnesses and, like the muse, modeled sympathetic feelings toward Africans. Offering a strategy with which colonial planters and managers could themselves improve slaves' conditions without potentially "abus[ive]" imperial intervention, Grainger simultaneously defended planters' economic interest and characterized their actions as humane (4.233). Plantation medical science thus healed not only slaves' illnesses but also planters' inhumane or unsympathetic actions.[107]

The *Essay* constructed plantation "medical science" as a technology of health, discipline, and order that maintained the hierarchical structure of Caribbean society and increased planters' profits even while allowing colonists to express sympathy for slaves.[108] Acknowledging planters' continuously unstable financial situation, Grainger admitted that his recommendations, such as his plan for a hospital, "would doubtless cost money; but if we must have slaves, our own interest should methinks, teach us to take all imaginable care of them when they become sickly."[109] He insisted that the cost of medical care would be repaid by slaves' renewed efficiency and longevity. Slaves "deserve[d] the utmost attention of the master" on a "principle of profit": by showing humanity, Grainger suggested, planters would also protect their interests.[110] Plantation medical science improved slaves' efficiency even while merging humanitarian and financial concerns, for as Grainger wrote, "I repeat again, the health of the gang will fully repay this expense."[111] Indeed, the "power of medical science" to facilitate the "pursuit of riches" united plantation medicine and sympathy and showed that both were useful to planters.[112]

Creolizing Obeah in Plantation Medical Treatises

The connections between practical and humanitarian concerns that the *Essay* accomplished were extended by nineteenth-century medical practitioners, who developed the prose style and practical subject matter of Grainger's medical treatise to defend the colonial policy of "legislative amelioration."[113] Amelioration allowed planters to resist, at least temporarily, a complete ban on the slave trade, for West Indian planters argued that the trade should continue until humanitarian policies could sufficiently increase the slave population. Citing planters' medical care and treatment for slaves as proof of their ability to improve slaves' conditions without metropolitan intervention, Caribbean physicians defended colonial laws "formed to protect the negroes against oppression" as "wise," if sometimes imperfect.[114] These medical writers explicitly defended the slave trade by reproducing Grainger's arguments that, with better treatment, slaves would not only work more willingly, but would also reproduce more quickly, with the result that this reproduction would eventually and naturally alleviate planters' reliance on the African trade. Far from devising original methods, these medical treatises provided "wise rules" that were quite similar to those Grainger had outlined thirty to forty years earlier in the *Essay*.[115] The physician and planter David Collins wrote, in a comment resembling Grainger's articulation of the connections between profit and medical care, that "calculation very clearly coincides with duty, and tells us, that it is much cheaper to breed than to purchase."[116] As planters presented it, amelioration would permit a gradual decline of the slave trade while allowing planters to maintain control of their interests—their ability to expand sugar production by buying slaves as long as they were needed. In reality, however, amelioration permitted planters to codify medical practices already outlined by Grainger and to avoid radically changing the social and economic structure in the West Indies.[117]

Plantation medical treatises also continued Grainger's process of describing slaves as irrational and uncivilized, a process that developed Grainger's representations of obeah and proposed new methods for controlling it. Caribbean physicians reproduced Grainger's explanation of obeah as a consequence of slaves' inferior intellectual faculties. They began to define belief in obeah as a mental disease, not just the result of strong faculties of the imagination but a "perversion of every rational exercise of the mind."[118] Obeah practitioners' "supernatural powers" continued to be coded as actions of resistance, and colonial medical practitioners sought to discover and control the "designing crafty people"[119] who caused slaves' "mental disease, despondency, and death."[120] Admitting that slaves' "assent, approbation, and confidence [in] such ignorant pretenders," made it difficult for a physician to "do his duty,"[121] medical practitioners advised planters to counteract the "unaccountable confidence which negroes put in old women, and persons who, they imagine, are gifted with supernatural powers" with the counter-magic of Christianity.[122] They wrote that "unless the mental disease is relieved or palliated, it is in vain to try the power of medicine."[123] These medical treatises developed Grainger's analysis of the symptoms and causes of obeah, while also marking obeah as a mental disease that attacked the reason and pathologizing slaves' belief in obeah men or women.

In addition to solidifying descriptions of Africans' minds as irrational and diseased, medical practitioners increasingly equated obeah with witchcraft, slowly erasing earlier colonial observations of obeah as composed of interconnected herbal and spiritual elements and accounts of its benefits. Representations of obeah published after *The Sugar-Cane* increasingly divided Africans' network of medical practices into categories that differentiated between religious and medical knowledge.[124] As Jerome S. Handler and Kenneth M. Bilby have argued, post-colonial anthropologists developed these conceptions by beginning their search for the African definition of the term "obeah" with the claim, made by such colonists as Grainger, that obeah was a socially malevolent magical practice with origins in Africa. In contrast to such interpretations, Handler and Bilby offer an alternate, New World etymology and history for "obeah."[125] Citing recent linguistic studies, they suggest that the word and its meanings were constructed in the New World and specifically in the Caribbean. They write:

> One can imagine a scenario in which native English-speakers in the British Caribbean, in Barbados or another early English col-

> ony, adopted the term from some African language (Igbo or Igbo related?) without being aware of its full meaning in that language group. The adopted term referred, or was related, to a type of slave healer who was involved with spiritual or magical practices, or the practices themselves which, although not fully understood by Europeans, were known to be of non-European origin.[126]

Obeah, Handler and Bilby contend, is best understood as a term that emerged in the West Indies, constructed in the rhetorical practices with which colonists mistranslated African words and supplied them with new meanings.[127]

Yet while Handler and Bilby suggest that "obeah" and its meanings were primarily colonial constructions, *The Sugar-Cane*'s texture—its fractured narrative and its footnotes—suggest that African medical knowledge was a far more active influence on colonists' interpretations and subsequent misperceptions of obeah than scholars have heretofore recognized. Enslaved Africans creatively adapted to colonists' strategies for keeping obeah in "proper subordination," and in this way, they contributed to the various meanings that obeah assumed, both before and after Tacky's Rebellion (144). To Africans, Grainger's medical philosophies and treatments for slaves' so-called imaginary ills could have seemed another powerful form of medicine, evidence that colonial physicians, similar to obeah men, possessed special access to the non-human forces that controlled disease.[128] Physicians often recommended controlling obeah by requiring that slaves change their religious beliefs, and Grainger himself suggested that "Negroes [should be] instructed in the practical principles of Christianity" to make them "better," more obedient servants.[129] However, slaves often responded to forced conversions by adding elements of Afro-Caribbean medical knowledge to European religions. In the Christmas Rebellion of 1831, for instance, slaves swore on a Bible and called on the Baptist religion for inspiration and protection, thereby revising their traditional source of inspiration from the obeah man to incorporate Christianity.[130] By practicing both obeah and European religions, enslaved people adapted African or Afro-Caribbean practices to colonists' conceptions of obeah as magical, and they continued to plan rebellions even while incorporating physicians' "practical principles of Christianity."[131]

New World Africans also responded to colonists' reliance on their medicinal knowledge of Caribbean herbs by continuing to incorporate African and New World remedies into plantation medical practices. In this way, they maintained and even improved their status as valued sources of medical knowledge.

Collins wrote that slave women were often appointed as nurses after they learned "the use of the simples of the country, . . . the dressing of sores, and the doses of different purges and vomits; and with such qualifications, I will venture to assure you, that you will receive infinitely more advantage from having her in that station than from her service in the field, or any where else."[132] Planters often depended on African nurses and on slaves trained as dentists to administer medicines in physicians' absence or in non-life-threatening cases. While Collins's account focused on improving plantation medicine for the planters' benefit, his description of the nurse's "qualifications" indicates that slaves continued to employ their herbal medical knowledge and that they achieved a level of autonomy and respect for such expertise, even after events such as Tacky's Rebellion led to increased scrutiny of African medical knowledge.[133] As a result of their adaptation to colonists' positive perceptions of their herbal knowledge, Africans maintained the spaces in which obeah men had practiced. This appropriation of colonial medical knowledge complicated colonists' subordination of obeah and required colonists to employ additional strategies, such as the prose styles and strategies of Grainger's *Essay* and subsequent medical treatises, to control African medical knowledge. As Edward Brathwaite has argued, "Action to alter the basis of the society and the disposition of its two main cultural groups in relation to each other could have come only from some new positive move (probably revolution by the slaves) by one or other of them."[134] Far from abandoning obeah or permitting colonists to control entirely its meanings, slaves responded to the proliferating views of obeah as magical knowledge and to the new methods for subordinating obeah with creative strategies of their own.

Roger Bastide has explained colonists' perception of obeah as witchcraft by arguing that African medical knowledge, "being too remote from white religious attitudes, declines into magic."[135] However, when we trace colonial representations of obeah from their earliest appearances, in Hughes's and Kalm's texts of the 1750s, through the accounts following Tacky's Rebellion and into the nineteenth century, we see that obeah's status as witchcraft was constructed in a rhetorical process, involving a variety of literary forms and texts that colonists formed and refashioned as they attempted to interpret and, later, to erase African medical knowledge. *The Sugar-Cane* and *Essay* occupy key positions in this trajectory, for Grainger's turn to describe African medical knowledge in footnotes acknowledged obeah's power over slaves and planters but also sought to address the threat of slave rebellion and metropolitan intervention.[136] Far from representing a purely African practice too "remote" for colonists to understand, the various meanings of "obeah" were constructed in Grainger's poem, the footnotes to *The Sugar-Cane,* his subsequent classification of Africans' illnesses, and, importantly, in Africans' responses to colonists' perceptions of their medical knowledge.[137] The new meanings that obeah accrued were less the result of a "decline . . . into magic" than the consequence of colonists' attempts to determine the meaning and significance of obeah and to avoid suggestions that their minds had degenerated in the tropical environment.[138]

When we consider *The Sugar-Cane*'s representation of multiple views on obeah and the *Essay*'s construction of plantation medical science in an intercultural and a transatlantic context, we see that Grainger's medical writing attempted to resolve colonists' anxieties regarding slave rebellion, to order relations between slaves and planters, and to reconcile socio-political tensions between planters and Europeans in the metropolis. Grainger's medical writing responded to pressing conflicts by establishing colonists' relation to obeah while also defending plantation medical science to metropolitan audiences. Moreover, nineteenth-century prose medical treatises developed and naturalized Grainger's classification of obeah as magical practices belonging to peoples with irrational mental faculties. Many Romantic writers developed Grainger's description of obeah as the result of misguided imaginations in poems, sensational and gothic novels, and melodramas. For example, a number of late eighteenth- and early nineteenth-century texts, from John Gabriel Stedman's *Narrative of a Five Years Expedition against the Revolted Negroes of Surinam* to Maria Edgeworth's *Belinda,* exoticized obeah as a superstitious irrational practice that preyed on credulous slaves until benevolent masters saved them.[139]

The connections that *The Sugar-Cane* and the *Essay* drew between slaves' medical practices and intellectual faculties show that plantation medical science not only provided strategies for preventing slaves' illnesses but also contributed to theories regarding differences between colonial and African knowledge and, eventually, physical and intellectual characteristics. In *The Sugar-Cane,* Grainger described obeah as effective and useful, but he then distanced himself from his encounters with it in the *Essay* by classifying it as witchcraft and by attributing obeah to Africans' mental faculties. Moreover, he modified earlier accounts of African knowledge as both poison and witchcraft, for Grainger suggested that practices of obeah and their apparent efficacy were based entirely on Africans' deluded minds and faculties of the imagination, rather than on knowledge of natural poisons or communications with the devil, as Douglass had postulated of African medical knowledge. By the nineteenth century, physicians began to posit that Africans' inferior intellectual faculties were unchangeable. James Thomson, a European physician who also practiced in the West Indies and who cited Grainger as an authority on tropical medicines, explicitly associated culture and climate, writing in 1820: "Every region on this earth has its own climate, men, morals, and religion. In vain would the ambitious self-love of some persuade us that one system should be common to all."[140] Physicians developed the boundaries that Grainger's medical writing had established between colonial and African medicine to contrast slaves' civilization and education with those of European cultures and to justify racial theories regarding slaves' minds and bodies.

As colonists attributed slaves' mental faculties to their Old World, African environment, they developed different cultural categories for themselves and for Africans, despite the fact that they shared the same environment and were both subject to its influences. Ultimately, colonists began to theorize that mental and physical traits were the result of national characteristics that resisted environmental alteration. The racial theories that would eventually posit immutable differences among colonists, Natives, and Africans were initially developed in literary forms that attempted both to interpret and to classify Native and African medical knowledge. Moreover, as the *Essay* shows, colonial medical discourse coexisted with and even relied on sympathetic humanitarian attitudes; slavery and progressive medical practices were not mutually exclusive.[141]

However, just as Africans continued to practice obeah by adapting to colonists' new definitions of their knowledge and finding new contexts in which to practice it, so Native Americans also employed medical knowledge to respond to conceptions of intellectual and physical traits as stable, national characteristics. Chapter 5 concludes *Medical Encounters*'s study of colonial representations of Native and African medical knowledge by focusing on medical writing authored by Samson Occom, a Mohegan Indian. In this chapter, I investigate the ways in which Occom employed his diagnoses of moral and physical illnesses in order to complicate colonists' classificatory forms, to collapse the distance colonists had constructed between themselves and Native and African peoples, and to suggest new strategies for healing bodies and minds.

CHAPTER 5

Drunkenness, Syphilis, and History in Samson Occom's Medical Writing

Moral "Illness" in Atlantic and Pacific Worlds

LATE IN 1765, Mohegan Samson Occom boarded a ship in Boston and traveled to London with Nathaniel Whitaker, who, like Occom, was a Presbyterian minister. For the next two and a half years, Occom toured Great Britain, raising funds for his mentor Eleazar Wheelock's mission school for Native children. In the course of his transatlantic travels, Occom met minister George Whitfield and King George II, was inoculated against smallpox, and preached throughout England, Scotland, and Ireland. As he embarked on his return voyage to America in the spring of 1768, a second expedition was preparing to set sail, albeit in a different direction: Captain James Cook set out on a voyage to the South Seas, with the goal of charting the transit of Venus, the point when the planet would cross in front of the sun. The travelers aboard Cook's ship, the *Endeavour,* included Joseph Banks, a budding botanist and supporter of Carl Linnaeus's new system of classification, who hoped to find undiscovered flora and fauna in the Pacific and who would later become president of the British Royal Society.

Banks did discover previously unknown plants, insects, and animals, and his discoveries were well publicized upon the expedition's return in 1771. However, his botanical investigations claimed only part of the public's interest.

Stories of the explorers' sexual exploits in Tahiti and accounts of the Tahitians' sexual freedom circulated widely in England. Popular satires drew analogies between Banks's botanical investigations of plants' reproductive parts—the foundation of Linnaean classification—and his sexual encounters with Native women who allegedly lacked inhibitions.[1] A 1773 compilation of Banks's and Cook's journals by John Hawkesworth reported that the sexual encounters in Tahiti resulted in an outbreak of syphilis among the Tahitians and the sailors, although the English explorers claimed to be uncertain regarding its origin.[2]

Meanwhile, Occom had returned to New England, where he faced a series of personal, professional, and tribal challenges: in 1769, Wheelock circulated letters chastising Occom in harsh terms for public drunkenness. Occom first denied the charges, then reversed himself and repented, but he was ultimately absolved by the Long Island Presbytery. In 1772, Occom once again confronted colonial accusations regarding Natives' alcohol abuse, when he preached the execution sermon for Moses Paul, a Wampanoag Indian who was convicted of murdering a colonist while intoxicated.[3]

In addition to facing colonial stereotypes of Indian drunkenness, Occom engaged in debates over land rights between the Mohegans and Connecticut Colony. Ongoing since the 1630s, these debates culminated in 1773, when the colony was awarded rights to a large section of Mohegan land. This loss was only the latest in a series of periodic dispossessions resulting from colonial expansion, dispossessions that disrupted Natives' political leadership, subsistence patterns, and relation to the land. Finally, Occom's transatlantic travel and fundraising efforts seemed to result in little of consequence for Native communities in New England. Wheelock decided to remove his school for Native children, Moor's Charity School, to Hanover, New Hampshire, a location Occom believed was purposely inconvenient for Native students and evidence that Wheelock wished to educate Anglo-American boys and men only.[4] Additionally, Occom struggled to support his own family, despite his successful fundraising for Wheelock. David Maccluer, a missionary ordained at Dartmouth, warned Wheelock in 1772 that some of the funds ought to be used for Occom's salary, "So that he might be cut off from any occasion to repeat what he says Mr. Whitfield told him when he left England; that they had made him a fool to collect monies for them in England, but when he got to America they would cut him *adrift*."[5] Occom eventually broke off correspondence with Wheelock in 1774.[6]

Some time thereafter, Occom wrote a sermon in which he commented on the experiences and challenges of these years by discussing encounters between British colonists and indigenous people in both New England and Tahiti.[7] Although no record exists of a meeting between Occom and Cook, Occom quoted Hawkesworth's compilation of Banks's and Cook's travel narratives in order to comment on the connections between disease, particularly syphilis, and colonialism and on the categories the explorers used to describe the Tahitians in their writings. Occom's sermon addressed several sins of intemperance, but he dwelt in particular on alcohol abuse and sexual promiscuity, behaviors that colonists cited as evidence of Natives' inferiority despite the fact that both British colonists and Natives were guilty of such sins. In doing so, Occom addressed emergent conceptions of inherent racial difference. In the late eighteenth century, colonists began to repurpose the categories of irrationality in which they had classified Native and African minds and medical knowledge in order to support interpretations of Natives' intoxication and promiscuity as evidence of natural appetites and passions. Although religious beliefs and environmental influences still played a key role in marking differences among colonists, Native Americans, and Africans, as they had during the first centuries of settlement, cultural differences were increasingly attributed to inherent physical and mental traits.

I examine Occom's sermon as medical writing that drew on Native and Christian conceptions of illness and healing in order to cure both Natives' and colonists' unhealthy spiritual and physical states. In doing so, I turn to investigate the relation between Native and colonial medical knowledge in the writings of a Native American who drew on both Native views of the body and its maladies and Protestant conceptions of illness and healing. Indeed, as a Native writer, minister, and medical practitioner, Occom complicated the boundaries between Native and colonial medical knowledge that colonists had erected in their classificatory forms. Recent scholarship has complicated older views of Occom as entirely embracing colonial Christian culture as well as descriptions of him as occupying a hybrid or liminal space between cultures. For example, Joanna Brooks argues that New England Natives who adopted Christianity were not assimilating to European culture but rather employed Christianity as "another venue through which indigenous peoples continue their ongoing struggle for self-determination."[8] Meanwhile, Lisa Brooks has shown that Occom drew on a range of inscriptive and non-alphabetic communication practices long employed by Natives as well as on printed media in order to serve the interests of his community.[9] Thus, neither models of acculturation nor those of hybridity fully capture the ways in which Occom and other Natives employed a variety of strategies—including, but not limited to Christianity and printed media—to engage and respond to colonialism. As Joanna Brooks argues of Occom, "It is more productive to read his writings not primarily as a record of the troubles of individual acculturation but as part of an ongoing indigenous intellectual history of engagement and survival against the epic crimes of colonialism."[10] I engage this framework to consider Occom's writings about medicine in particular, and I situate the sermon as part of and as responding to a larger genre of medical writing from the Americas. As Natives and Africans throughout the Americas used stories, performances, healings, and publications to respond to epidemics and to colonists' medical knowledge, so Occom employed narratives of disease and colonization to offer a cure for diseases that infected both Natives and colonists.

Occom employed medical writing to engage colonial explanations of behaviors and maladies that Europeans claimed were natural to indigenous peoples. Moreover, he engaged the classificatory strategies with which colonists in the Americas and the South Seas constructed differences between their bodies and minds and those of indigenous peoples. As previous chapters have shown, classificatory forms distanced colonists from encounters with Native and African medical knowledge, and they allowed colonists to deny connections between their mental faculties and those belonging to Natives and Africans. In Tahiti, Cook and Banks denied responsibility for the Tahitians' illness by rhetorically distancing themselves from the encounter and by analyzing the Tahitians' sexual practices as the likely cause of disease. By contrast, Occom's sermon removed indigenous peoples from the classificatory forms in which colonists placed them by elucidating the relations between colonial encounters and illness and by describing colonists' participation in such exchanges. In this way, he identified imperial exploration and expansion, rather than traits inherent in indigenous peoples, African peoples, or their environments, as the source of diseases. Finally, Occom presented love as a cure for diseases of the body and the soul, thus proposing what Carlos Fausto and Michael Heckenberger have called a model of "transformative action" with which to reform behavior and restore rationality and health to Natives and colonists alike.[11]

This chapter suggests new rhetorical and geo-historical contexts in which to understand Occom's writing, first by attending to his sermon as medical writing and second by considering the sermon in the context of medical exchanges in both New England and the South Seas. At the same time, this chapter looks at the narrative and classificatory forms of colonial medical writing from the perspective of a Mohegan Christian who critically evaluated the rhetorical strategies with which colonists described indigenous people's illnesses and medical knowledge. It departs methodologically from prior chapters by focusing primarily on the Native medical and religious practices on which Occom drew as he intervened in colonists' classifications of indigenous bodies and minds as irrational and inferior. In particular, it shows that Occom revised colonists' classificatory practices using both rhetorical strategies and healing practices, which he employed in the course of his duties as a minister. Occom's sermon provided a revisionary history of colonial encounters that illuminated the connections between contact and disease and that revised colonists' classification of indigenous bodies and minds as inferior.

"Voluntary Madness": Alcohol Abuse and Race in New England

Occom began his sermon by discussing alcohol abuse, a practice to which Native Americans were seen as especially susceptible and one that colonists presented as evidence that Natives had irrational minds that inclined them toward heathenism. Although both European colonists and Natives drank liquor, Natives' alcohol abuse was attributed to characteristics unique to them. Colonial ministers, in particular, suggested that Natives lacked the rationality and self-control necessary to moderate their desire for and consumption of alcohol; consequently, Natives were believed to display their true, savage natures when they became intoxicated. Yet Occom did not openly critique colonial biases regarding Natives' alleged propensity for alcohol; instead, he presented a description of a drunken man that seemed quite similar to colonial ministers' diagnoses of Indian drunkenness. Then, he connected alcohol abuse to other forms of promiscuous behavior that, as he showed, were not caused by Natives' inferior bodies and minds but by colonial expansion and exploration.

Occom described a man—significantly, the sermon does not specify whether he is Native or Euro-American—who seeks out alcohol and becomes intoxicated, a process that results in a loss of rationality and a concomitant turn to serving the devil. Occom wrote,

> When he [the drunkard] drowned his Reason he loses all that Time and he is fit for no Service at all, either for him Self, for his Family, for his Country, and how much more is he unfit to Serve God,—And yet, (to astonishment) he is just fit to Serve the Devil, Yea Drink itself is the Service of the Devil, and This fits him for all manner of service to the old Greedy, and many has undone themselves, and their families by Drunkenness.[12]

Alcohol, Occom claimed, transformed one's mental faculties, for alcohol abuse turned "a Rational Man [in]to worse than a Natural fool" (226). The resulting state of irrationality rendered the man suitable only for diabolic practices and heathen beliefs.

Occom had employed the same language of "drowning" the reason and of mental degeneration in his execution sermon for Moses Paul, in which he described a "drunkard . . . when he has drowned his reason" in graphic, detailed language that depicted the stages by which a man lost his rational faculties.[13] He wrote:

> how deformed and shameful does he appear. . . . He appears with awful deformity, and his whole visage is disfigured; if he attempts to speak he cannot bring out his words distinct, so as to be understood; if he walks he reels and staggers to and fro, and tumbles down. And see how he behaves, he is now laughing, and then he is crying; he is singing and the next minute he is mourning.[14]

Not only is the drunkard's body deformed and disfigured, leaving him unable to walk, but his speech is likewise disordered as his words become incomprehensible, and he loses the power to communicate. Moreover, alcohol upset his control over the passions, leaving the drunkard to swing from one emotional extreme to another. As Occom made clear, drinking degenerated the mind and body, subsequently leaving the man in an irrational state, in which he was unable either to control his passions or to speak "as to be understood."[15]

Occom also discussed the connections between intoxication and devilish behavior in "Moses Paul." He explained that one's mental faculties began to mirror those of beasts and of devils in the state of irrationality induced by intoxication. Occom wrote: "when we are intoxicated with strong drink we drown our rational powers, by which we are distinguished from the brutal creation; we unman ourselves, and bring ourselves not only level with the beasts of the field, but seven degrees beneath them; yea we bring ourselves level with the devils; I don't know but we make ourselves worse than devils, for I never heard of drunken devils."[16] Alcohol acted on the mind by transforming formerly rational mental faculties into an irrational state that rendered one's mind similar to that of a beast, resulting in a loss of the rational faculties that defined one as human. Accompanying this degeneration into irrationality was a connection with and likeness to devils, or worse. Those who drank, Occom argued, served Satan as his devils did and themselves took on characteristics that made them "level with the devils."[17]

Occom's description of drunkenness echoed statements about the consequences of drinking made by colonial ministers, who also linked alcohol abuse to irrationality and devil worship. However, unlike Occom, who represented the series of decisions that a person, Native or Euro-American, made in order to become intoxicated, Anglo-colonial ministers attributed such practices to traits that, they argued, were specific to Natives. Indeed, in the eighteenth century, colonists began to define Indians' intoxication as an "indelible mark of racial inferiority" that signified their great passion for alcohol and their inability to control those desires.[18] In a 1710 sermon delivered at the execution of two Indians who had murdered several colonists while intoxicated, minister Samuel Danforth pointed out that intoxication transformed the mind and behavior by allowing "the Will and Passions [to] get head above the Reason, and Understanding, *Prov. 20.21.* Hereby the Soul is debased, and immersed into sensuality."[19] Drinking disordered the proper natural hierarchy by which the understanding governed the passions, thus allowing irrational desires to overwhelm the reason. In a point quite similar to those Occom later made, Danforth explained that alcohol transformed people from thinking, rational beings into beast-like creatures: "Drunkenness is justly termed a brutish Sin, and a voluntary Madness; Sense & Reason being laid asleep thereby, nothing remains in exercise, but that part of man wherein he resembles a Beast, which produces beastly actions and behaviour."[20] Like Occom, Danforth identified "madness" and a degrading irrationality as the consequences of alcohol abuse.

However, unlike Occom, who represented the series of decisions that a person, Native or Euro-American, made in order to become intoxicated, Danforth attributed Natives' desire for alcohol to inferior physical and mental characteristics. Danforth connected the Indian men's drunkenness to natural features that rendered them unable to determine when they reached a state of intoxication and irrationality. As he explained later in the sermon, "We are not ignorant of their [Natives'] natural extraordinary craving Appetite after Strong Drink: We are not ignorant that most of them are very unmeet judges to determine when they have drank enough."[21] Danforth's references to Indians' "natural extraordinary craving Appetite" suggested that, although alcohol transformed Natives into beasts who lacked reason, they were already irrational and thus lacked the reason necessary to resist their "Appetite" for alcohol.[22] The "voluntary madness" into which drunkards slipped was therefore not truly voluntary, for Natives' actions were prescribed by powerful appetites.[23]

Ministers and colonial travelers drew connections between Natives' religious beliefs and their "madness" while intoxicated.[24] In this way, they contributed to classifications of Natives' minds as irrational and their religious practices as heathen, even while also stabilizing these categories as natural and innate characteristics. They likened Natives' "madness" while drunk to superstitious practices, and they described Natives' state of intoxication as similar to possession by diabolic forces. The missionary David Brainerd wrote of the Delaware Indians when they were drunk that: "I could not but hope that God would bring in these miserable, wicked Indians; though there appeared little human probability of it; for they were then dancing and revelling, as if possessed by the devil."[25] Colonists also described intoxicated Natives as devils themselves, a description that Occom echoed when he noted that drink made one level with or worse than a devil. As John Hays wrote of the Delaware in his journal, "Sume of them Wanted to have Rosted us for they Like as Maney Raiging Divels and Sum of the chiefes would not Taast of the Rum or We would have had A Bad time of hit."[26] In colonial accounts, Natives' intoxication was the consequence of an irrational mind that did not know its own weaknesses; the same mental weakness facilitated Natives' transformation into irrational states in which they communicated with, worshipped, and resembled the devil.

Colonists drew further connections between drinking and diabolic practices by aligning these actions with Native medical practitioners. Brainerd described a *powah* who was also a drunkard and who was cured of both his "sins" when he converted. He wrote: "Another man advanced in years, who had been a murderer, a *pawaw* or conjurer, and a notorious drunkard, was likewise brought now to cry for mercy with many tears, and to complain much that he could be no more concerned when he saw his danger so very great."[27] Places in which Satan had a foothold were also places where alcohol use and intoxication were frequent, as Brainerd complained: "The Indians of this place, are accounted the most drunken, mischievous, and ruffianlike fellows, of any in these parts; and satan seems to have his seat in this town in an eminent manner."[28] Colonists such as Brainerd described the causes and effects of alcohol by incorporating pre-existing descriptions of Native Americans as irrational and as devil worshippers into accounts of Natives' alcohol abuse. They aligned intemperance with Natives' allegedly heathen medical and religious practices, such that drunkenness operated as another symptom or sign of Indians' irrational mental faculties and, by extension, of their trust in diabolic forces. The same irrational mental faculties that allowed the devil to dupe Natives into believing he had special powers—as Nicolás Monardes had speculated—also led Natives to drink so much that they entered alternate states in which the devil controlled their actions. In this way, colonists drew on prior classifications of Natives' bodies and minds as disordered and irrational, and they employed these classifications to support descriptions of Natives as devil-worshipers and as characterized by irrational mental faculties.[29]

But colonists also began to modify previous accounts of Natives' mental faculties and religious practices by locating the origins of Natives' desire for alcohol in innate characteristics rather than in environmental factors. Minister Samuel Kirkland wrote in a 1772 letter:

> By searching more into Indian traditions—National temper, past conduct under Providence—with the present state of the different Nations and tribes—I am ready to conclude they are in a peculiar sense and manner under the curse of Heaven—yea, I can resolve the paradox no other way—They appear, as a body, to be given over to strong delusions . . . as they do not like to retain God in their knowledge—they are left to a reprobate or injudicious mind.[30]

Kirkland's turn to "Indian traditions" to discover causes for Natives' "present state" suggested that irrational mental faculties and heathen beliefs—or "strong delusions" and a resistance to Christianity—were shared by all Natives, regardless of time or place.[31] Other colonists shared Kirkland's views: Peter Chester, governor of West Florida, pointed out in his account of Natives' use of rum that although both birth and education were significant influences on Natives, education did not alter the state they received at birth. He wrote that they were "born in savage ignorance and brought up in the same way."[32] Meanwhile, Eleazar Wheelock commented that Natives' "ungovernable appetites, . . . will prescribe no bounds, nor admit any restrains, till a total inability to purchase more liquor, does it for them."[33] Only the absence of liquor, rather than rational actions or religious conversion, would keep Natives from alcohol.

Many colonists admitted that European settlers and traders were responsible for introducing liquor to the Americas, and many colonial writers chastised those who supplied Natives with alcohol. But rather than citing intercultural trade as the ultimate cause of Indians' alcohol abuse, colonists positioned Indians' intoxication as a consequence of natural characteristics of irrationality and savagery. As Peter Mancall and Ava Chamberlain have each pointed out, Indians' drinking was the aspect of Native life that seemed most barbaric to colonists. Although colonists regularly drank far more than Natives did, colonists did not become intoxicated as often as Natives, and they consequently concluded that Natives had a natural desire for and susceptibility to alcohol.[34] As Mancall explains:

> At the end of the colonial period many colonists believed that Indians' inability to control their thirst for rum signaled deep-seated, permanent inferiority. Nothing else could explain their continued demand for a commodity that so palpably destroyed their communities. After all, since colonists themselves drank alcohol in prodigious quantities and did not suffer greatly from it, Indians' intemperance and its associated risks must have been proof of something forever alien about America's natives, a confirmation of their savagery.[35]

In Kirkland's comment, the physical and mental qualities that explained Natives' weakness for alcohol were simultaneously indicative of their "traditions" and perpetually present in their "National temper."[36] By conflating the past and present and suggesting that Natives existed in an unchanging state of savagery, colonists placed Natives in a timeless space in which "past conduct" continued to define present behavior.[37] From their place within this temporal category, Natives lacked the ability to change their behavior and thus to alter their national history or their future actions. Similarly, Wheelock claimed that most Natives lacked minds and souls receptive to civilization and conversion. Rather, Natives would remain in a state of barbarity and irrationality "unless the Arm of the Lord should be revealed in an eminent Manner, to cure them of such savage and sordid Practices, as they have been inured to from their Mother's Womb, and form their Minds and Manners to proper Rules of Virtue, Decency and Humanity, while they are daily under the pernicious Influence of their Parents Example, and their many Vices made familiar thereby."[38] Even Christianized Indians did not completely escape these categories of irrationality and paganism, for they "could at any moment revert to their original savage state by falling into the sin of intemperance."[39] Colonists began to define Indians' intoxication as a sign of their inability to control their desire for alcohol, regardless of environmental or religious influences.[40]

Although Natives' irrational mental faculties had formerly been attributed to climatological factors that also influenced colonists' minds, colonists began to suggest that Natives possessed irrational mental faculties from birth onwards. As we have seen in James Grainger's attribution of slaves' belief in obeah to mental traits formed in Africa, so in the late eighteenth century, characteristics that had previously been defined as the product of environmental factors began to be attributed to Natives' innate racial and national characteristics. As Roxann Wheeler points out, characteristics of mind and body that had been "considered *effects* of climate or of differing stages of civilization during the eighteenth century became *causes* of European superiority and of other races' inferiority."[41] During the nineteenth century, these traits would be further solidified, as a "controlling power of the will."[42] Attributing Natives' desire for alcohol to a "National temper," as Kirkland did, contributed to the process of transforming formerly environmentally constructed features of irrationality and appetite into natural traits belonging to all Natives.[43] In this way, ministers erected differences between colonists and Natives that effaced the fact that they shared the same climate.[44]

The Great Pox: Place, Promiscuity, and the American Origins of Syphilis

Occom engaged descriptions of Natives' irrationality and diabolism as national traits by offering an alternate history of moral and physical illnesses. To do so, he drew connections between drunkenness and another malady that also possessed moral and physiological elements and that was believed to be caused by traits inherent to Native Americans: syphilis, or the great pox, the so-called American disease. Many Europeans claimed that syphilis originated in the Americas, and accounts of Natives as naturally lascivious and passionate supported theories of an American origin for the disease and its circulation. Many medical practitioners and historians agreed that the disease had been transmitted from Hispaniola to Spain and throughout Europe by Columbus's men, who were said to have contracted the pox in sexual encounters with Native women.[45] Furthermore, eighteenth-century natural historians revived sixteenth- and seventeenth-century arguments about America's climate and cultures in order to articulate differences among plants, animals, and people in various climates.

Occom incorporated a discussion of syphilis and "Whoredom" into his sermon by drawing on news of the recent outbreak of syphilis in Tahiti (227). He described the transmission of syphilis in the Pacific by quoting from John Hawkesworth's account of Cook's voyage. Occom explained that "Captain Cook in his Voige Round the World, Says that there was a Vesel in a Place Called Otaheite, about fifteen months before him, and had leff that a Cursed ~~disease~~ Common among the poor Indians, Which they were utterly Ignorant of before" (227). Occom directly referenced Hawkesworth's compilation by citing the volume and page number in a "Voige Round the World," where the account of syphilis appeared. Although it is possible that Occom himself purchased a copy of Hawkesworth's book on one of his travels throughout New England, it is also quite likely that he encountered news of Cook's voyage while in England or in conversations once he had returned to New England. Finally, some of Occom's acquaintances, including the minister John Seargant and his son, are listed as subscribers to the American edition of *A New Voyage,* making it possible that Occom had obtained the text from them.[46]

Occom's citation of Hawkesworth's text referenced a colonial history of disease transmission and sexual encounters in which indigenous peoples were figured both as the victims and the sources of venereal disease. In order to understand the ways in which Occom engaged this history, it is first necessary to examine documents from Cook's voyage to Tahiti and the theories of syphilis that shaped eighteenth-century ideas about indigenous bodies and behaviors. Hawkesworth wrote that sexual exchanges between Europeans and Tahitians had transmitted syphilis to the island, although he claimed that it was not clear which European nation was to blame, since Cook had attempted to ensure that none of his men carried the disease before setting sail. Hawkesworth echoed Banks's comment that "When first we discoverd this distemper among these people we were much alarmd, fearing that we ourselves had notwithstanding our many precautions brought it among them; but upon strict inquiry we found that one of our people had been infected within 5 days after our arrival and when we a little better understood the Language the natives explained the matter fully to us."[47] Despite their initial concern that the English had brought syphilis with them, Banks, Cook, and Hawkesworth all concluded that the disease had existed in Tahiti before the English arrived.

Hawkesworth further distanced the English explorers from accusations that they were the cause of the illness by reminding readers that syphilis had originated among Native peoples in the Americas, where it first diseased Spanish colonists. He referenced Columbus's men's role in the transmission of syphilis by explaining that the Tahitians' "commerce with the inhabitants of Europe has, however, already entailed upon them that dreadful curse which avenged the inhumanities committed by the Spaniards in America, the venereal disease."[48] This reference to the Spanish conquest of America reinvigorated the Black Legend, stereotypes of Spanish colonists as greedy and violent and of syphilis as a punishment for such behavior.[49] In the same way that colonial promoters such as Thomas Harriot argued that English colonists departed from the violence of Spanish conquistadors, so Hawkesworth's references to exchanges of disease in Spanish America shifted the blame for transmitting syphilis away from English explorers and toward unnamed European travelers whose "commerce" with the Tahitians resulted in the transmission of disease.[50] Further, Hawkesworth drew on Banks's journal to write:

> it is certain that no European vessel besides our own, except the Dolphin, and the two that were under the command of Mons. Bougainville, ever visited this island, it must have been brought either by one of them or by us. That it was not brought by the Dolphin, Captain Wallis has demonstrated in the account of her voyage, and nothing is more certain than that when we arrived it had made most dreadful ravages in the island.[51]

Both Banks and Hawkesworth attempted to rule out the possibility that the Tahitians could have caught syphilis from the English men by suggesting that the disease preceded the arrival of Cook's ship and that Captain Wallis had given sufficient counterarguments waiving the *Dolphin's* responsibility.

The English writers' anxiety about the source of syphilis participated in an ongoing debate about the disease and its origins, a debate that involved ideas about indigenous bodies and minds as well as about the connections between climate and disease. In the eighteenth century, medical and natural philosophers added to centuries-old arguments about syphilis by supporting claims that the disease originated in particular places, which acted on bodies and behavior in special ways, to produce diseases unique to those places. In this way, they combined older, environmental theories of disease and identity with emerging conceptions of physical and moral characteristics as inherent. The French medical philosopher Jean Astruc wrote that countries characterized by hot climates, which he identified as Asia, Africa, and America, were "formerly so many seed-plots of the *Venereal Disease*. For as these were all situate [*sic*] in the Torrid Zone, there must have been in them the like heat of the air as in *Hispaniola,* a like disposition to impurity, and the same propensity to a promiscuous copulation. Every one knows what the first Writers of *America* have said concerning the warmer *American* climates."[52] Astruc's medical geography suggested that the "warmer *American* climates" fostered diseases unique to "Torrid" regions and produced certain immoral "disposition[s]" in people.[53] Promiscuous behavior was to be expected of Native men and women, and so, medical philosophers argued, was venereal disease.

Men and women exposed to hot climates were said to possess different fluids than people from more temperate regions, and these fluids were the cause of syphilis. Astruc argued that women's "menstrual Blood [was] so virulent in the hotter climates"[54] and that, when mixed with the "different, acrid, and heterogenous seed of several Men," the "first seeds of the *Venereal Disease*" formed in the "over-heated Wombs of very filthy Women."[55] Astruc warned:

> even here in our milder regions of *Europe,* if any one has to do with a menstrous Woman, the Glans and Prepuce shall for the most part be affected with a slight inflammation or superficial Pustules, which will soon pass off. How much more grievous consequences therefore in a hot and burning climate must attend such as are not asham'd to converse with Women under the circumstance of so sharp, and, in a manner venomous flux?[56]

Hot climates inclined Native women and men to engage in promiscuous behavior, but such behavior rendered female bodies shaped by these climates extremely dangerous. Sexual encounters, especially if they were excessive or aberrant and involved multiple partners, held more risk in hot climates than in Europe's ideal "milder regions." As Astruc explained: "the *Venereal Disease* seems to have been formerly endemial, the like heat of the climate was joyn'd with the like incontinence of the inhabitants."[57] Native Americans' sexual appetites, along with the effect of the hot climate on the fluids in women's wombs, allowed syphilis to take root and spread throughout the Atlantic world.

As indicated by his reference to "what the first Writers of *America* have said concerning the warmer *American* climates," Astruc's etiology of syphilis drew on histories of the discovery and conquest of the Americas.[58] These "first Writers of *America*" described America's climate as hot, and they likewise identified people from the Americas as promiscuous.[59] Gonzalo Fernández de Oviedo y Valdés, whom Astruc cited multiple times, wrote that "The landes and regions that are neare about the clymes of the Equinoctiall lyne, are naturally hotte, althowghe they bee otherwyse temperate by the divine providence."[60] Similarly, José de Acosta explained that although the ancients claimed that the "burning Zone was hotte and exceeding drie, the which is not so, for it is hote and moist, and in the greatest part, the heat is not excessive but rather moderate."[61] Oviedo's and Acosta's histories of America were translated and reprinted myriad times throughout the sixteenth and seventeenth centuries, and they shaped Europeans' expectations and conceptions of the American climate as hot and humid. In the English context, for example, James I referenced the "intemperate heate of [America's] Climat" to explain why Native Americans had an "uncleanly and adust constitution" that made them subject to the "Pockes."[62]

Astruc's theory of the pox's origins also drew on descriptions of Native women as lascivious, a trait allegedly produced by the hot climate. Early explorers of the Americas, such as Oviedo and Amerigo Vespucci, established conceptions of Native women as passionate and as possessing dangerous sexual desires. Oviedo explained that the Natives had many sexual partners throughout their lives: "Sum of them take as many wyues as them lyste, and other lyue with one wyfe whome they forsake not without consent of both parties, which chauncethe especially when they have no chyldren."[63] Similarly, Vespucci wrote that the Natives enjoyed liberty in their sexual practices, claiming that they not only went naked but also did not practice marriage and took as many partners as they liked. He explained that the Natives were "lascivious beyond measure, the women much more so than the men."[64] Such passion was also directed at the European travelers, for whose "company" the women showed "excessive desire."[65] This desire was dangerous, as Vespucci noted. "Another custom among them is sufficiently shameful, and beyond all

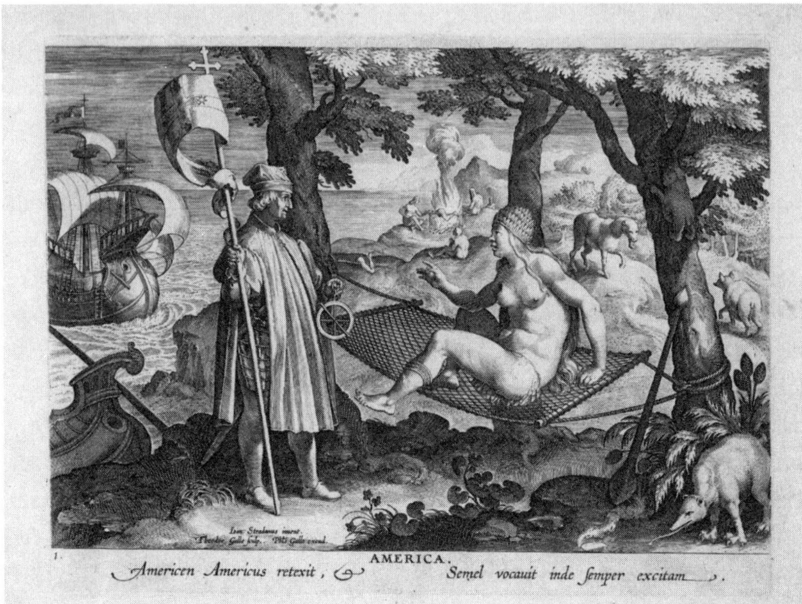

Figure 6. "Vespucci Landing in America," Jan van der Straet (1575). Reproduced by permission of The Huntington Library, San Marino, California.

human credibility," he wrote. "Their women, being very libidinous, make the penis of their husbands swell to such a size as to appear deformed; and this is accomplished by a certain artifice, being the bite of some poisonous animal, and by reason of this many lose their virile organ and remain eunuchs."[66] Native women's frightening sexuality was made apparent in visual representations of encounter as well. Images of America as a naked women open to the gaze of Europeans were juxtaposed with scenes of cannibalism, in this way representing Native women's dangerous passion and sexual freedom as capable of consuming male European bodies (Figures 6 and 7).[67]

Descriptions of the hot American climate and dangerously passionate indigenous women coalesced in the earliest accounts of syphilis. The Spanish historians who first attributed syphilis to America claimed that Columbus's men had had sexual encounters with local women and returned infected with syphilis, after which they spread the disease throughout Europe. Oviedo assured Charles V of Spain that "this horrible disease came from the Indies. Although it is quite common among the natives, it is not so dangerous there as it is here in Europe" due to the difference in climate.[68] As the Spanish phy-

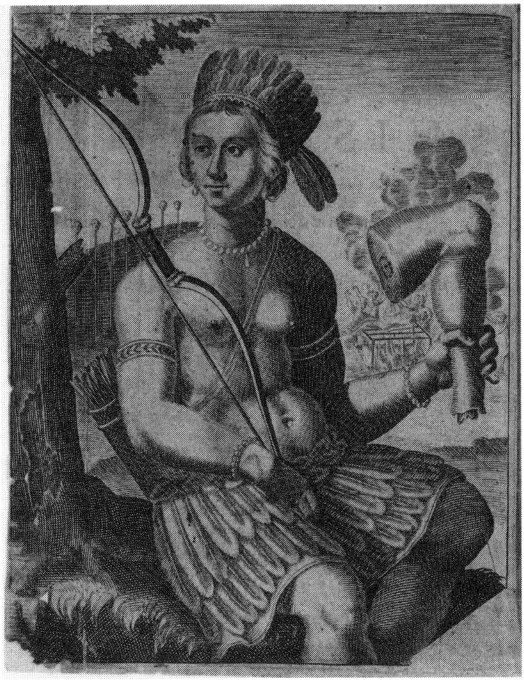

Figure 7. Ferdinando Gorges, *America Painted to the Life* (London, 1659). Courtesy of the John Carter Brown Library at Brown University.

sician Ruy Diaz de Ysla commented, "This disease appeared in Spain in the Year of our Lord 1493, in the city of Barcelona and as this city was infected, it followed that all Europe, and all parts of the Universe which are known and accessible became infected too. This disease had its origin and birthplace in the island which is now called Hispaniola, as was concluded from a long and sound experience."[69] The Dominican priest Bartolomé de las Casas likewise attributed syphilis to the New World, writing that despite being called the French disease, the pox "came from this island with the first Indians when the Admiral Christopher Columbus returned with the news of the discovery of the Indies. The Indians I saw afterwards in Seville, and they may have brought the disease into Spain either by infecting the air or in some other way; or it was brought by some Spaniards already infected, in the first return voyage to Seville."[70] Las Casas's comment that the Indians "infect[ed] the air" marked their bodies and the New World climate as unhealthy and suggested that encounters with Natives had polluted Spanish bodies and lands.

As these comments suggest, America's climate was at the center of arguments that syphilis had a non-European origin. Many early modern medical practitioners believed that diseases were place-specific, determined by environmental features that characterized different places and acted on bodies in particular ways. Moreover, when roots and barks specific to the Americas, such as guaiacum and sassafras, were discovered to abate the symptoms of venereal disease, European medical practitioners concluded that the pox, like its cures, originated in the Americas. In his providence, God was thought to provide cures in the same place that a disease originated, so that the country devastated by an illness would not be devoid of a cure. Nicolás Monardes explained in his herbal:

> Our Lord God would from whence the euill of the Poxe came, from thence should come the remedy for them. Since it is known that they came into these parts from the Indias, and first of all from *Santo Domingo*. The Poxe bee as common amongst the Indians, and as familiare, as the Measelles bee unto us, and well neere the most part of the Indians, both men and women have them, without making thereof any scruple, and they came first in this sorte.[71]

As Monardes's claim that God willed that "from whence the evil of the Poxe came, from thence should come the remedy for them" suggests, the presence of remedies for the "euill of the Pox" seemed to provide evidence that the disease did indeed originate in the Americas.[72] The American climate thus produced the infected air and bodies that Natives transmitted to Spain as well as the plants that cured syphilis.

The connections between syphilis and the Americas were so established by the seventeenth century that colonists in New England expected to find Natives infected with the illness there. As John Josselyn wrote in *An Account of Two Voyages to New-England,* "There are Diseases that are proper to certain climates, as the Leprosie to *AEygpt,* swelling of the Throat or *Mentegra* to *Asia,* the sweating sickness to the Inhabitants of the North; to the *Portugals* the Phthisick, to *Savoy* the mumps; So the *West-Indies* the Pox."[73] Josselyn added to his consideration of climate and disease the fact that the Natives in New England were alleged to be "*Man-eaters*"; this combination of inappropriate behavior and inhospitable climate made the "great pox . . . proper to them."[74] His account of North American cannibals infected with the pox hearkened back to Spanish histories, for Oviedo's natural history is full of descriptions of warlike Natives who consumed human flesh, and Vespucci likewise described Natives as savage cannibals who lusted after flesh.

Eighteenth-century writers employed such histories of New World disease to support arguments that the American climate had a degenerative effect on bodies and morals. Like Astruc, the Dutch writer Cornelius de Pauw commented that America's climate prevented its people from building an advanced civilization: "noxious vapours, corrupt juices, and vitiated qualities of the plants and aliments, will account for that feebleness of complexion, that aversion from labour, and general unfitness for improvements of every kind, which have prevented the Americans from emerging out of savage life."[75] He described the inferiority of American nature by referencing Oviedo's description of the Iuanna, or iguana, a reptile believed to activate the symptoms of the great pox. Oviedo explained that the iguana "hurteth none but onely such as haue had the frenshe poxe. In so much that if they haue onely byn touched of that infyrmitie, although they have byn hole of longe tyme, nevertheless they feele burnte and complayne of the eatynge of these *Iuannas,* as hath byn often tymes proved by experience."[76] De Pauw revived this account by reporting that the pox would be contracted by anyone "eating the meat of the American iguana."[77] America's nature—both animals and people—was degenerate and diseased, de Pauw suggested, and the climate was to blame.

The physical and moral degeneration characterizing the morals and bodies of those native to America was reflected as well in their minds. As de Pauw claimed, "The Europeans who pass into America degenerate, as do the animals; a proof that the climate is unfavourable to the improvement of either men or animals. . . . This degradation of humanity must be imputed to the vitiated qualities of the air stagnated in their immense forests, and corrupted by noxious vapours from standing waters and uncultivated grounds."[78] Just as Natives from Hispaniola passed syphilis to Spanish explorers by infecting the air, so in the eighteenth century America's air was to blame for the irrational behavior and degenerated bodies of people and animals exposed or native to the New World's climate. As Marie E. McAllister writes, even Thomas Jefferson's "Enlightenment arguments about diet could not stop readers from suspecting that New World degeneracy—either the outsize lusts of older myths or the impotence in Buffon—had played some role in the origins of syphilis."[79] Thus despite Grainger's and other plantation physicians' moves to subordinate the environment as a cause of difference, environmental theories were still powerful explanations for disease and for identity at the end of the eighteenth century. They were particularly compelling for European philosophers because these theories allowed writers to group all people from the Americas into an inferior category due to their shared exposure to America's climate.[80]

Syphilis, Classification, and Indigenous Bodies in Tahiti

English explorers in Tahiti transferred descriptions of the American and tropical origins of syphilis to the South Seas to describe indigenous women's sexual practices and illnesses. In particular, the men attributed the Tahitians' sexual behavior to the island's tropical climate. An unnamed "gentleman"[81] who traveled on board the *Endeavour* commented that the English men "married with their women, and enjoyed a felicity amongst them [the Tahitian women] peculiar to the salubrity of so sweet a clime."[82] A letter by another expedition member explained that the Tahitian women "are not very decent in their amours, having little regard to either place or person; this is not general amongst them, though it is often done and seen. Upon occasions of festivity the women dance in the most indecent manner, performing a thousand gesticulations, like the Indostan dancing girls."[83]

Hawkesworth and Banks likewise followed eighteenth-century natural philosophers and medical practitioners for whom place and behavior explained syphilis's origin and circulation. They presented the Tahitians' sexual practices and medical knowledge as evidence that they were already acquainted with the disease, even before the English arrived.[84] Hawkesworth commented on the Tahitians' open sexual behavior, writing that the women, "drawing [the men] down upon them, left us no room to doubt of their being much less jealous of observation than we were."[85] He went on to explain: "A very considerable number of the principal people of Otaheite, of both sexes, have formed themselves into a society, in which every woman is common to every man; thus securing a perpetual variety as often as their inclination prompts them to seek it, which is so frequent, that the same man and woman seldom cohabit together more than two or three days."[86] Such accounts of the Tahitians' sexual intemperance seemed to confirm their familiarity with syphilis.

Hawkesworth's descriptions of the Tahitians' medical knowledge and of the island's medicinal plants likewise supported the suggestion that the Tahitians were familiar with venereal diseases and their cures. Hawkesworth wrote that despite the "universal terror and consternation" that syphilis produced among the Tahitians, the English explorers "had some reason, however, to hope that they [the Tahitians] had found out a specific to cure it: during our stay upon the island we saw none in whom it had made a great progress, and one who went from us infected, returned after a short time in perfect health; and by this it appeared either that the disease had cured itself, or that they were not unacquainted with the virtues of simples."[87] In Banks's journal, on which Hawkesworth likely based this account of the Tahitians' medical knowledge, Banks noted: "Yet shocking as these symptoms were they had even at the time when we came there found a method of cure and that I should suppose not of a despicable nature, as we saw no one during the whole of our stay in whoom the distemper arrivd to any hight and some who went from us for their cure returnd in a short time perfectly recover'd."[88] Observations that the Tahitians seemed capable of curing an illness that had perplexed European physicians for centuries identified the island as a site both of the pox's origin and of its cure, just as Native Americans' knowledge of the healing virtues of herbs such as sassafras and guaiacum supported arguments that the Americas' climate fostered syphilis.

Banks further ruled out the colonists as the source of syphilis by employing classificatory forms to separate the Tahitians' behavior from colonists' actions. He removed his description of the Tahitians' cultural practices, including their medical knowledge of cures for syphilis, from his narrative of the men's travels by placing this description in a separate section, "Manners and Customs of S. Sea Islands."[89] Banks provided a moral history of Tahitian political, religious, domestic, and agricultural practices, and he detailed the Tahitians' appearance, behavior, and history. By removing descriptions of the islanders from the narrative of the voyage, Banks—and later Hawkesworth—presented them as exotic objects of scrutiny, similar to the new flowers and insects that the explorers named and classified. The form of the "manners and customs" section "suggested that indigenous people were, like flowers and insects, less than human. Like Tahitian flora and fauna, it suggested, indigenous peoples could properly be assessed *en masse,* displaying the characteristics of a species rather than the complexities of human character and society."[90]

As with Kirkland's attribution of Natives' intoxication to a national temper, so Banks's "manners and customs" section constructed separate categories and, consequently, separate histories for European observers and their Tahitian objects of observation. This section posited features that had previously been seen as environmentally constructed as natural to the Tahitians instead, by presenting the people as possessing unchanging traits that determined their actions and knowledge. As Mary Louise Pratt writes, "The portrait of manners and customs is a normalizing discourse, whose work is to codify difference, to fix the Other in a timeless present where all 'his' actions and reactions are repetitions of 'his' normal habits. Thus, it textually produces the Other without an explicit anchoring either in an observing self or in a particular encounter in which contact with the Other takes place."[91] Just as colonists understood Natives' alcohol abuse as the consequence of timeless appetites and traditions, so Banks's "manners and customs" section fixed promiscuous behavior on the Tahitians. Moreover, by effacing the contexts of encounter in which the men collected information about indigenous peoples, the manners and customs section allowed colonists to distance themselves from the experiences of disease and sexual encounter they shared with the Tahitians. This rhetorical distance fixed the explorers and Tahitians in different histories by presenting the Tahitians in a "timeless present" in which they could always be preserved as they had once been observed.[92] As Johannes Fabian has pointed out, such "temporal distancing" allowed observers to deny their "coevalness," that is, the fact that they shared the same time and experiences as indigenous peoples, and subsequently to remove the objects of their observation from the "dialogic situation."[93] The objects of anthropological discourse, as Fabian argues, are always located in the past "in relation to the acts of recording, interpreting, and writing" performed by observers.[94]

In Banks's and, by extension, in Hawkesworth's account, placing the Tahitians' illnesses and medicines in the "manners and customs" section constructed temporal distance and cultural difference between islanders and English colonists. The "manners and customs" section classified the Tahitians in a separate textual space in which their illness was attributed to physical characteristics and to behavior that remained fixed in time. English explorers used their reports to position themselves outside this space, as observers and recorders who did not share experiences, illnesses, or physical characteristics with their objects of observation. In this way, Banks's classificatory strategies supported conceptions of differences between European and tropical locales as well as differences between European and Tahitian bodies, minds, and morals. Like the catalogs, moral histories, and footnotes that, as previous chapters have shown, colonists in the Americas attached to their medical writing, so Banks's classificatory forms placed him in a separate category from the one the Tahitians occupied. He held a position of observational authority even as he showed that he maintained English mental and physical features in colonial encounters.[95]

Narrative and Colonial Encounters

Although Occom closely followed *A New Voyage* by citing Hawkesworth directly, he also departed from Banks's and Hawkesworth's accounts in ways that altered Europeans' classifications of Natives as naturally irrational, passionate, and promiscuous and of Native American or Tahitian peoples as the origin of syphilis. Occom repeated the colonists' speculation that syphilis already existed in Tahiti before the British ship arrived, and he incorporated the explorers' statement that the Tahitians told the British men of a previous ship that had brought the disease. But Occom then revised Banks's and Hawkesworth's accounts of the pox's origin by rewriting the sequence of events that led to the transmission of syphilis in Tahiti. In contrast to Hawkesworth's reference to Spanish colonization and the American origins of syphilis, Occom presented an alternate narrative by repeating that the Natives were "intirely" and "utterly Ignorant" of the pox before Europeans arrived (227). Moreover, he intervened in the debate regarding how syphilis arrived in Tahiti, for he did not identify one European nation as responsible for bringing the pox. In this way, Occom left open the possibility that the English ship had transferred syphilis to the island. He thus reinterpreted Hawkesworth's statement that "Their commerce with the inhabitants of Europe has, however, already entailed upon them that dreadful curse which avenged the inhumanities committed by the Spaniards in America."[96] Hawkesworth's convoluted formulation of revenge suggested that the Tahitians, as the originators of syphilis, transferred the "dreadful curse" to "them"—meaning the Europeans who preceded Cook—in recompense for apparently inhumane behavior, just as Natives in Spanish America repaid Spanish conquistadors for their actions by giving them syphilis. But Occom redirected this narrative of disease transmission, so that the curse of disease was transmitted to the Tahitians, not, as the English travelers would have it, from the Tahitians to the English sailors.

Occom further revised Hawkesworth's account of syphilis by making visible several elisions in *A New Voyage,* a move that allowed him to restore the context of sexual encounters in which the transmission of disease had occurred. He pointed out that if the Tahitians had actually infected Cook's men, they were only "returning the Compliment" that the English had first given to them (227). This comment suggests that Occom was aware of theories that syphilis originated in tropical climates and the bodies shaped by those environments, but he also amended these theories by making the Tahitians recipients of the "Compliment" of disease (227). He extended his subtle suggestion that the English might have been the source of syphilis by pointing out that Cook himself "was not quite so Honest as to Say whether he had it [the pox] himself" (227). Occom noted that Cook did not comment on his own medical condition or sexual practices but rather was presented (and presented himself) as a distanced observer of events, rather than as a participant. As Beth Fowkes Tobin has pointed out, Cook, like Banks, employed rhetorical strategies of distancing by removing his "bodily pleasure from the printed account of the voyage."[97] When revising his daily logs for publication as a travel narrative, he deleted words that referred to physical experiences such as tasting and feeling; these excisions acted "as an epistemological tool to produce a line that reads as if it is reporting simply a fact."[98] In contrast to the English explorers who employed such rhetorical strategies to position themselves as observers rather than as participants in sexual exchanges with Tahitian women, Occom suggested that Cook himself might have participated in the sexual exchanges he tried to regulate among his own men. Occom's account of exchanges in Tahiti thus restored the shared experiences of physical contact that the classificatory form of the "manners and customs" section elided.

Occom further revised the classificatory rhetorical strategies by which English writers placed the Tahitians and their medical knowledge by pointing out that Native medical knowledge could not always be framed in European categories. He wrote, "If he [Cook] Could have learnt their Specific for the Venereal Disease, if Such they have *any* it would have been of great advantage to us" (227). Yet, as Occom suggested and Hawkesworth admitted, although the men—certainly Banks, whose botanical interests would have facilitated his interest in discovering flora that would cure syphilis—attempted to locate this plant, they were ultimately unable to obtain the cure. Hawkesworth admitted that "our knowledge of their language was too imperfect" for the English to discover the "medical qualities" that might have healed syphilis.[99] His note points to the fact that communication was not transparent in cross-cultural encounters in Tahiti, but it also raised the possibility that the Tahitians deliberately obfuscated their explanation of medicinal plants, perhaps in order to protect them from the English. Regardless, the English colonists' failure to find the specific, or cure, marked a gap in the project of collecting and classifying that both Cook and Banks undertook. Although, as Londa L. Schiebinger has pointed out, European botanical nomenclature, such as the Linnaean system Banks used, "served as an instrument of empire detaching plants from their native cultural moorings and placing them within schema comprehensible first and foremost to Europeans," the Tahitians' specific for syphilis resisted being "swallowed" into such botanical schema, remaining beyond the colonists' knowledge.[100] The specific for syphilis marked the boundary of the European taxonomizing project, the point past which European knowledge did not extend and objects remained unclassified.

Occom's sermon undercut both the catalog of plants and the classificatory practices with which Banks, Cook, and Hawkesworth had placed the bodies and behavior of English travelers and Tahitians in separate categories. Specifically, Occom refuted theories of a climatological cause for syphilis by undoing the connections among place, disease, and its cure. In the sermon, the Tahitians' specific for syphilis did not operate as a sign that the disease was native to the island or even as an indication that the Tahitians were familiar with the specific because they already had the pox. Instead, Occom's comment that the Tahitians had "no difficulty in returning" the "Compliment" of disease shifted the focus from the Tahitians' medical knowledge as evidence for an indigenous source of syphilis to English sailors' behavior and to colonization as the causes of the disease's transmission and circulation (227). In Occom's sermon, the Tahitians' medical knowledge remained powerful and effective against syphilis without becoming evidence that their environment or their bodies manufactured disease or that syphilis was native to the island. Occom's sermon revised theories that syphilis originated in hot climates among indigenous peoples construed as lascivious by making behavior, rather than climate, the key feature determining health.

Finally, then, Occom's account of syphilis in Tahiti collapsed the distance that the "manners and customs" section had erected between European observers and indigenous people. He revised the categories of promiscuity and irrationality in which Europeans positioned Tahitian and American indigenous peoples. Occom's references to Cook's behavior restored contexts of encounter, and of sexual encounter in particular, responsible for the transmission of disease in Tahiti. Occom's commentary thus exposed the fact that the stance of distanced observation that Banks adopted and that Hawkesworth reproduced was constructed through rhetorical acts, such as placing the Tahitians' illness in the "manners and customs" form. Moreover, Occom contested representations of indigenous women as unhealthy, morally depraved, and irrational by pointing out that Europeans also practiced immoral behavior and participated in the same experiences of sexual encounter as the Tahitian women. He repositioned English explorers and their behavior inside the narrative of disease and encounter, and he complicated claims regarding environmental and cultural differences between tropical locales such as Tahiti or America and Europe's temperate regions by showing that Europeans were promiscuous. As a result, in Occom's sermon the Tahitians' bodies were not defined by their position in classificatory forms: they remain actors in the narrative of exploration, in which they interacted with the English.

Occom applied the same rhetorical strategies with which he restored narrative to accounts of colonial encounters in Tahiti to his representation of drunkenness and its causes. Just as he represented the practices that resulted in the outbreak of syphilis in Tahiti, so Occom also detailed the choices that one made to obtain alcohol and to become intoxicated. He placed the drunkard's actions into a narrative that showed the series of decisions—not inherent desires or weaknesses for alcohol—that resulted in intoxication. He wrote:

> does not the Drunkard Use that natural Power & understanding Which god has given him in his persute after Strong Drink? Dont he think and Consider Where he can get Liquor; and when he has found a Place in his Mind, he will use them Legs, which God has given him, and direct his Course to the Place Where he expects to get Liquor, and When he is got there, he will [use] that Tongue and Speech, Which God has given him, and Call for Liquor, and When it is granted; he takes the Cup with his own Hands, and he pours it down his own Throat, and he Uses the power of Swallowing and Swallows down his Liquor. (226)

Occom's narrative of intoxication restored the process whereby reason was "drowned" without assuming that drunkards were inherently characterized by irrationality (226). He related each step involved in getting drunk, and his language of choice showed that even drunkards used their "natural Power" and "Mind" to "Consider" how to find alcohol (226). In Occom's account, the man's intoxication was not already determined by innate appetites or delusions but rather was the result of a series of decisions.

Reason was slowly drowned by drink, but Occom's narrative asserts that it was present as the man used rational consideration to find liquor and begin drinking.[101]

Occom's medical writing, particularly his narratives of disease, intervened in colonists' practice of employing classificatory forms to construct differences between their bodies and minds and those of Native Americans, Africans, and Tahitians. Furthermore, Occom diagnosed moral ills by presenting the process whereby people were rendered irrational, or "level with the devils," and his narratives illuminated as well the ways in which these practices were not exclusive to non-European peoples.[102] For example, as Occom removed the Tahitians from classificatory spaces that positioned them as objects of study, he also revised the histories of Tahitians' irrationality and promiscuity circulated by colonists in the South Seas and in New England. As I note above, he represented syphilis as a disease of which "Natives" were "intirely ignorant" prior to their encounters with Europeans (227). Occom's reference to Natives' ignorance played on Euro-colonial descriptions of Natives as naturally uncivilized and irrational. He admitted that Natives were indeed ignorant—ignorant, that is, of sexually immoral behavior and the maladies transmitted by such behavior. By contrast, Europeans were capable of promiscuous, diseased behavior, as Occom pointed out by asking: "How many Baudy or Whore Houses are there in that Nation [England], and I suppose it is just so among the French, these are Calld Christian Nations and the most Learned Nations in the World" (227–28). Occom had viewed such behavior firsthand, as a journal entry describing the London streets showed: "in the Streets some Cursing, Swaring & Damning one another, others was loud hollowing, Whrestling, talking gigling, & Laughing, & Coaches and footmen passing and repassing, Crossing and Cross-Crossing, and the poor Begars [*sic*] Praying, Crying and Beging upon their knees."[103] By defining "ignorance" as a state of health and of right behavior that existed prior to colonial encounters, Occom reclaimed ignorance as a state that was indeed "native" to indigenous peoples in Tahiti and in America. In this way, he represented Natives' "National temper" as healthy, or moral, and suggested that it was corrupted when European colonists transmitted immoral behavior and illnesses.[104] Finally, he made spiritual and behavioral, rather than physical or environmental, factors the causes of the illnesses of intoxication and of syphilis.

Occom's critique of Banks's and Cook's classificatory forms contributed to his ongoing efforts to revise the categories through which colonists interpreted Natives' behavior. In a short prose piece written in 1783, he recounted the practices that colonists, beginning with the first explorers of the Americas, had cited as evidence of Natives' inferior status. Occom mentioned Natives' poverty and seeming failure to save for the future; their reliance on hunting, fishing, and fowling rather than on agriculture; the women's "Drudgery"—the agricultural work that Europeans considered men's labor; and their failure to learn trades.[105] This list of uncivilized behavior includes the categories with which colonists defined Natives as uncivilized and barbaric in classificatory forms, especially in moral or cultural histories such as the ones Edward Winslow and Joseph Banks wrote of New England and Tahiti, respectively. Yet Occom also pointed out that Natives appeared uncivilized only from one perspective; if one looked closer, their behavior was characterized by kindness and morality. In fact, he argued, Natives' practice of being "kind to one another" and of not "Lying, Cheating, and Steeling" was natural to them, not an effect of education or conversion.[106] By invoking and then critiquing the categories that Europeans employed to classify Natives and to distance themselves from cross-cultural encounters, Occom de-naturalized the behaviors that Euro-colonists defined as inferior and as inherent to Natives: their response to colonial trades and education and their methods of providing for their families appeared unusual only if one agreed that European conceptions of civilization were the norm. In this way, he showed that Natives' "Most Remarkable and Strange State Situation and Appearence [*sic*]" was only strange from a European perspective that privileged certain forms of knowledge over others. As he redefined what was "natural," Occom detached the practices of moral and rational behavior from Euro-colonial knowledge and signs of civility, and he privileged Native forms of interaction, knowledge, and behavior. As the next section shows, he also suggested a cure for diseased bodies and minds that drew on Native conceptions of illness, of behavior, and of bodies and minds.

Transformative Cures: Love and Rationality

Occom's reference to indigenous peoples' ignorance of syphilis and moral ills prior to colonial encounters offered a new history of colonization that included non-human entities and causes and that illuminated the ways in which diseases—both physical and moral—were consequences of colonization. European exploration and settlement disrupted the practices whereby Natives maintained their relationships with one another and with non-human beings, and colonists took possession of the land that grounded these relationships. The resulting imbalance between human and non-human realms was manifested in maladies, including syphilis and alcohol abuse, as well as in Natives' forced departure from the everyday practices that maintained their connections with the non-human forces responsible for causing such diseases. Natives' ill and intoxicated bodies signaled these altered, or "diseased," relationships between individuals and metaphysical realms. Like Occom, other Native medical practitioners represented these diseased relations in histories of colonialism and illness. As a Delaware physician pointed out: "In ancient times there was but little sickness among the Indians. The Delaware were greatly blessed because we always kept up our ceremonies and observed the rules of right living. The Indian was healthy because he ate only clean, pure food and lived closed [*sic*] to nature. Then came the new people with their strange ways and food, and dreadful diseases."[107] Although Natives' ignorance of "strange ways and food, and dreadful diseases" had been accompanied by "right living," colonization disrupted Natives' ability to follow "the rules of right living," consequently altering their relationship to the forces to whom ceremonies and right living appealed.[108] The consequences of colonization were physical and spiritual, meaning that "suffering bodies and the suffering world become interchangeable; thus, to experience pain is to perceive a shift in the texture of the world wherein the proper balance between the seen and the felt or heard is upset."[109]

Occom's sermon provided a cure for diseased bodies and souls by restoring appropriate relationships between individuals and non-human beings. He recommended love as a cure for physical and spiritual illnesses, writing that "Love is every where Commend[ed] and Command[ed] [by] the Holy Scriptures, and it is Certainly Beutiful [*sic*] and agreable amongst Rational Creatures" (229). Occom's cure of love healed diseases such as syphilis and alcohol abuse by restoring relationships with divine forces and with one's fellow humans. This cure had to be performed in order for it to take effect; it was manifested in right living, and it was enacted in conversations, in interpersonal exchanges, and in actions. As Occom wrote: "is man, a Rational Man, unable to turn from this detestable, Filthy, Shameful, and Beastly Practice? or Can he desist, and become a Chaste Creature? I immagine [*sic*] to hear an Answere Universaly from all Rational Men, Saying, O! Yes O! Yes" (228).

Occom's statement might appear to be circular: he questioned whether men were rational and therefore capable of turning from moral illness, but he also expected to hear from all rational men that they could indeed repent. The action of "Saying, O! Yes" confirmed his audience members as rational by developing and displaying their rationality (228). Occom's sermon thus made the transformative power of rationality available to any one who would take action by saying "Yes."

Occom presented Native traditions of hospitality and kindness as a model for actions grounded in love. In another sermon, he critiqued people who claimed to be Christians yet treated their neighbors poorly, writing that they:

> dont Love God, and consequently they have Religion, they are no Christians, let their pretentions be what they will in Religion, —they are worse than the Heathen, Heathen in general manifest more Humanity, than such degenerate Christians. The Savage Indians, as these are so calld, are very kind to one another, and they are kind to strangers—But I find amongst these who are Calld Christians, Void of Natural affection, according to their Conduct in the world.[110]

Occom called for his audience to "truely Love their Neighbors,"[111] regardless of their nation or spiritual condition, and he pointed out that people known as "Savage Indians" exhibited more kindness and natural affection than those Europeans who called themselves Christian yet failed to behave as such.[112] He urged that his call for actions of love be extended to enslaved Africans in particular, for he wrote in the same sermon: "I think I have made out by the Bible, that the poor Negroes are your Neighbours, and if you can prove it from the Bible that Negroes are not the Race of Adam, then you may keep them as Slaves, Otherwise you have no more right to keep them as slaves as they have to keep you as Slaves."[113] In addition to arguing that Africans were of the same "Race" as European colonists and Native Americans, Occom defined the lack of neighborly behavior, particularly slaveholding, as antithetical to reason, writing that "Slavekeepers must keep Slaves against their own Light and understanding."[114] In this way, he defined colonists who held slaves as irrational, not because of the environment or deficient mental faculties, but because of their behavior toward and treatment of Africans.

Occom extended his revision of categories in which colonists placed Natives and Africans by replacing these categories with definitions of identity founded on right actions and on practices of establishing relationships with others. Just as being "kind to one another"[115] was part of Natives' "State Situation and Appearence," so their actions were full of kindness even before they had been civilized.[116] Indeed, Occom connected the refusal to love one's neighbor with colonization, dispossession, and slavery, saying that such a choice was the "Language of the Practice of all oppressors, over reachers, Defrauders, Extortioners with holders of Corn and other Necessaries that they have to Sell."[117] Natives' traditions for interacting with others, rather than "Religion," or hypocritical claims to belief and moral actions, formed the foundation for Occom's cure of love. In this context, "healthy" actions were not limited to people with bodies and minds defined as rational by certain innate qualities or environmental features; instead, health could be claimed by taking rational actions. Adopting a cure of love could restore individuals and the community to a state characterized by physical, interpersonal, and spiritual health, a state that many Natives, such as the Delaware physician, identified with the time before colonization or with a return to Native practices.[118] Occom's diagnoses of Natives' ills thus reconnected the body and soul, and they reestablished the soul and sin as potential causes of disease, notwithstanding colonists' attempts to attribute illness only to natural phenomena. This move certainly participated in conceptions of sin and grace as having physical manifestations shared by colonial ministers, but, as Occom's sermons show, it derived in large part from his critique of colonialism.[119] If they were sometimes manifested in Christianity, Natives' actions of love pre-existed their contact with colonists and with Christianity.

In addition to preaching about the importance of actions founded in love as a cure for diseases of the body and soul, Occom worked consistently to heal both ill bodies and the behavior that caused illness by urging his audience to healthy actions. In his journal for 1785, for example, he noted that he preached a sermon in which he argued that rational actions could counter sin. He wrote that he urged the "Stockbridge Indians" to "Use their Natural Powers and Conduct as becomes Rational Creatures, and to break off from all out breakings of Sin, and Especially to break off from that abominable Sin of Drunkenness and give themselves to watching and Prayer."[120] Rationality, as realized in conduct, would heal sins of drunkenness and enable people to replace alcohol with self-examination and prayer. In Occom's sermons, rationality was defined not by the climate or by innate characteristics shaping one's mind but by actions, performed with help from divine powers.

Like these rational actions, Occom's words had transformative effects, for they brought about the health to which he urged his audience. He explained in the sermon's conclusion that "what has been Said is quite Sufficient to Lead the minds of men, to Consider the Conduct of their fellow men, and also their own Conduct" (229). Occom's words, or "what has been Said," motivated men to better conduct and, by extension, to better health. Similarly, Occom noted in his journal that he "gave them [the Stockbridge Indians] a Word of Exhortation" in order to help them to become "Rational Creatures" and to turn away from drinking.[121] Such words did not simply reflect the situation or context of which Occom spoke: the diseased state of his audience's souls and of the relations between colonists and indigenous peoples. Instead, his words interpreted this situation and changed that situation by transforming his listeners' actions and souls. Occom's words performed the cure for intemperance by transforming his listeners' behavior, and his words simultaneously displayed Occom's own rationality.[122]

The performative nature of Occom's words further confirmed action and behavior, rather than climate or nation, as the basis of health—both moral and physical. Moreover, Occom prescribed the same cure for Natives and Europeans alike by calling the cure of love a "Universal Doctrine," not one possessed by either Natives or Europeans but known to both (229). Just as sins such as "Whoredome" and alcohol abuse were "Universal" practices, so rationality could likewise be possessed by those who acted in love, regardless of their nation or place of birth (227). By making actions of love the basis of rationality and health, Occom's sermon refuted arguments that innate characteristics determined the behavior of people indigenous to the Americas. He revised Euro-colonial conceptions of mental faculties as determined by birth and national traditions to make right action the foundation of rational intellectual faculties.

Occom himself drew on practices of love to effect social and spiritual change by ministering to bodies even as he cared for souls. In doing so, he took on the role that Native *powahs* and colonial ministers had both traditionally held: the responsibility to restore balance to relationships between people and the divine beings responsible for illness and to employ prayers in order to appease divine beings and bring about healing. His sermons reflect his understanding of medical and religious duties as interconnected: on the back page of a sermon on 2 Corinthians 5:17, Occom included a recipe for a mixture of roses and balsam to be taken morning and night.[123] In his best-known sermon, the execution sermon for Moses Paul, Occom directly addressed colonial ministers, or "reverend gentlemen," saying, "You are to declare the whole counsel of God, and to give a portion to every soul in due season; as a physician gives a portion to his patients, according to their diseases, so you are to give a portion to every soul in due season, according to their spiritual maladies."[124] The medical rhetoric with which Occom described ministers' responsibilities collapsed the distance that colonists had begun to posit between spiritual and medical realms and between ministers and physicians, for Occom suggested that both the soul and the body were the concern of spiritual leaders. Unlike colonial physicians such as Douglass and Grainger, who limited their investigations of disease and healing to natural causes, Occom acknowledged supernatural causes of disease, such as sin and judgment, and he included treatment aimed at addressing the natural and supernatural causes of illness. His writings and actions corresponded with conceptions of disease, long shared by Natives and colonists, as having both physical and spiritual dimensions.

Occom made concrete his comments regarding the connections between religious and medical duties in the course of his travels throughout New England. He was well acquainted with local herbs and their medicinal remedies, as indicated by his 1754 manuscript titled "Herbs and Roots." An herbal, Occom's manuscript lists about fifty herbs, the maladies they cured, and instructions for their preparation. In his journals, he records that he combined his medicinal and spiritual knowledge: he provided prayer and spiritual council for ill Natives, but he also bled invalids on several occasions.[125] For example, he wrote that one night in October 1787, he offered medical care to a woman who was "exceedingly distrest with uncommon Difficulties in her Pregnancy."[126] In the middle of the night, Occom "was Calld up, to the other House, and Bleed Mrs Dean and I went directly, and found her much distrest and took Blood from her foot, and Bleed exceeding Well,—and her distreses began to mitigate directly."[127] Occom's herbal indicates that he knew of remedies for women in labor, specifically, "an herb boild in 2 gallon of water and boil it about half away and then Cool it, and the[n] Put about 3 Quts of Pound it flax Sead good for to Ease Women that are in Traval."[128]

Occom accompanied such medical care with assistance for his patients' spiritual well-being. He frequently visited bedsides to examine the souls of invalids and to pray with them. As he related in a journal entry for July 16, 1787, he was called to attend a woman who "was taken very Strangely at once her Breath was most gone all of a Sudden."[129] He asked her: "What then is the matter with you, and She Said, with Tears, I want to Love god more, and

Serve him better; and I Said to her, if She really Desired and Askd for it She Shud have her desire granted, for it was a good Desire, & gave her Some further advice and Councel."[130] He addressed both the spiritual and physical manifestations of illness by ministering to patients' bodies and by inquiring after their souls. In this way, Occom mediated between patients and the non-human forces responsible for disease, and he fused the duties of a Native medical practitioner, who mediated between the community and metaphysical forces, and a "reverend Gentleman" or colonial minister, who had each traditionally considered body and soul his rightful province.[131]

Occom drew as well on Native conceptions of herbal knowledge as "partly pharmacological and partly psychological."[132] Even when a practitioner did not directly address the spiritual powers believed to give herbs their powers, she or he nonetheless maintained an awareness of the metaphysical forces at work. As Gladys Tantaquidgeon (Mohegan) has pointed out of Algonquian medicine: "where the action of the herbs, if not other substances, is mechanical or chemical, there is always the dependence upon the spiritual power of the healer with the deep emotional attributes from which the Delaware mind is never free when operating in these channels of thought."[133] Occom's herbal knowledge prepared him to provide medicinal cures to ill people he encountered on his travels, and his training by the Montaukett healer Ocus would also have made Occom aware of the spiritual power of which Native healers remained constantly cognizant.[134] Medical practitioners acted as instruments of healing power, for: "practitioners are the media through whom the Creator sends his healing power to alleviate distress caused by the physical and mental ills which attack the frail bodies of mankind."[135] In this context, Occom's religious training with Wheelock would have supported his pre-existing understanding of the medical and spiritual duties of religious practitioners and of healers as intermediaries between patients and divine entities. Occom's Christian education did not so much displace as build on his prior understanding of the relation between body and soul and of healers as divine agents. The long-standing correspondences between Native and colonial medical knowledges facilitated Occom's ability to integrate these two traditions into his practice, colonists' attempts to deny such parallels notwithstanding.

In his sermon on alcohol abuse and syphilis and, more broadly, in his medical writing and practices, Occom revised the categories of irrationality and promiscuity in which colonists placed Natives, and he foregrounded the ways in which colonization had introduced corrupt behaviors and physical maladies into Native history. In place of the "timeless present" in which colonists had fixed Natives' bodies, minds, and actions with classificatory forms, Occom constructed narratives of disease that charted the connections among indigenous experiences of colonization in the Atlantic and Pacific worlds.[136] We might think of Occom's medical writing as a statement of intellectual sovereignty, which, as Robert Warrior points out, is "not a struggle to be free from the influence of anything outside ourselves, but a process of asserting the power we possess as communities and individuals to make decisions that affect our lives."[137] Rather than cutting oneself off from the world, intellectual sovereignty involves a consideration of the "material circumstances of colonization that require of American Indians creativity and adaptability."[138] Occom exercised intellectual sovereignty as he engaged the very real consequences of colonialism for indigenous peoples, including his tribe and his family, and as he restored the connections between encounter and illness. Finally, he proposed a transformative cure that allowed Natives to adapt to the "material circumstances of colonization" while affirming their pre-existing knowledge and traditions.[139]

Occom included colonists' actions in this history, in this way presenting a point of view that acknowledged the medical consequences of encounter for both Natives and Europeans. He thus restored to medical writing the contexts of encounter and exchange in which it was composed, and he created what scholars have recently described as a global history, defined by the "complex weaving together of all coexisting histories."[140] Occom's account of medical exchanges acknowledged the multiple histories that emerged from colonial encounters in the Americas and in the Pacific by representing the "series of histories sharing space, relating to one another, often with causal consequences, but not assimilating one to another."[141] Quoting Hawkesworth's account of Cook's voyage, stating that Natives were ignorant of syphilis before colonization, and representing the process of intoxication, Occom presented the various histories of disease and encounter that "share[ed] space" in accounts of colonial exchange, and he showed how English explorers played key roles in the circulation of disease.[142]

Several scholars have argued that Atlantic world frameworks occlude Native Americans because their focus on "transatlantic commerce, seaborne migration, the circulation of commodities, capital flows, colonial settlement,

European geopolitics, the African slave trade, and the plantation complex" leaves little room for Native histories.[143] Occom's medical writing provides a view of the Atlantic world that acknowledges the histories of Native American, Tahitian, and European peoples, and this engagement with Atlantic and Pacific colonization shows that Natives themselves wrote the history of the Atlantic world in their own terms.[144] We might compare Occom with Tisquantum, whose transatlantic travels included time in England, Newfoundland, and possibly Spain (his exact route is unknown). In Tisquantum's history of the plague that virtually eradicated his community at Patuxet, he critiqued providential explanations for disease by representing the Plimouth colonists as playing an active role in circulating disease. In Occom's case, the results of a global perspective were not merely more stories of contact and exchange, or an expanded understanding of the Atlantic or Pacific worlds or of global or transatlantic networks. Rather, Occom's history of disease was transformative; it required new ways of acting and of interacting with others on the part of Natives and Euro-colonists alike.

Conclusion

Early American Studies and Deep Literary Histories

TEXTURE—THE NARRATIVE FRAGMENTATION and formal inconsistencies that signal colonists' transcriptions of Native and African knowledge and the influence of that knowledge on colonial writing—is a key feature of colonial American literatures. Furthermore, a focus on texture and the cross-cultural communications it signals presents an opportunity to reconceptualize early American literary study: its definition, its materials, and its methods. Following William Spengemann, scholars have pointed out that the colonial Americas lacked any uniquely national literature because colonists' language and nationality were defined by their Old World origins. Early American literatures were thus traditionally viewed as an inferior version of European writing that lagged behind its Old World counterparts.[1] However, Spengemann proposed a new definition by examining how writing about travels to and experiences in the New World altered European literary strategies by introducing new words and descriptions. Focusing on the British Americas, he redefined early American literature as all texts, written in English, that attempted to adapt Old World languages to account for the discovery of the New World, and he focused particularly on the linguistic repercussions of this discovery, which he called an "Americanization of English."[2] Literary historians of early America have expanded Spengemann's study by further decentering the nation as a container of culture and identity; they now regularly investigate colonial literatures in transatlantic and hemispheric contexts in order to trace the appropriations of European literary strategies—from poetry to natural history—with which colonists in the Americas verified, promoted, and defended their experiences and culture.[3]

Medical Encounters both expands and reorients these scholarly projects by investigating the material, performative, and inscriptive communications that circulated in cross-cultural contexts. These communications were made possible not only by epistemological commensurability but also by Natives', Africans', and colonists' corporeal commensurability: the belief that the New World would produce similar bodies and minds among the people who were born and lived in its environment. In the case of medical writing, fractured narratives point to the fact that Natives, Africans, and colonists alike were the objects of illness as well as the agents of healing and information. At the same time, colonial medical writing displays the strategies whereby colonists attempted to limit and eventually to deny the medical knowledge they shared with Natives and Africans in order to protect themselves from accusations that their bodies and minds had degenerated in the New World. Colonial literatures developed out of the actions, conversations, and writing that represented and processed encounters and exchanges of knowledge among colonists, Natives, and Africans. In this way, this book directs early American literary studies toward the cross-cultural origins of colonial writing even while contributing to efforts to expand what counts as literature in early America.[4]

From this perspective, what might seem anomalies or imperfections in colonial writing instead signals Natives' and Africans' contributions to the literary history of early America. Birgit Brander Rasmussen has argued that "fragmented form in [the colonial] archive is not a deficiency but a symptom of colonial violence."[5] I agree with Rasmussen that "fragmented form" in early American literatures is not a sign of their deficiency and with her efforts to expand early American literary studies to include non-alphabetic literatures by indigenous peoples. But I would also argue that narrative fragments and rhetorical inconsistencies do not signal colonial violence alone but also colonial uncertainty and the knowledge that circulated in cross-cultural encounters as Natives, Africans, and colonists attempted to explain unfamiliar phenomena. Violence was undoubtedly present in colonial encounters, in the form both of dispossession and enslavement and of colonists' rhetorical classification and subordination of Native and African knowledge. But this violence did not overwhelm or drown out Native and African communications and medical expertise, and it did not mean that colonists ignored Native and African knowledge. Indeed, Natives and Africans continued to circulate medical knowledge and to employ healing practices, sometimes including colonists in these exchanges and sometimes conducting them secretly. For their part, colonists continued to value and to represent Native and African knowledge in their medical writing.

Texture offers scholars an opening through which to consider the deep literary histories of early America, histories that do not simply include Native and African paradigms and communications but that take account of how colonial literatures were actively shaped by Natives' and Africans' perspectives and actions.[6] European epistemologies and literary strategies were far from dominant in early America, and colonial writing attests to the significance and relevance of Native and African forms of communication and knowledge for everyone involved in cross-cultural encounters. The rhetorical inconsistencies and fragmented narratives of colonial literatures thus require scholars to resist reading Native and African knowledge and communications back into colonial ideologies or generic conventions. Discourses of colonialism certainly influenced colonial encounters and colonists' representations of those encounters, but they were not the only interpretive resources available to colonists nor were they always the most compelling. Texture requires attention to the specific, materially located knowledge and practices that circulated in colonial encounters as well as to the shared and divergent histories of Natives, Africans, and colonists.

Analyzing deep literary histories of early America requires an interdisciplinary methodology that positions Native and African knowledge and communications as central and Natives and Africans as active participants in the construction of colonial writing. Many challenges confront scholars seeking to analyze Native and African knowledge and histories in colonial literatures, especially because many of the sources available were written by colonists and because they contain biases that privilege colonial perspectives. But as *Medical Encounters* shows, incorporating resources from multiple disciplines can illuminate the knowledge that circulated in colonial encounters, the strategies with which it was communicated, and various people's responses to that knowledge. This interdisciplinary research illuminates the moments when early American literatures did not foreground colonial frameworks but incorporated and relied on Native and African ways of thinking and interacting. This move does not include the claim, sometimes made by colonists, that one can fully understand or recover Native and African knowledge or that a transparent translation of Native and African words and actions is possible. Instead, the absence of perfect knowledge should not deter scholars from considering how Native and African knowledge shaped colonial writing and how Natives and Africans participated not only in colonial history but also in colonial literary history, while simultaneously maintaining their own beliefs and practices and adapting new knowledge to advance their goals. Early American literatures are not only able to illuminate colonial strategies of representing the New World and its peoples; they also provide insight into the perspectives and communicative strategies of the various people who contributed to colonial writing.

Finally, then, conceptualizing early American literatures as composed of deep literary histories revises the terms with which early American literary history is defined and differentiated from other disciplines. As a number of literary scholars have pointed out, one key disciplinary difference between histories and literary studies of early America is the "status of literature as evidence," that is, whether scholars read texts as documentary sources or whether they examine how form and genre shape how colonists represented their experiences.[7] *Medical Encounters* alters the terms of this debate by showing that Natives and Africans were not only objects of description in colonial writing but also co-producers of those texts. They circulated medical knowledge that motivated colonists to depart from conventional literary strategies and to adopt alternate methods of communicating medical knowledge from colonial encounters; they also engaged colonial literatures to create their own histories of encounter. Deep literary histories should expand scholars' focus from what information early American literatures can reflect about Natives and Africans to include the ways in which Natives and Africans influenced the performative, oral, manuscript, and printed forms of writing that constitute early American literatures. As such, deep literary histories require a methodology that draws on multiple disciplinary approaches and insights; they necessarily bridge the "trade gap" between history and literature by utilizing literary and historicist—as well as anthropological and ethnohistorical—methods and evidence in order to uncover Natives' and Africans' specific knowledge and practices and how they acted on colonial literatures.[8]

The Imagination and Cross-Cultural Encounters

Near the end of the eighteenth century, the political and epistemological conditions that had allowed medical knowledge to act as a shared form of communication underwent significant changes. Euro-American physicians and lay people expanded eighteenth-century skepticism about the non-human or supernatural causes of disease by repudiating the connections between bodies and souls and between material and immaterial realms that had made the medical knowledge of Natives, Africans, and colonists (and later, U.S. Americans) commensurable. Illness was separated from sin and from the soul, and it was defined as an entity in nature that was could be studied on patients' bodies and that was most fully manifested in death.[9] Physicians diagnosed disease by correlating the visible signs of illness with internal natural causes, a process founded on the idea that bodies were orderly mechanical entities governed by natural laws.[10] Thus, physicians privileged a professional, penetrating gaze, rather than the ability to identify or influence the non-human or supernatural causes of disease, and they examined not the spiritual causes of illness but the inner states and conditions that they posited as its source. Moreover, the responsibility for diagnosing and curing illness was increasingly claimed as unique to professional physicians, rather than ministers, plantation owners, and lay people, while medical societies and schools offered distinct elite spaces in which physicians could learn and discuss medical knowledge.[11] Finally, the confined space of the hospital replaced the home, the slave hut, and the *wetu* as the ideal site of medical investigation, a space where illness could be supervised and controlled and where practitioners could develop theories of disease causation and prevention.[12]

At the same time that the body became the center of medical investigations and the primary site of disease, new understandings of the mental faculty of the imagination began to emerge. As previous chapters have shown, the imagination was known as a paradoxically productive and dangerous faculty: it could inspire poetry but could also delude the mind with irrational ideas, wild dreams, and superstitious beliefs. By the 1780s, the imagination began to assume more positive meanings as the creative faculty that inspired writers. As James Engell has argued, in its new manifestation the imagination governed "the interrelated activities of perception, experience, aesthetic appreciation, and the crown of all, artistic creativity. The imagination was also viewed as a cosmic power, responsible for bringing forth and organizing the unity of all creation and for implanting the divine in man."[13] For Euro-Americans, using one's imagination to create representations of the Americas could now figure as a positive, desirable action of creativity and inspiration rather than as a potential sign of degenerated mental faculties.

Medicine and literature subsequently developed along separate trajectories: imaginative writings were separated from medical literatures, as professional physicians assumed responsibility for medical writing and professional authors the responsibility for literatures inspired by the imagination, from novels to poems. As scholars have argued, this reconfiguration of the long-standing connections between medicine and writing was less the result of a new regard for reason or empiricism than a "purification" and separation of previously overlapping spheres that came about by making nature, particularly illness, an inert object of study, separate from humans.[14] Euro-Americans posited nature and culture as two separate entities, and their insistence upon this split provided the foundation for articulating the relationship between the west, or modern society, and other, allegedly premodern, cultures, which were accused of holding inaccurate conceptions of nature. As Bruno Latour has argued, the double divide between nature and culture and between "us" and "them" defined the "particular way Westerners had of establishing their relations with others as long as they felt modern."[15]

Euro-Americans also began to revise older characterizations of Natives and Africans as possessing strong faculties of the imagination due to their location in hot climates. Physicians such as Juan Huarte had argued in the sixteenth century that people whose wits were shaped by hot climates had strong faculties of the imagination and consequently could write poetry and song but were also superstitious. Travelers to the Americas such as Thomas Harriot and Edward Winslow applied theories connecting southern climates and the imagination to speculate that Natives possessed strong faculties of the imagination that opened their minds to communications from the devil. In the eighteenth century, physicians such as William Douglass and James Grainger developed the connections between hot climates and superstition by arguing that New World Africans possessed strong imaginations that misled them by inclining them to accept irrational knowledge or to attribute mysterious phenomena to supernatural causes. By the end of the eighteenth and early nineteenth centuries, colonists began to posit that the mental faculties belonging to different peoples differed in kind rather than in degree. They claimed the positive traits of imagination for themselves and argued that Natives and Africans did not possess the same capacity for creativity, sensation, and thought that Euro-Americans did. And, rather than attributing different mental faculties to differences in climate, Euro-Americans began to make these contrasting mental traits the origins of superiority and inferiority. They connected mental and physical attributes to external appearance or features, in this way making internal characteristics the cause of appearance rather than the effect of climate.[16] U.S. Americans consequently participated in efforts throughout the Atlantic World to "establish rigid differences between whites and others that biological racism will supplement and nineteenth-century colonial imperialism will capitalize on."[17]

Euro-Americans accordingly began to deny that Natives and Africans possessed any useful medical knowledge. In striking contrast to colonists from Harriot to Grainger, Benjamin Rush commented in 1774: "We have no discoveries in the materia medica to hope for from the Indians in North-America."[18] Edward Long drew similar conclusions regarding Africans in the Caribbean, writing that the "Negroes generally apply them [medicines] at random, without any regard to the particular symptoms of the disease; concerning which, or the operation of their *materia medica,* they have formed no theory."[19] Native and African knowledge was increasingly identified only with witchcraft, while colonial and U.S. American medical knowledge was opposed to such illegitimate knowledge and defined as founded on reason and empirical investigation.

Such denials that Natives and Africans possessed useful medical knowledge and the faculties necessary to apply medicines effectively were part of the larger practice of positing discrete differences among the mental faculties of U.S. Americans, Africans, and Natives. Furthermore, conceptions of Natives' and Africans' irrationality, savagery, and lack of civilization developed alongside, but not always parallel to, the continuation and intensification of plantation slavery as well as policies of Native removal and dispossession.[20] For example, colonists argued that Africans' mental faculties did not process stimuli in the same way that Anglo-Americans' minds did. The planter David Collins stated in 1803 that the African did "not sublime misery in the laboratory of the imagination. His powers are corporeal only."[21] Meanwhile, writers such as Thomas Jefferson argued that access to learning did not significantly affect Africans' minds. Jefferson's infamous statement that "Religion has produced a Phillis Whatley [*sic*] but it could not produce a poet" suggests that despite Wheatley's education, conversion to Christianity, and the fact that she had been taken from Africa to Boston, her mind still lacked mental faculties of the imagination that would inspire her to write poetry.[22] Like the enslaved Africans in Jamaica who did not process their suffering in the "laboratory of the imagination" but experienced it as physical sensations only, Wheatley had a mind limited to irrational and inferior sensations and thoughts, notwithstanding the education and climate she shared with Euro-Americans. As U.S. Americans began to define mental abilities as natural and unchanging, they solidified earlier suggestions that Africans could not alter or improve their inferior mental faculties even when transported to or born in the Americas.[23]

Meanwhile, Native Americans were defined as a "barbarous people" whose heathen religious practices made them amazingly strong and noble even while they obstructed their capacity for civilization.[24] As Jefferson explained, Native warriors' ability to withstand pain exemplified a "firmness unknown almost to religious enthusiasm with us."[25] At the same time that their strength and nobility were celebrated, Natives were described in political speeches, in legislation, and in novels as vanishing from the United States in the wake of American expansion—seen as bringing civilization to the rest of the continent.[26] Schools and missions took up the project of civilizing Native children; they required the pupils' transformation, assimilation, and passive acceptance of their inferior status.[27] Although these projects rested on the assumption that Native minds could be trained to repudiate their heathen, superstitious beliefs, Anglo-Americans also denied that Natives could completely erase the savagery that allegedly defined them. For example, Native ministers faced skepticism about the legitimacy of their religious convictions and abilities. How, colonists asked, could divinely inspired words come out of the mouths of men who looked Native—and who were thus associated with barbarism and savagery? Samson Occom faced scrutiny before he traveled to Britain on his fundraising trip for Eleazar Wheelock over the question of whether he could embody Christian and Native identities at the same time.[28] Meanwhile, Methodist minister William Apess (Pequot) discovered that crowds of people flocked to see him preach, only to pelt him with vegetables and ridicule him. As Robert Warrior has stated, the "last thing people in the northeast probably imagined when they pictured Indians was an articulate Methodist minister writing books."[29] Thus, Natives were figured both as capable of change—and as needing to change completely their traditional practices and ways of living if they were to survive—and as incapable of being anything but savage.

Many Natives and Africans, however, critiqued Euro-Americans' assessment of their medical knowledge as diabolic and their imaginations as producing irrational, inferior ideas. For example, Phillis Wheatley directly addressed the question of Africans' mental faculties of the imagination and their capacities by connecting heat, blackness, and poetry. As Katy L. Chiles has pointed out, Wheatley explicitly associated the imagination with the sun by referencing Aurora, the mythological goddess of the dawn, in her poem "On Imagination."[30] In this way, Wheatley drew on earlier conceptions of hot climates as producing strong faculties of the imagination and, consequently, songs and poetry. She described the imagination as a capacious faculty that creates new knowledge by associating separate ideas or sensations:

> From star to star the mental optics rove,
> Measure the skies, and range the realms above.
> There in one view we grasp the mighty whole,
> Or with new worlds amaze th' unbounded soul.[31]

For Wheatley, the imagination was a faculty—or "force"[32]—capable of collecting wide-ranging images and ideas in order to create "new worlds." Far from being foreign to Africans, the imagination was associated with hot places, and, as Wheatley's own poetry attested, it inspired creativity and song from people who were also associated with hot climates.

Meanwhile, William Apess, a Methodist minister of white, African American, and Pequot ancestry, critiqued the discrete boundaries that Anglo-Americans erected to divide their minds and knowledge from those of Natives and Africans. Apess concluded his "Eulogy on King Philip" by reciting the Lord's Prayer in Algonquian. In a speech praising the leader of a war in which a pan-Indian alliance opposed the New England colonies and that fueled anti-Indian sentiments among colonists, Apess insisted on the shared histories and belief systems that had characterized cross-cultural encounters, even while challenging his audience's understanding of those belief systems. He pointed out that Native Americans had already possessed the "Christian" virtues of hospitality and kindness before Europeans arrived in the Americas; in this way, he not only claimed commensurability between Native and Christian religious practices but asked his audience to reconceptualize Christianity. Rather than following a westward trajectory from Europe to the Americas, Christianity and civilization existed in the

Americas before Europeans' arrival, as displayed by Natives' kind actions and "virtues."[33] Apess reminded his audience that the Wampanoags had offered such kindness to the Pilgrims during their first difficult winter, stating that "In their sickness, too, the Indians were as tender to them as to their own children; and for all this, they were denounced as savages by those who had received all the acts of kindness they possibly could show them."[34] Natives' state as "savages" was a repercussion of colonization, not a pre-existing, inherent condition.

In the speech, Apess insisted on the commensurability not only of religion and medicine—for example, the Natives' natural virtues manifested in the medical care they provided for New England colonists—but also of Native and Euro-American belief systems, as attested to in his Algonquian-language version of the Lord's Prayer. Against Euro-Americans' claims that Native and African medicine was of no interest and against biological theories of race, Apess's "Eulogy" offers an alternate history, one that acknowledged the long tradition of shared medical knowledge and of employing medical knowledge as a form of communication in cross-cultural encounters. Apess's and Wheatley's actions and writings model the deep histories of early American encounters and writing that illuminate instances of shared knowledge and of cross-cultural communications.

NOTES

Introduction

1. Samson Occom, "Account of the Montauk Indians, on Long Island (1761)," in *The Collected Writings of Samson Occom, Mohegan: Leadership and Literature in Eighteenth-Century America,* ed. Joanna Brooks (Oxford: Oxford University Press, 2006), 49.
2. Ibid.
3. Ibid.
4. On Native American religious and medical knowledge and its similarities to colonial knowledge, see Dane Morrison, *A Praying People: Massachusett Acculturation and the Failure of the Puritan Mission, 1600–1690* (New York: Peter Lang, 1995); Kathleen J. Bragdon, *Native People of Southern New England, 1500–1650* (Norman: University of Oklahoma Press, 1996), 224; Karen Ordahl Kupperman, *Indians and English: Facing Off in Early America* (Ithaca: Cornell University Press, 2000); and Paula Gunn Allen, *Pocahontas: Medicine Woman, Spy, Entrepreneur, Diplomat* (New York: HarperCollins, 2006), 30. For the same subject in an African context, see James H. Sweet, *Domingos Álvares, African Healing, and the Intellectual History of the Atlantic World* (Chapel Hill: University of North Carolina Press, 2011); John Thornton, *Africa and Africans in the Making of the Atlantic World, 1400–1800,* 2nd ed. (Cambridge: Cambridge University Press, 1998); Yvonne P. Chireau, *Black Magic: Religion and the African American Conjuring Tradition* (Berkeley: University of California Press, 2003); and Dianne M. Stewart, *Three Eyes for the Journey: African Dimensions of the Jamaican Religious Experience* (Oxford: Oxford University Press, 2005), esp. xv.
5. On the classical connections between medicine and poetry, see Raymond A. Anselment, *The Realms of Apollo: Literature and Healing in Seventeenth-Century England* (Newark: University of Delaware Press, 1995), esp. introduction and chap. 1.
6. See Ernest B. Gilman, *Plague Writing in Early Modern England* (Chicago: University of Chicago Press, 2009).
7. David D. Hall makes a similar point regarding religion when he writes, "The people of seventeenth-century New England lived in an enchanted universe." Colonists believed they lived in a world of wonders, in which supernatural forces were responsible for events and in which ritual, prayer, and dreams could provide insight into the meaning of

unusual phenomenon. See Hall, *Worlds of Wonder, Days of Judgment: Popular Religious Belief in Early New England* (Cambridge: Harvard University Press, 1990), 71 and chap. 2.

8. See Patricia A. Watson, *The Angelical Conjunction: The Preacher-Physicians of Colonial New England* (Knoxville: University of Tennessee Press, 1991).
9. See James Grainger, *The Sugar-Cane* (London, 1764); Alexander Hamilton, "Itinerarium," in *Colonial American Travel Narratives*, ed. Wendy Martin (New York: Penguin, 1994), 173–327; Hamilton, *The History of the Ancient and Honorable Tuesday Club* (Chapel Hill: University of North Carolina Press, 2011); and James Kirkpatrick, *The Sea-Piece; A Narrative, Philosophical and Descriptive Poem. In Five Cantos* (London, 1750).
10. See, for example, David S. Shields, *Oracles of Empire: Poetry, Politics, and Commerce in British America, 1690–1750* (Chicago: University of Chicago Press, 1990); William Spengemann, *A New World of Words: Redefining Early American Literature* (New Haven: Yale University Press, 1994); Ralph Bauer, *The Cultural Geography of Colonial American Literatures: Empire, Travel, Modernity* (Cambridge: Cambridge University Press, 2003); Susan Scott Parrish, *American Curiosity: Cultures of Natural History in the Colonial British Atlantic World* (Chapel Hill: University of North Carolina Press, 2006); and Christopher P. Iannini, *Fatal Revolutions: Natural History, West Indian Slavery, and the Routes of American Literature* (Chapel Hill: University of North Carolina Press, 2012).
11. Alfred Crosby, *The Columbian Exchange: Biological and Cultural Consequences of 1492* (Westport, CT: Greenwood Press, 1972), esp. chaps. 2 and 4. The question of where syphilis originated has been a matter of debate since the fifteenth century. For just a few references on this matter, see Brenda J. Baker and George J. Armelagos, "The Origin and Antiquity of Syphilis: Paleopatholgical Diagnoses and Interpretation," in vol. 26 of *Biological Consequences of the European Expansion, 1450–1800*, ed. Kenneth F. Kiple and Stephen V. Beck (Variorum: Ashgate, 1997), 1–35; and Amy G. Carmichael, "Syphilis and the Columbian Exchange: Was the New Disease Really New?," in *The Great Maritime Discoveries and World Health*, ed. Mario Gomes Marques and John Clue (Lisbon: Escola Nacional de Saude Publica Ordem Dos Medicos Instituto De Sintra, 1991), 187–200.
12. Joyce E. Chaplin, *Subject Matter: Technology, the Body, and Science on the Anglo-American Frontier, 1500–1676* (Cambridge: Harvard University Press, 2003), 160.
13. Ibid., 27.
14. Ibid., 28.
15. Cristobal Silva, *Miraculous Plagues: An Epidemiology of Early New England Narrative* (Oxford: Oxford University Press, 2011), 11.
16. Ibid., 32.
17. Ibid., 18.
18. Ibid., 59.
19. Ibid., 57.
20. Colin G. Calloway, *New Worlds for All: Indians, Europeans, and the Remaking of Early America* (Baltimore: Johns Hopkins University Press, 1998), 41.
21. The most influential of such studies include Peter Hulme, *Colonial Encounters: Europe and the Native Caribbean, 1492–1797* (London: Methuen, 1986); Stephen Greenblatt, *Marvelous Possessions: The Wonder of the New World* (Chicago: University of Chicago Press, 1991); Anthony Pagden, *European Encounters with the New World* (New Haven:

Yale University Press, 1993); and Eric Cheyfitz, *The Poetics of Imperialism: Translation and Colonization from The Tempest to Tarzan*, 2nd ed. (Philadelphia: University of Pennsylvania Press, 1997). One important exception to these studies, which I discuss in more detail below, is Mary Louise Pratt, *Imperial Eyes: Travel Writing and Transculturation* (London: Routledge, 1992).

22. The reaction against straightforward readings of colonial texts was indebted both to postcolonial critiques of anthropology and to the Foucauldian turn to examine the inextricable relation between knowledge (especially of the "other") and power. Peter Mason draws on both critiques in his *Deconstructing America: Representations of the Other* (London: Routledge, 1990). For just a few examples of postcolonial critiques of anthropology, see Talal Asad, ed., *Anthropology and the Colonial Encounter* (London: Ithaca Press, 1973); George Marcus and Michael Fischer, *Anthropology as Cultural Critique: An Experimental Moment in the Human Sciences* (Chicago: University of Chicago Press, 1986); and James Clifford and George Marcus, eds., *Writing Culture: The Poetics and Politics of Ethnography* (Berkeley: University of California Press, 1986). See also Michel Foucault, *The Archaeology of Knowledge and the Discourse on Language*, trans. A. M. Sheridan Smith (New York: Pantheon Books, 1972).
23. Ed White, "Invisible Tagkanysough," *PMLA* 120, no. 3 (2005), 756. For one statement of the relation between postcolonial studies of the early Americas and decolonization, see Hulme's discussion of his "radical history" and critique of colonialism in *Colonial Encounters*, 8–10 (quote on page 8).
24. Greenblatt, *Marvelous Possessions*, 56. See also Pagden, *European Encounters*, chaps. 1 and 2, and Cheyfitz, *Poetics of Imperialism*, esp. chap. 2.
25. Pagden, *European Encounters*, 21. See also 21–27; 34–36.
26. Hulme, *Colonial Encounters*, 2. For critiques of new historicist and postcolonial studies of encounter, see Myra Jehlen, "History Before the Fact; or, Captain John Smith's Unfinished Symphony," *Critical Inquiry* 19 (1993): 677–92; Daniel Carey, "Questioning Incommensurability in Early Modern Cultural Exchange," *Common Knowledge* 6 (1997): 32–50; Neil L. Whitehead, "The *Discoverie* as enchanted text" and "The *Discoverie* as ethnological text" in *The Discoverie of the Large, Rich and Bewtiful Empyre of Guiana*, ed. Whitehead (Manchester: Manchester University Press, 1997), 1–116; and White, "Invisible Tagkanysough." See also Peter Hulme, "Critical Response: Making No Bones: A Response to Myra Jehlen," *Critical Inquiry* 20 (1993): 179–86; Myra Jehlen, "Critical Response II. Response to Peter Hulme," *Critical Inquiry* 20 (1993): 187–91.
27. White, "Invisible Tagkanysough," 764.
28. Greenblatt, *Marvelous Possessions*, 12–13.
29. See ibid., 7; Chaplin, *Subject Matter*, 26–27; Silva, *Miraculous Plagues*, 18, and afterword.
30. Nancy G. Siraisi, *The Clock and the Mirror: Girolamo Cardano and Renaissance Medicine* (Princeton: Princeton University Press, 1997), 196.
31. Ibid., 195. See also Andrew Wear, *Knowledge and Practice in English Medicine, 1550–1680* (Cambridge: Cambridge University Press, 2000), 133. There are many studies of narrative and medicine; for just a few, see Cheryl Mattingly and Linda C. Garro, eds., *Narrative and the Cultural Construction of Illness and Healing* (Berkeley: University of California Press, 2000), and Kathryn Montgomery Hunter, *Doctors' Stories: The Narrative Structure of Medical Knowledge* (Princeton: Princeton University Press,

1991). On narrative and medicine in a history of medicine context, see David Harley, "Rhetoric and the Social Construction of Sickness and Healing," *Social History of Medicine* 12, no. 3 (1999), esp. 420–24.

32. Wear, *Knowledge and Practice,* 135.
33. See Gianna Pomata and Nancy G. Siraisi, "Introduction," in *Historia: Empiricism and Erudition in Early Modern Europe,* ed. Pomata and Siraisi (Cambridge: MIT Press, 2005), 13.
34. Siraisi, *The Clock and the Mirror* 200. For examples of early modern *historia,* see Nicolás Monardes, *Joyfull Newes Out of the Newe Founde Worlde,* trans. John Frampton (London, 1577), fol. 39; Hans Sloane, vol. 1 of *A Voyage To the Islands Madera, Barbados, Nieves, S. Christophers and Jamaica, With the Natural History of the Herbs and Trees, Four-footed Beasts, Fishes, Birds, Insects, Reptiles, &c. of the Last of Those Islands . . . In Two Volumes* (London, 1707), esp. the introduction; and Thomas Sydenham, *The Compleat Method of Curing Almost All Diseases . . . Written in* Latin, *by Dr.* Thomas Sydenham, *and now faithfully Englished* (London, 1694), esp. 14–15, 17–18. On Monardes's use of *historia,* see Daniela Bleichmar, "Books, Bodies, and Fields: Sixteenth-Century Transatlantic Encounters with New World Materia Medica," in *Colonial Botany: Science, Commerce, and Politics in the Early Modern World,* ed. Londa Shiebinger and Claudia Swan (Philadelphia: University of Pennsylvania Press, 2005), 83–99.
35. On the widespread use of *historia,* see Nancy G. Siraisi, "Girolamo Cardano and the Art of Medical Narrative," *Journal of the History of Ideas* 52, no. 4 (1991): 581–602.
36. Susan P. Mattern, *Galen and the Rhetoric of Healing* (Baltimore: Johns Hopkins University Press, 2008), 68. On the multiple uses for *historia* in medieval and early modern medical practice, see Pomata and Siraisi, *Historia: Empiricism and Erudition,* esp. the introduction and chap. 3.
37. Whitehead, "*Discoverie* as enchanted text," 35.
38. Ibid., 36.
39. Ibid., 34.
40. Jehlen, "History Before the Fact," 692. Jehlen's analysis concludes with the insight that textual ruptures are signs of "underdetermined" narratives; however, she does not consider Natives' specific interpretations of colonists. Ed White applies Jehlen's conclusion to a different context by considering Roanoke Algonquian responses to British colonists. See White, "Invisible Tagkanysough."
41. Hulme, *Colonial Encounters,* 12.
42. Greenblatt, *Marvelous Possessions,* 19.
43. Hulme, *Colonial Encounters,* 12. Hulme examines how oriental and Herodotean discourses produced European conceptions of the Caribbean and of cannibals, and Greenblatt examines how colonists drew on classical and European discourses of wonder.
44. Greenblatt, *Marvelous Possessions,* 7.
45. Ibid. The choice is not between reading colonial literatures as transparent accounts of Natives or a focus only on European representations. Colonial texts are certainly imperfect accounts of encounter, but they may still offer some insight into those encounters and the multiple responses to them. For example, Gordon M. Sayre has called for a "more holistic approach" to colonial travel and ethnographic writing, in order to avoid what he describes as a "hermeneutic dilemma," in which scholars must

decide between a skeptical approach to colonial literatures that emphasizes absolute differences between the cultures that met in the New World and a focus on European stereotypes and their transfer to the Americas. Sayre draws on a "rhetorical and historicist" methodology that utilizes ethnohistorical methods of comparing sources against one another to locate a probable account of events while also taking into account the "shape" of colonists' texts. Sayre focuses on what scholars can learn about Natives from colonial texts; *Medical Encounters* extends his insights to examine the ways in which Native and African knowledge actively shaped the structure and content of colonial literatures. See Gordon M. Sayre, *Les Sauvages Américains: Representations of Native Americans in French and English Colonial Literature* (Chapel Hill: University of North Carolina Press, 1997), 28–29.

46. Nicholas Thomas, *Entangled Objects: Exchange, Material Culture, and Colonialism in the Pacific* (Cambridge: Harvard University Press, 1991).
47. Whitehead, "*Discoverie* as enchanted text," 38.
48. See Sandra M. Gustafson, *Eloquence Is Power: Oratory and Performance in Early America* (Chapel Hill: University of North Carolina Press, 2000); Hilary E. Wyss, *Writing Indians: Literacy, Christianity, and Native Community in Early America* (Amherst: University of Massachusetts Press, 2000); Kristina Bross, *Dry Bones and Indian Sermons: Praying Indians in Colonial America* (Ithaca: Cornell University Press, 2004); Gustafson, "American Literature and the Public Sphere," *American Literary History* 20, no. 3 (2008): 465–78; Lisa Brooks, *The Common Pot: The Recovery of Native Space in the Northeast* (Minneapolis: University of Minnesota Press, 2008); Matt Cohen, *The Networked Wilderness: Communicating in Early New England* (Minneapolis: University of Minnesota Press, 2010); Joshua David Bellin and Laura L. Mielke, eds., *Native Acts: Indian Performance, 1603–1832* (Lincoln: University of Nebraska Press, 2011); Birgit Brander Rasmussen, *Queequeg's Coffin: Indigenous Literacies and Early American Literature* (Durham: Duke University Press, 2012); and Hilary E. Wyss, *English Letters and Indian Literacies: Reading, Writing, and New England Missionary Schools, 1750–1830* (Philadelphia: University of Pennsylvania Press, 2012).
49. See Gustafson, *Eloquence Is Power,* esp. the introduction. See also Lisa Brooks, *Common Pot,* introduction and chap. 1.
50. Cohen, *Networked Wilderness,* 2.
51. See Chaplin, *Subject Matter,* 24, where she states that scholars cannot know how Natives responded to colonization because "we lack Indian texts for the earlier period," by which she seems to mean only written or printed texts.
52. See William A. Starna, "The Biological Encounter: Disease and the Ideological Domain," *American Indian Quarterly* 16, no. 4 (1992): 511–19.
53. See Calloway, *New Worlds,* 41, and Joanna Brooks, *American Lazarus: Religion and the Rise of African-American and Native American Literatures* (Oxford: Oxford University Press, 2003), 56.
54. See Sweet, *Domingos Álvares;* Thornton, *Africa and Africans;* Chireau, *Black Magic;* and Sharla M. Fett, *Working Cures: Healing, Health, and Power on Southern Slave Plantations* (Chapel Hill: University of North Carolina Press, 2002).
55. Joshua David Bellin, *The Demon of the Continent: Indians and the Shaping of American Literature* (Philadelphia: University of Pennsylvania Press, 2001), 5.
56. Ibid., 3.
57. Pratt, *Imperial Eyes,* 7. As Rolena Adorno points out, she first used the term "contact

zone" or "zona de contacto" in her study of Guaman Poma. Adorno defines the contact zone as a "colonial society in which the simple line between Spaniard and Andean that defined native experience at the moment of conquest no longer existed with such clarity." See Adorno, *The Polemics of Possession in Spanish American Narrative* (New Haven: Yale University Press, 2007), 23.

58. Pratt, *Imperial Eyes,* 90.
59. Ibid., 136.
60. Ibid. For one study that productively adopts some of Pratt's terms to consider Native American writing, see Wyss, *Writing Indians.*
61. Pallabi Chakravorty, "From Interculturalism to Historicism: Reflections on Classical Indian Dance," *Dance Research Journal* 32, no. 2 (2000–2001): 109.
62. Julie Stone Peters, "Intercultural Performance, Theatre Anthropology, and the Imperialist Critique: Identities, Inheritances, and Neo-Orthodoxies," in *Imperialism and Theatre: Essays on World Theatre, Drama and Performance,* ed. J. Ellen Gainor (Routledge: London, 1995), 206. The improvisation necessary to apply pre-existing knowledge in new situations is a characteristic of performance as Joseph Roach discusses it in *Cities of the Dead.* Roach focuses on the ways in which cultures are reproduced through surrogation: the process of replacing absences created by death or departure. Although I do not focus extensively on surrogation, I find that as colonists, Natives, and Africans attempted to meet challenging experiences and phenomena, their epistemological and rhetorical practices were altered in the process. See Joseph Roach, *Cities of the Dead: Circum-Atlantic Performance* (New York: Columbia University Press, 1996), esp. chap. 1.
63. For a study of how Natives, Africans, and colonists alike attempted to regain pre-contact stability in colonial Mexico, see Serge Gruzinski, *The Mestizo Mind: The Intellectual Dynamics of Colonization and Globalization,* trans. Deke Dusinberre (New York: Routledge, 2002), esp. 17–63.
64. Carey, "Questioning Incommensurability," 49. He argues that travelers' concerns that they would become like the people with whom they interacted—that is, travelers' fears of *commensurability*—played a key role in early modern travel literature. See ibid., esp. 40–49.
65. See Antonello Gerbi, *The Dispute of the New World: The History of a Polemic, 1750–1900,* trans. Jeremy Moyle (Pittsburgh: University of Pittsburgh Press, 1973). For studies of race as a response to accusations of colonial degeneration, see Jorge Cañizares-Esguerra, "New World, New Stars: Patriotic Astrology and the Invention of Indian and Creole Bodies in Colonial Spanish America, 1600–1650," *American Historical Review* 104, no. 1 (1999): 33–68; and Cañizares-Esguerra, *How to Write the History of the New World: Histories, Epistemologies, and Identities in the Eighteenth-Century Atlantic World* (Stanford: Stanford University Press, 2001); Ralph Bauer, "The Hemispheric Genealogies of 'Race': Creolization and the Cultural Geography of Colonial Difference across the Eighteenth-Century Americas," in *Hemispheric American Studies,* ed. Robert Levine and Caroline Levander (New Brunswick: Rutgers University Press, 2007), 36–56; and Ralph Bauer and José Antonio Mazzotti, "Introduction," in *Creole Subjects in the Colonial Americas: Empires, Texts, Identities,* ed. Bauer and Mazzotti (Chapel Hill: University of North Carolina Press, 2009), 1–51.
66. For studies of race as responses to Africans' unusual appearance and culture, see Winthrop D. Jordan, *White Over Black: American Attitudes toward the Negro, 1550–1812,*

2nd ed. (Chapel Hill: University of North Carolina Press, 2012). For studies that have reconsidered "race" as a strategy designed to privilege Englishness and whiteness, see Kim F. Hall, *Things of Darkness: Economies of Race and Gender in Early Modern England* (Ithaca: Cornell University Press, 1995) and Mary Floyd-Wilson, *English Ethnicity and Race in Early Modern Drama* (Cambridge: Cambridge University Press, 2003).

67. On multiple markers of difference, see Roxann Wheeler, *The Complexion of Race: Categories of Difference in Eighteenth-Century British Culture* (Philadelphia: University of Pennsylvania Press, 2000).

68. On environmental theories of physical and cultural degeneration in the British context, see Karen Ordahl Kupperman, "Fear of Hot Climates in the Anglo-American Colonial Experience," *William and Mary Quarterly* 3d. ser., 41, no. 2 (1984): 213–40; Kupperman, "The Puzzle of the American Climate in the Early Colonial Period," *American Historical Review* 87, no. 5 (1982): 1262–89; Joyce E. Chaplin, "Natural Philosophy and an Early Racial Idiom in North America: Comparing English and Indian Bodies," *William and Mary Quarterly* 3d. ser., 54, no. 1 (1997): 229–52; James Egan, *Authorizing Experience: Refigurations of the Body Politic in Seventeenth-Century New England Writing* (Princeton: Princeton University Press, 1999), esp. chap. 1; and Floyd-Wilson, *English Ethnicity.* On these theories in Iberian contexts, see Cañizares-Esguerra, "New World," and, for a comparative perspective, Bauer, "Hemispheric Genealogies"; and the essays in Bauer and Mazotti, eds., *Creole Subjects.*

69. See Wear, *Knowledge and Practice,* 34.

70. Egan, *Authorizing Experience,* 17.

71. Baptist Goodall, *The Tryall of Travell* (London, 1630), E1r.

72. Sir Kenelm Digby, *Two Treatises: in the One of Which, the Nature of Bodies, in the Other, the Nature of Mans Soule is Looked Into, in Way of Discovery of the Immortality of Reasonable Soules* (London, 1665), 304–5.

73. For one description of the mental faculties and their various roles, see Pierre Charron, *Of Wisdom: Three Books written in French by Peter Charro[n] Doctr of Lawe in Paris,* trans. Samson Lennard (London, 1615), 47–72.

74. Juan Huarte, *The Examination of Mens Wits. In Which, by Discovering the Varietie of Natures, is Shewed for what Profession Each One is Apt, and How Far He Shall Profit Therein,* trans. R.C. (London, 1594), 21–22. Francis Bacon likewise divided knowledge into three parts corresponding to the three mental faculties: the memory produced history; the imagination, poetry; and the reason, philosophy. See, for example, Sachiko Kusukawa, "Bacon's Classification of Knowledge," in *The Cambridge Companion to Bacon,* ed. Markku Peltonen (New York: Cambridge University Press, 1996), 51–52.

75. Huarte, *Examination of Mens Wits,* 21–22.

76. Steven Shapin, *A Social History of Truth: Civility and Science in Seventeenth-Century England* (Chicago: University of Chicago Press, 1994), 77.

77. Ibid.

78. See Floyd-Wilson, *English Ethnicity,* chaps. 1–3, and Nicolás Wey-Gómez, *The Tropics of Empire: Why Columbus Sailed South to the Indies* (Cambridge: MIT Press, 2008), chap. 1.

79. Wey-Gómez, *Tropics of Empire,* xiv.

80. See Floyd-Wilson, *English Ethnicity,* esp. chaps. 1–3, and Wheeler, *Complexion of Race,* 23–24.

81. Kupperman, "Fear of Hot Climates," 215.

82. Edward Winslow, *Good Newes From New England: OR, A True Relation of Things Very Remarkable at the Plantation of* Plimoth *in New-England* . . . *As also What Commodities are There to be Raysed for the Maintenance of That and Other Plantations in the Said Country* (London, 1624), 62.
83. See George Best, "The First Booke of the First Voyage of *Martin Frobisher* Esquire, Captayne Generall for the Discouerie of the Passage to Cataya and the East India, by the Northweast, First Attempted in *Anno Dom.* 1576. The 15 of May," in *A True Discourse of the Late Voyages of Discoverie for Finding of a Passage to Cathaya, by the North-West, under the Conduct of* Martin Frobisher *General* (London, 1578), 19–46.
84. John Astruc, vol. 1 of *A Treatise of the Venereal Disease, in Six Books; Containing An Account of the Original, Propagation, and Contagion of this Distemper in General,* trans. William Barrowby (London, 1737), 95.
85. Martin Brückner, *The Geographic Revolution in Early America: Maps, Literacy, and National Identity* (Chapel Hill: University of North Carolina Press, 2006), 77. On eighteenth-century fears of America's hot climates, see also Bauer, "Hemispheric Genealogies"; Parrish, *American Curiosity,* 83; and Iannini, *Fatal Revolutions.*
86. Alden T. Vaughan, "From White Man to Redskin: Changing Anglo-American Perceptions of the American Indian," *American Historical Review* 87, no. 4 (1982): 921.
87. Dionyse Settle, *A True Report of the Laste Voyage into the West and Northwest Regions, &c. 1577, Worthily Achieved by Capteine Frobisher of the Sayde Voyage the First Finder and Generall* (London, 1577), 25.
88. William Wood, *New Englands Prospect· A True, Lively, and Experimentall Description of that Part of America, Commonly Called New England* . . . *Laying Downe That Which may Both Enrich the Knowledge of the Mind-Travelling Reader, or Benefit the Future Voyager. By William Wood* (London, 1634), 63.
89. Gonzalo Fernández de Oviedo y Valdés, "The Hystorie of the Weste Indies," in *The Decades of the Newe Worlde or West India Conteynyng the Nauigations and Conquestes of the Spanyardes, with the Particular Description of the Moste Ryche and Large Landes and Ilandes lately Founde in the West Ocean* . . . *Wrytten in the Latine Tounge by Peter Martyr of Angleria, and Translated into Englysshe by Rycharde Eden* (London, 1555), 181v.
90. Ibid., 181r–v.
91. Charron, *Of Wisdom,* 50 and 171.
92. Wood, *New Englands Prospect,* 6.
93. Ibid.
94. Ibid.
95. See Huarte, *Examination of Mens Wits,* 44.
96. William Vaughan, *The Newlanders Cure. As well of Those Violent Sicknesses which Distemper Most* Minds *in these Latter Dayes* . . . *Published for the weale of Great Brittaine, by Sir William Vaughan, Knight* (London, 1630), 13.
97. E. Ruth Harvey, *The Inward Wits: Psychological Theory in the Middle Ages and the Renaissance* (London: Warburg Institute, 1975), 49. Sarah Rivett examines the problem of forbidden knowledge and the possibility of faulty or imagined interpretations in the context of early modern natural philosophy and colonial testimonies of faith. See Sarah Rivett, *The Science of the Soul in Colonial New England* (Chapel Hill: University of North Carolina Press, 2012), esp. pages 14–18.
98. Sloane, vol. 1 of *Voyage to the Islands,* xxxi.
99. Ibid.

100. Ibid.
101. Daniel Webb, *A General History Of The Americans, Of Their Customs, Manners, And Colours An History Of The Patago, Selected From M. Pauw, By Daniel Webb, Esq.* (Rochdale, UK, 1806), 7.
102. Ibid.
103. Several recent studies have employed postcolonial approaches to examine British Americans' position as colonized peoples subject to metropolitan policies. However, some of these studies (Watts, Tennenhouse) focus on the North American shift from colony to nation but occlude a consideration of colonists' relation with Natives and Africans before American independence. See Edward Watts, *Writing and Postcolonialism in the Early Republic* (Charlottesville: University Press of Virginia, 1998); Robert Blair St. George, ed., *Possible Pasts: Becoming Colonial in Early America* (Ithaca: Cornell University Press, 2000); Bauer, *Cultural Geography;* Sean Goudie, *Creole America: The West Indies and the Formation of Literature and Culture in the New Republic* (Philadelphia: University of Pennsylvania Press, 2006); and Leonard Tennenhouse, *The Importance of Feeling English: American Literature and the British Diaspora, 1750–1850* (Princeton: Princeton University Press, 2007).
104. Michel de Certeau, *The Writing of History,* trans. Tom Conley (New York: Columbia University Press, 1988), 3.
105. Ibid.
106. Thomas Wright, *The Passions of the Minde in Generall . . . With a treatise thereto adjoining of the clymatericall yeare, occasioned by the death of Queene Elizabeth* (London, 1604), 124–25.
107. Thomas Walkington, *The Optick Glasse of Humors. Or The Touchstone of a Golden Temperature, or the Philosophers Stone to make a Golden Temper . . . by which every one may judge of what complection he is, and answerably learne what is most sutable to his nature* (London, 1607), 15r.
108. Ibid., 59v.
109. Wright, *Passions of the Minde,* 125.
110. On classificatory forms in imperial contexts see Mary Louise Pratt, "Scratches on the Face of the Country; Or, What Mr. Barrow Saw in the Land of the Bushmen," *Critical Inquiry* 12, no. 1 (1985): 119–43, and Pamela Regis, *Describing Early America: Bartram, Jefferson, Crevecoeur, and the Rhetoric of Natural History* (DeKalb: Northern Illinois University Press, 1992). Pratt and Regis focus on the ways in which "manners and customs" sections in travel narratives (Pratt) and natural histories (Regis) identified differences between indigenous peoples and Europeans or U.S. Americans. See also Johannes Fabian, *Time and the Other: How Anthropology Makes Its Object* (New York: Columbia University Press, 1983).
111. John Wilson, *The Day-breaking, If Not The Sun-Rising, of the Gospell With the Indians in New England* (London, 1647), 21.
112. John Heckewelder, *An Account of the History, Manners, and Customs of the Indian Nations: Who Once Inhabited Pennsylvania and the Neighbouring States. Communicated to the Historical and Literary Committee of the American Philosophical Society, Held at Philadelphia, for Promoting Useful Knowledge* (Philadelphia: Abraham Small, 1818), 228.
113. Ibid.
114. Ibid., 217.

115. I discuss Chaplin's and Parrish's influential studies of colonial natural knowledge and the Enlightenment in detail below. Although I focus here on the relation between Enlightenment views of the supernatural and colonial views of Native and African knowledge, many scholars have connected colonists' use of so-called modern scientific discourses, more generally, with the construction of differences between Euro-colonial knowledge and that of Natives and Africans. See, for a few examples, Pratik Chakrabarti, *Materials and Medicine: Trade, Conquest, and Therapeutics in the Eighteenth Century* (Manchester: Manchester University Press, 2010); Pratt, *Imperial Eyes;* Regis, *Describing Early America;* Londa L. Schiebinger, *Plants and Empire: Colonial Bioprospecting in the Atlantic World* (Cambridge: Harvard University Press, 2004), chap. 5; and Beth Fowkes Tobin, *Colonizing Nature: The Tropics in British Arts and Letters, 1760–1820* (Philadelphia: University of Pennsylvania Press, 2005).
116. Chaplin, *Subject Matter,* 283.
117. Parrish, *American Curiosity,* 43.
118. Ibid., 217.
119. See studies by Charles Webster, *From Paracelsus to Newton: Magic and the Making of Modern Science* (Cambridge: Cambridge University Press, 1982) and his *Paracelsus: Medicine, Magic and Mission at the End of Time* (New Haven: Yale University Press, 2008). See also the forum on alchemy in *Isis:* "Alchemy and the History of Science," *Isis* 102, no. 2 (2011): 300–337.
120. Brian Vickers, "Introduction," in *Occult and Scientific Mentalities in the Renaissance,* ed. Vickers (Cambridge: Cambridge University Press, 1984).
121. See Walter W. Woodward, *Prospero's America: John Winthrop, Jr., Alchemy, and the Creation of New England Culture, 1606–1676* (Chapel Hill: University of North Carolina Press, 2010). On the Enlightenment engagement with invisible realms, see James Delbourgo, *A Most Amazing Scene of Wonders: Electricity and Enlightenment in Early America* (Cambridge: Harvard University Press, 2006), and Rivett, *Science of the Soul.*
122. For an argument that racial conceptions of difference were a defense against metropolitan bias, see Bauer, "Hemispheric Genealogies."
123. Keith Thomas, *Religion and the Decline of Magic* (New York: Charles Scribner's Sons, 1971).
124. Chaplin, "Natural Philosophy and an Early Racial Idiom."
125. Wheeler, *Complexion of Race,* 5.
126. Whitehead, "*Discoverie* as enchanted text," 35.

1. Epidemic, Encounter, and Colonial Promotion in Virginia

1. Thomas Harriot, *A Briefe and True Report of the New Found Land of Virginia . . . By Thomas Harriot, seruant to the aboue named Sir Walter, a member of the Colony, and there employed in discouering* (Frankfurt, 1590), title page. Future references to this text will be cited parenthetically. "Virginia" was in present-day North Carolina.
2. As Michael Leroy Oberg points out, Ossomocomuck may be translated as "*the land that we inhabit, the dwelling house, or the house site.*" See Oberg, *The Head in Edward Nugent's Hand: Roanoke's Forgotten Indians* (Philadelphia: University of Pennsylvania Press, 2008), 3.
3. Wingina was also known as Pemisipan; he changed his name to Wingina after his brother Granganimeo died.

4. On the publication history of Harriot's *Report* and the engravings based on John White's watercolors, see Michael Gaudio, *Engraving the Savage: The New World and the Techniques of Civilization* (Minneapolis: University of Minnesota Press, 2008), esp. chaps. 1 and 2; the essays in Kim Sloan, ed., *A New World: England's First View of America* (Chapel Hill: University of North Carolina Press, 2007), and Peter Stallybrass, "*Admiranda narratio:* A European Best Seller," in *A briefe and true report of the new found land of Virginia: The 1590 Theodor de Bry Latin Edition* (Charlottesville: University of Virginia Press, 2007), 9–30. For historical studies of the colony, see Karen Ordahl Kupperman, *Roanoke: The Abandoned Colony* (Totowa, NJ: Rowman & Allanheld, 1984), and David B. Quinn, *Set Fair for Roanoke: Voyages and Colonies, 1584–1606* (Chapel Hill: University of North Carolina Press, 1985).
5. The colonists settled near Roanoke Algonquians, who comprised several autonomous villages united under the *werowance* Wingina. On the Carolina Algonquians, see Christian F. Feest, "North Carolina Algonquians," and "Virginia Algonquians," in vol. 15 of *Handbook of North American Indians,* ed. Bruce G. Trigger (Washington, DC: Smithsonian Institution, 1978), 270–81 and 253–70, respectively; and Michael Leroy Oberg, "Gods and Men: The Meeting of Indian and White Worlds on the Carolina Outer Banks, 1584–1596," *North Carolina Historical Review* 76 (1999): 367–90. Although I follow contemporary scholars in using the terms "Algonquian" and "Roanoke Algonquian" to refer to the Native American peoples Harriot met, these words would have been anachronistic for both Harriot and indigenous peoples in Virginia.
6. See Stephen Greenblatt, *Shakespearean Negotiations* (Berkeley: University of California Press, 1988), 21–39, and Joyce Chaplin, *Subject Matter: Technology, the Body, and Science on the Anglo-American Frontier, 1500–1676* (Cambridge: Harvard University Press, 2003), 28–35. Greenblatt published an earlier version of the "invisible bullets" essay, which is more dismissive of Algonquian culture and which concludes with a reading of *Henry IV.* See Greenblatt, "Invisible Bullets: Renaissance Authority and Its Subversion," *Glyph* 8 (1981): 40–61. Although he does not examine the account of "invisible bullets," Eric Cheyfitz also reads the *Report* as providing insight into Harriot's own religion. See Cheyfitz, *The Poetics of Imperialism: Translation and Colonization from The Tempest to Tarzan,* 2nd ed. (Philadelphia: University of Pennsylvania Press, 1997), 196. Sixteenth-century European medical philosophies did not include a germ theory of disease. On Galenic medical philosophies and theories of disease, see Nancy Siraisi, *Medieval and Early Renaissance Medicine: An Introduction to Knowledge and Practice* (Chicago: University of Chicago Press, 1990), chap. 5.
7. Greenblatt, *Shakespearean Negotiations,* 35.
8. Ibid., 28.
9. Chaplin, *Subject Matter,* 29.
10. Ibid., 31.
11. Ed White's article, which recovers Native responses to contact, is a notable exception to most interpretations of Harriot's *Report.* However, White does not examine either the Roanoke Algonquians' or Harriot's medical knowledge. See White, "Invisible Tagkanysough," *PMLA* 120, no. 3 (2005): 751–67.
12. Greenblatt, *Shakespearean Negotiations,* 35.
13. On Wanchese and Manteo, see Oberg, *Head in Edward Nugent's Hand,* 50–55.
14. The extent to which Harriot learned Algonquian has been a matter of debate. Virginia colonist William Strachey noted in 1612 that Harriot "spake the Indian Language." See

Strachey, *Historie of Travaile Into Virginia Britannia; expressing the Cosmographie and Comodities of the Country Together with the Manners and Customs of the People* (London: Hakluyt Society, 1849), 15. David Beers Quinn suggests that Harriot had a "working knowledge" of Algonquian by 1585, thanks to his work with Manteo and Wanchese, and most scholars agree with this assessment. See Quinn, "Thomas Harriot and the New World," in *Thomas Harriot: Renaissance Scientist,* ed. John W. Shirley (Oxford: Oxford University Press, 1974), 39, and Quinn, *Set Fair for Roanoke,* 49. See also John W. Shirley, *Thomas Harriot: A Biography* (Oxford: Clarendon Press, 1983), 107, and Vivian Salmon, "Thomas Harriot (1560–1621) and the Origins of Algonkian Linguistics," in *Language and Society in Early Modern England: Selected Essays, 1981–1994,* ed. Konrad Koerner (Amsterdam: J. Benjamins, 1996), 143–72. On correspondences between Harriot's linguistic and mathematical interests, see Michael Booth, "Thomas Harriot's Translations," *Yale Journal of Criticism* 16, no. 2 (2003): 345–61. For a linguistic analysis of Carolina Algonquin and the words in Harriot's and Lane's accounts, see James A. Geary, "The Language of the Carolina Algonkian Tribes," in vol. 2 of *The Roanoke Voyages, 1584–1590: Documents to Illustrate the English Voyages to North America Under the Patent Granted to Walter Raleigh in 1584,* ed. David Beers Quinn (London: Hakluyt Society, 1995), 873–900. For opposing views of Harriot's linguistic abilities and knowledge that insist on fluency and focus on Harriot's mistranslation of an Algonquian phrase, see Chaplin, *Subject Matter,* 32 and Cheyfitz, *Poetics of Imperialism,* 173–215.

15. George Best, "A True Reporte of Such Things as Hapned in the Second Voyage of Captayne Frobysher, Pretended for the Discouerie of a New Passage to Cataya, China, and the East Indies, by the Northwest. *Anno Do.* 1577," in *A True Discourse of the Late Voyages of Discouerie, for the Finding of a Passage to Cathaya, by the Northweast, vnder the Conduct of Martin Frobisher Generall Deuided into Three Books . . . With a particular Card therevnto adjoined of* Meta Incognita, *so farre forth as the secretes of the voyage may permit* (London, 1578), 12. There are many variant spellings of the Inuits' names. Egnock and Nutioc correspond to "Baffin Eskimo" words for woman and child. See Neil Cheshire, Tony Waldron, Alison Quinn, and David Quinn, "Frobisher's Eskimos in England," *Archivaria* 10 (1980): 38.
16. On Frobisher's captives, see Cheshire, "Frobisher's Eskimos," and Alden T. Vaughan, *Transatlantic Encounters: American Indians in Britain, 1500–1776* (Cambridge: Cambridge University Press, 2006), chap. 1. On Harriot's engagement with New World ventures, see Quinn, "Thomas Harriot."
17. Allen G. Debus, "The Paracelsian Aerial Niter," *Isis* 55, no. 1 (1964): 49.
18. On Lane's leadership in Virginia, see Michael Leroy Oberg, *Dominion and Civility: English Imperialism and Native America, 1585–1685* (Ithaca: Cornell University Press, 1999), chap. 1.
19. Ralph Lane, "An Account of the Particularities of the Imployments of the *English Men Left in Virginia by Sir Richard Greeneuill Vnder the Charge of* Master Ralfe Lane Generall of the Same, From the 17. of August, 1585, vntill the 18. of June 1586, At Which Time They Departed the Countrie: Sent, and Directed to Sir Walter Ralegh," in *Principall Navigations, Voyages and Discoveries of the English Nation . . . By Richard Hakluyt, Master of Artes, and Student sometime at Christ-church in Oxford,* ed. Richard Hakluyt (London, 1589), 737.
20. Ibid., 739. Mary Fuller argues that Lane discovered his "sincere intentions" rather than natural resources on his "hypothetical voyage." See Fuller, *Voyages in Print: English*

Travel to America, 1576–1624 (Cambridge: Cambridge University Press, 1995), 53. On the ways in which colonial narratives presented experiences in terms of future potential, see Wayne Franklin, *Discoverers, Explorers, Settlers: The Diligent Writers of Early America* (Chicago: University of Chicago Press, 1979), 77.

21. Lane, "Account of the Particularities," 739.
22. Ibid., 743. On tensions between Lane and Wingina, see Quinn, *Set Fair for Roanoke,* chap. 8, and Oberg, *Dominion and Civility.*
23. Oberg argues that Manteo's attitude toward the English may be attributed to the fact that he had been Anglicized. See Oberg, *Dominion and Civility,* 78. It is possible that Manteo did adopt elements of English culture, but it is also possible that he recommended assisting the colonists because he had concluded that the English had power that could be appropriated for the Roanokes' benefit. The decision of how to respond to English colonists was less one of assimilation versus resistance than one of determining how to respond to the newcomers and their power.
24. Lane, "Account of the Particularities," 740.
25. Ibid., 741.
26. Ibid., 743.
27. Ibid.
28. Harriot writes that the colonists ran out of "English victuall" after twenty days, in part because some of their food stores were ruined in their landing at Roanoke. See Harriot, *Briefe and True Report,* 29, and Kupperman, *Roanoke,* 22.
29. Lane, "Account of the Particularities," 746.
30. Ibid.
31. Anthony Pagden, *European Encounters with the New World: From Renaissance to Romanticism* (New Haven: Yale University Press, 1993), 21.
32. See Shirley, *Thomas Harriot,* esp. pages 38–69.
33. Harriot does not explain what he meant by "subtile device." Perhaps he was referencing the misinformation that Lane received from Wingina.
34. *Oxford English Dictionary,* 2nd ed., s.v. "Accident," 1b.
35. Little ethnohistorical information regarding the Roanoke Algonquians is available, so I have consulted histories of the colony that attend to the Roanokes' experiences and actions; firsthand colonial accounts of the Carolina Algonquians; and ethnohistorical and linguistic studies of the Algonquians. I have also drawn on studies of southeastern Native Americans, but I do not mean my use of these studies to suggest that Roanoke Algonquian peoples may be folded into other Native groups.
36. See Virgil J. Vogel, *American Indian Medicine* (Norman: University of Oklahoma Press, 1970), 16–18. Ed White suggests that the Algonquians' explanation of the illness may be read as an interpretation of the colonists that was similar to stories of the Cherokee "Little People," who were invisible beings who caused disease. See White, "Invisible Tagkanysough," 759.
37. See Kathleen J. Bragdon, *Native People of Southern New England, 1500–1650* (Norman: University of Oklahoma Press, 1996), 184–90.
38. Charles Hudson, *The Southeastern Indians* (Nashville: University of Tennessee Press, 1976), 363. See also Vogel, *American Indian Medicine,* 16. On animals as the cause of disease, see Kupperman, *Roanoke,* 57.
39. Samuel Purchas, *Purchas his Pilgrimage, or Relations of the World and the Religions Obserued in al Ages and Places Discouered, from the Creation vnto this Present In Foure*

Parts . . . The third edition, much enlarged with additions through the whole worke; by Samuel Purchas, parson of St. Martins by Ludgate London (London, 1617), 954. Okeeus is probably a reference to Okeus, the Powhatans' most important deity. This name seems to be a cognate of the Roanokes' name for their deity, Kiwasa. See Helen C. Rountree, *The Powhatan Indians of Virginia: Their Traditional Culture* (Norman: University of Oklahoma Press, 1992), 136.

40. Purchas, *Purchas his Pilgrimage,* 954.
41. Ibid.
42. John Lawson, *A New Voyage to Carolina; Containing the Exact Description and Natural History of that Country: Together with the Present State Thereof. And a Journal of a Thousand Miles, Travel'd Thro' Several Nations of Indians. Giving a Particular Account of their Customs, Manners, &c.* (London, 1709), 20.
43. Ibid., 18 and 223.
44. Oberg, "Gods and Men," 379. On the question of whether indigenous peoples interpreted Europeans as gods and whether, in taking these interpretations as evidence of indigenous peoples' responses to Europeans, western scholars reproduce European colonists' irrational belief in their own power, see the debate in Marshall Sahlins, *Islands of History* (Chicago: University of Chicago Press, 1985); Gananath Obeyesekere, *The Apotheosis of Captain Cook: European Mythmaking in the Pacific* (Princeton: Princeton University Press, 1997); and Sahlins, *How 'Natives' Think: About Captain Cook, For Example* (Chicago: University of Chicago Press, 1995).
45. On connections between trade goods and *mantoac* in a French-Ojibwa context, see Bruce White, "Encounters with Spirits: Ojibwa and Dakota Theories about the French and Their Merchandise," *Ethnohistory* 41, no. 3 (1994): 369–405. On Iroquois interest in guns for their " 'power' (especially their thunder and lightning) rather than for any practical reason," see James W. Bradley, *Evolution of the Onondaga Iroquois: Accommodating Change, 1500–1655* (Syracuse: Syracuse University Press, 1987), 142.
46. Arthur Barlowe, "The First Voyage Made to the Coastes of America, With Two *Barkes, Wherein were Captaines Master Philip Amadas, and* Master Arthur Barlowe, Who Discouered Part of the Countrey, now Called Virginia, Anno 1584; Written by One of the Said Captaines, and Sent to Sir Walter Raleigh, Knight, at Whose Charge and Direction, the Said Voyage was Set Forth," in *Principall Navigations,* 729.
47. "Bullet" dates from 1557, when it was used to describe cannonballs, developing from the older term "ball," which was also employed to describe a "missile" projected from firearms or cannons. See *Oxford English Dictionary,* 2nd ed., s.v. "Ball," 5a, and "Bullet," 1a, 2, 3a. This definition of "ball," its earliest, dates from 1387. Since "bullet" referred to small projectiles in both English and Native vocabularies, the word as used in Roanoke would have represented the small objects that the invisible spirits shot rather than the larger cannonballs referenced by the English word "ball."
48. Ives Goddard, "More on the Nasalization of PA *a- in Eastern Algonquian," *International Journal of Linguistics* 37, no. 3 (1971): 144. Narragansett and Carolina Algonquian languages were closely related. See also Ives Goddard, "The Description of the Native Languages of North America Before Boas," vol. 17 of *Handbook of North American Indians,* ed. Goddard (Washington: Smithsonian Institution, 1996), 19. On thunder-beings, see Hudson, *Southeastern Indians,* 127, and Bragdon, *Native People of Southern New England,* 188–89.
49. Robert Beverly, *The History and Present State of Virginia, in Four Parts . . . By a Native*

and Inhabitant of the Place (London, 1705), 33. See also Rountree, *Powhatan Indians of Virginia,* 136.

50. Beverly, *History and Present State of Virginia,* 33.
51. John Reed Swanton, *Religious Beliefs and Medicinal Practices of the Creek Indians* (Lincoln: University of Nebraska Press, 2000), 486.
52. Roger Williams, *A Key Into the Language of America: Or, An help to the* Language *of the* Natives *in that part of America, called New-England . . . By Roger Williams, of* Providence *in* New-England (London, 1643), 84.
53. Ibid., 176.
54. Ibid., 177.
55. Ibid., 84.
56. Titu Cusi Yupanqui, *An Inca Account of the Conquest of Peru by Titu Cusi Yupanqui,* trans. Ralph Bauer (Boulder: University Press of Colorado, 2005), 60.
57. Kelly Donahue-Wallace, *Art and Architecture of Viceregal Latin America, 1521–1821* (Albuquerque: University of New Mexico Press, 2008), 160. See also J. H. Elliott, *Empires of the Atlantic World: Britain and Spain in America, 1492–1830* (New Haven: Yale University Press, 2006), 198.
58. Lawson, *New Voyage to Carolina,* 214.
59. See John Duffy, "Medicine and Medical Practices among Aboriginal American Indians," in *History of American Medicine: A Symposium,* ed. Félix Martí-Ibáñez (New York: MD Publications, 1959), 25, and Vogel, *American Indian Medicine,* 129.
60. Swanton, *Religious Beliefs and Medicinal Practices,* 625.
61. See William A. Starna, "The Biological Encounter: Disease and the Ideological Domain," *American Indian Quarterly* 16, no. 4 (1992): 511–19.
62. John Clayton, "A Letter from the Reverend Mr. John Clayton Afterwards Dean of Kildare in Ireland to Dr. Grew, in Answer to Several Querys Sent to Him by that Learned Gentleman. A.D. 1687. Communicated by the Right Reverend Father in God Robert Lord Bishop of Corke to John Earle of Egmont F.R.S.," in *The Reverend John Clayton: A Parson with a Scientific Mind. His Scientific Writings and Other Related Papers,* ed. Edmund Berkeley and Dorothy Smith Berkeley (Charlottesville: University Press of Virginia, 1965), 27.
63. Jean Bossu, vol. 1 of *Travels through that Part of North America Formerly called Louisiana . . . Together with an Abstract of the most useful and necessary articles contained in Peter Loefling's Travels through Spain and Cumana in South America. Referred to the Pages of the Original Swedish Edition,* trans. John Reinhold Forster, F.A.S. (London, 1771), 301.
64. Antoine-Simon Le Page Du Pratz, *The History of Louisiana, or of the Western Parts of Virginia and Carolina . . . Translated from the French of M. Le Page du Pratz; with some Notes and Observations relating to our Colonies* (London, 1774), 29.
65. See Nicolás Monardes, *Joyfull Newes Out of the Newe Founde Worlde . . . Englished by Jhon Frampton, Marchant,* trans. John Frampton (London, 1577). The herbal was republished in several English editions in the sixteenth century alone, becoming the "most frequently issued book of overseas interest in the Elizabethan period." See John Parker, *Books to Build an Empire: A Bibliographical History of English Overseas Interests to 1620* (Amsterdam: Thieme-Nigmegen, 1965), 76.
66. On ideas regarding similarities among climates along lines of latitude, see Karen Ordahl Kupperman, "Fear of Hot Climates in the Anglo-American Colonial Experience," *William and Mary Quarterly* 3d. ser., 41, no. 2 (1984): 215.

67. On paradoxical descriptions of hot climates as sites of wealth and disease, see ibid. On early modern environmental theories and national characteristics, see Jim Egan, *Authorizing Experience: Refigurations of the Body Politic in Seventeenth-Century New England Writing* (Princeton: Princeton University Press, 1999), esp. the introduction and chap. 1; Mary Floyd-Wilson, *English Ethnicity and Race in Early Modern Drama* (Cambridge: Cambridge University Press, 2003), esp. chaps. 1 and 2; and Joyce E. Chaplin, "Natural Philosophy and an Early Racial Idiom in North America: Comparing English and Indian Bodies," *William and Mary Quarterly* 3d. ser., 54, no.1 (1997): 229–52.
68. In just one example, Apollo, the Greek god of poetry and medicine, was believed to send arrows that brought disease as a punishment for sin. See Raymond A. Anselment, *The Realms of Apollo: Literature and Healing in Seventeenth-Century England* (Newark: University of Delaware Press, 1995), 24.
69. Paracelsus, vol. 2 of *The Hermetic and Alchemical Writings of Aureolus Philippus Theophrastus Bombast, of Hohenheim, called Paracelsus the Great,* ed. Arthur Edward Waite (London: James Elliot and Co., 1894), 240. On the "seeds" of disease, see Walter Pagel, *Paracelsus: An Introduction to Philosophical Medicine in the Era of the Renaissance,* 2nd ed. (Basel: Karger, 1982), 240, and Vivian Nutton, "The Seeds of Disease: An Explanation of Contagion and Infection from the Greeks to the Renaissance," *Medical History* 27 (1983): 1–34. In some of his obscure writings, Galen had employed an analogy of "seeds" to explain the cause for fevers. However, as Nutton argues, for most Renaissance medical practitioners the "seeds of disease" offered a new metaphor for describing plague but did not affect their medical treatment or reliance on more prevalent theories of environmental factors and the humors.
70. See Walter Pagel, "Van Helmont's Concept of Disease—To Be or Not To Be? The Influence of Paracelsus," *Bulletin of the History of Medicine* 46, no. 5 (1972): 441.
71. Paracelsus, *Hermetic and Alchemical Writings,* 240. The "Alchemist" distilled nutritious from poisonous entities in food and ruled digestion. On the archei and Paracelsian philosophies of disease, see Allen G. Debus, *The English Paracelsians* (London: Olbourne, 1965), 30–31, and Debus, vol. 1 of *The Chemical Philosophy: Paracelsian Science and Medicine in the Sixteenth and Seventeenth Centuries* (New York: Science History Publications, 1977), 59 and 107.
72. Richard Bostocke, *Difference Between the Auncient Phisicke . . . And wherein the naturall Philosophie of Aristotle doth differ from the trueth of Gods worde, and is injurious to Christianitie and sound doctrine,* n.p., chap. 2.
73. Quoted in Pagel, *Paracelsus,* 180. See also Charles Webster, *Paracelsus: Medicine, Magic, and Mission at the End of Time* (New Haven: Yale University Press, 2008), 140.
74. Debus, "Paracelsian Aerial Niter," 49.
75. Ibid., 47.
76. Ibid., 49. Debus argues that Paracelsus's aerial niter would later be incorporated into theories of the role of oxygen in respiration and combustion.
77. Books on chemical therapies were published in England starting in 1527 and with increasing frequency through the rest of the century. See Charles Webster, "Alchemical and Paracelsian Medicine," in *Health, Medicine, and Mortality in the Sixteenth Century,* ed. Webster (Cambridge: Cambridge University Press, 1979), 301–34. Webster convincingly revises arguments by Allen Debus and Paul Kocher that English physicians and surgeons arrived at a compromise in which they employed chemical therapies but

did not incorporate Paracelsian theories until the mid-seventeenth century. Webster argues that in spite of official resistance to non-Galenic theories from the College of Physicians, the English interest in alchemy facilitated the reception of Paracelsus's ideas, which were accepted into English medical and alchemical practices toward the end of the sixteenth century. Paracelsian medical philosophies were accessible in Latin works published on the continent as well as in copies of Paracelsian writings in college and private libraries. Less educated people could read a few vernacular works published in English (though these were usually published only once and tended to focus mostly on chemical therapies). See Webster, "Alchemical and Paracelsian Medicine," 330; Debus, *English Paracelsians,* chap. 2; and Paul Kocher, "Paracelsian Medicine in England: (*ca.* 1570–1600)," *Journal of the History of Medicine* 2 (1957): 273–88.

78. Hilary Gatti notes that she has discovered references to "Gasto Claveus called Dulco" in Harriot's notes on alchemical experiments. See Gatti, "The Natural Philosophy of Thomas Harriot," in *Thomas Harriot: An Elizabethan Man of Science,* ed. Robert Fox (Burlington: Ashgate, 2000), 72. As Lawrence M. Principe has shown, Gasto Claveus called Dulco is more accurately known as Gaston DuClo; his name was misrepresented by typesetters' errors and mistranslations. See Principe, "Diversity in Alchemy: The Case of Gaston 'Claveus' DuClo, a Scholastic Mercurialist Chrysopoeian," in *Reading the Book of Nature: The Other Side of the Scientific Revolution,* ed. Allen G. Debus and Michael T. Walton (Kirksville, MO: Truman State University Press, 1998), 181–200. On Percy's library, see Webster, "Alchemical and Paracelsian Medicine," 321 n. 53, and G. R. Batho, "The Library of the 'Wizard' Earl: Henry Percy Ninth Earl of Northumberland (1564–1632)," *The Library,* 5th ser. 15 (1960), 259–61. On Ralegh's library, see W. Oakshott, "Sir Walter Ralegh's Library," *The Library,* 5th ser. 23 (1968), 285–327. On hypotheses regarding the timeframe in which Harriot conducted alchemical experiments, see Gatti, "Natural Philosophy of Thomas Harriot," 72, and Shirley, *Thomas Harriot,* 272. On the political implications of Harriot's associations with Ralegh and Percy, see Gatti, "Natural Philosophy of Thomas Harriot," 67.

79. Webster, *Paracelsus,* 142. Webster points out that Paracelsus generally adopted a Neoplatonic cosmology but disagreed with some ideas. See ibid., 143. On the connections between Paracelsian medical philosophies and Neoplatonic cosmology, see also Debus, *English Paracelsians,* chap. 1.

80. Brian Vickers, "Analogy Versus Identity: The Rejection of Occult Symbolism, 1580–1680," in *Occult and Scientific Mentalities in the Renaissance,* ed. Vickers (Cambridge, Cambridge University Press, 1984), 128.

81. Webster, *Paracelsus,* 142.

82. Vickers, "Analogy Versus Identity," 95. Although Vickers categorized Paracelsian ideas as "occult" philosophies and separated them from "scientific" mentalities, Webster has discovered continuities between Paracelsian and later "scientific" ideas. See Webster, *From Paracelsus to Newton: Magic and the Making of Modern Science* (Cambridge: Cambridge University Press, 1982).

83. See Gatti, "Natural Philosophy of Thomas Harriot," 64–65.

84. Salmon, "Thomas Harriot," 2.

85. Scott Mandelbrote, "The Religion of Thomas Harriot," in *Thomas Harriot: An Elizabethan Man of Science,* 268. On Harriot's reputation, see also Julie Robin Solomon, "'To Know, To Fly, To Conjure': Situating Baconian Science at the Juncture of Early Modern Modes of Reading," *Renaissance Quarterly* 44, no. 3 (1991): 543–45; Chaplin,

Subject Matter, 30–31; Jean Jacquot, "Thomas Harriot's Reputation for Impiety," *Notes and Records of the Royal Society* 9, no. 2 (1952): 164–87; and Robert Kargon, "Thomas Hariot, the Northumberland Circle, and Early Atomism in England," *Journal of the History of Ideas* 27, no. 1 (1966): 128–36.

86. Oberg, "Gods and Men," 367–90.
87. J. W. Springer, "An Ethnohistoric Study of the Smoking Complex in Eastern North America," *Ethnohistory* 28, no. 3 (1981): 219. See also Alexander von Gernet, "North American Indigenous *Nicotiana* Use and Tobacco Shamanism: The Early Documentary Record, 1520–1660," in *Tobacco Use by Native North Americans: Sacred Smoke and Silent Killer,* ed. Joseph C. Winter (Norman: University of Oklahoma Press, 2000), 59–80; and Joseph C. Winter, "Traditional Uses of Tobacco by Native Americans," in *Tobacco Use,* 9–58.
88. On Monardes's herbal, see Daniela Bleichmar, "Books, Bodies, and Fields: Sixteenth-Century Transatlantic Encounters with New World Materia Medica," in *Colonial Botany: Science, Commerce, and Politics in the Early Modern World,* ed. Londa Shiebinger and Claudia Swan (Philadelphia: University of Pennsylvania Press, 2005), 83–99. As Marcy Norton has shown, Monardes's herbal justified tobacco's use for medical consumption by separating the herb from the diabolic rituals in which Natives employed it. Interestingly, Harriot both described the Roanoke Algonquians' rituals for smoking tobacco and imbibed the herb himself in both Virginia and in England. See Norton, *Sacred Gifts, Profane Pleasures: A History of Tobacco and Chocolate in the Atlantic World* (Ithaca: Cornell University Press, 2008).
89. Harriot's concern regarding the implications of participating in the Algonquians' medical practices might explain his failure to cite Monardes explicitly. For another argument regarding this silence, see Jeffrey Knapp, who attributes it to Harriot's attempt to differentiate between English and Spanish colonization. Jeffrey Knapp, "Elizabethan Tobacco," *Representations* 21 (1988), esp. 32–40. On tobacco in early modern Europe, see Kristen G. Brookes, "Inhaling the Alien: Race and Tobacco in Early Modern England," in *Global Traffic: Discourses and Practices of Trade in English Literature and Culture from 1550 to 1700,* ed. Barbara Sebek and Stephen Deng (New York: Palgrave, 2008), 157–78, and Peter Mancall, "Tales Tobacco Told in Sixteenth-Century Europe," *Environmental History* 9, no. 4 (2004): 648–78.
90. Monardes, *Joyfull Newes Out of the Newe Founde Worlde,* fol. 39r.
91. Ibid.
92. Ibid.
93. Ibid.
94. See Brookes, "Inhaling the Alien," 169–70.
95. Barlowe, "First Voyage," 728.
96. On wonder, see Stephen Greenblatt, *Marvelous Possessions: The Wonder of the New World* (Chicago: University of Chicago Press, 1991), and Jonathan P. A. Sell, *Rhetoric and Wonder in English Travel Writing 1560–1613* (Burlington: Ashgate, 2006). Greenblatt argues of wonder that "what most matters takes place not 'out there' or along the receptive surfaces of the body where the self encounters the world, but deep within, at the vital, emotional center of the witness." As English writings from Roanoke show, colonists certainly drew on interior sensations, but their encounters with the environment and people of Ossomocomuck also influenced their written accounts. Greenblatt, *Marvelous Possessions,* 16.

97. Solomon, "To Know, To Fly, To Conjure," 526. My study of the rhetorical strategies Harriot employed in the *Report* complicates Solomon's argument that Harriot presented himself as someone who could influence the natural world and others in order to increase his own power.
98. Mandelbrote, "Religion of Thomas Harriot," 268.
99. Serge Gruzinski, *The Mestizo Mind: The Intellectual Dynamics of Colonization and Globalization,* trans. Deke Dusinberre (New York: Routledge, 2002), 25.
100. Ibid., 177.

2. *Healing, Medical Authority, and Moral Degeneration in New England*

1. Ferdinando Gorges, *America Painted to the Life. The True History of The Spaniards Proceedings in the Conquests of the Indians, and of their Civil Wars among themselves, from Columbus his First Discovery to These Later Times. . . .* More especially, an absolute *Narrative* of the North parts of *America,* and of the Discoveries and Plantations of our English in *Virginia, New England,* and *Berbadoes* (London, 1659), 27. Neal Salisbury suggests that the diseases were transferred by French traders and subsequently by tribes who traded directly with the French. See Salisbury, *Manitou and Providence: Indians, Europeans, and the Making of New England, 1500–1643* (New York: Oxford University Press, 1982), 102–3.
2. Thomas Dermer, "To his Worshipfull Friend M. Samuel Purchas, Preacher of the Word, at the Church a Little within Ludgate, London," in vol. 4 of *Hakluytus Posthumus or Purchas His Pilgrimes. Contayning a History of the World in Sea Voyages and Lande Travells by Englishmen and Others . . . in fower parts, Each containing fiue Bookes,* ed. Samuel Purchas (London, 1625), 1778.
3. Thomas Shepard, *The Clear Sun-shine of the Gospel Breaking Forth Upon the Indians in New-England, Or, An Historicall Narration of Gods Wonderfull Workings Upon Sundry of the Indians . . . By Mr. Thomas Shepard Minister of the Gospel of Jesus Christ at* Cambridge *in* New-England (London, 1648), 10.
4. Ibid.
5. Salisbury, *Manitou and Providence,* 105–6.
6. Edward Winslow, *Good Newes From New England: Or, A True Relation of Things Very Remarkable at the Plantation of* Plimoth *in New-England. Shewing the Wondrous Providence and Goodness of God, in their Preservation and Continuance,* Being Delivered from many Apparent Deaths and Dangers. *Together with a Relation of such Religious and Civill Lawes and Customs, as Are in Practice amongst the* Indians, *Adjoyning Them at this day. As also* What Commodities are There to be Raysed for the Maintenance of That and Other Plantations in the Said Country (London, 1624), title page. Future references to this text will appear parenthetically.
7. Massasoit seems to have been a title for the sachem, Ousemequin his personal name. Both names appear in writings by colonists. I refer to the sachem as Massasoit throughout this chapter because Winslow used it in *Good Newes.*
8. See Salisbury, *Manitou and Providence,* 125–40.
9. For a study of *Good Newes* from a literary historical perspective, see Matt Cohen, *The Networked Wilderness: Communicating in Early New England* (Minneapolis: University of Minnesota Press, 2009), chap. 2. I engage Cohen's study in more detail below. Although it focuses on colonists' religious practices, Martha L. Finch's recent *Dissenting Bodies* also

includes a chapter on *Good Newes.* See Finch, *Dissenting Bodies: Corporealities in Early New England* (New York: Columbia University Press, 2009), chap. 1.

10. Alfred A. Cave, *The Pequot War* (Amherst: University of Massachusetts Press, 1996), 21.
11. Dana Nelson, *The Word in Black and White: Reading 'Race' in American Literatures, 1638–1867* (Oxford: Oxford University Press, 1994), 6.
12. Ibid.
13. Robert Cushman, *A Sermon Preached at Plimmoth in New England . . . Written in the yeare 1621* (London, 1621), 10.
14. Ibid.
15. Ibid., 18.
16. Ibid.
17. Ibid., 11.
18. Ibid., A2v.
19. Ibid.
20. *A Relation or Journall of the Beginning and Proceedings of the English Plantation Setled at Plimouth in New England, by Certaine English Aduenturers both Merchants and Others . . . With an answer to all such objections as are in any way made against the lawfulnesse of English plantations in those parts* (London, 1622), 4.
21. Ibid., 14.
22. Ibid.
23. John Canup, *Out of the Wilderness: The Emergence of an American Identity in Colonial New England* (Middletown, CT: Wesleyan University Press, 1990), 97.
24. John Robinson to William Bradford, 1623, in *Of Plimouth Plantation,* ed. Samuel Eliot Morison (Franklin Center, PA: The Franklin Library, 1983), 375.
25. Ibid., 375–76.
26. Cohen, *Networked Wilderness,* 80.
27. On Winslow's education and apprenticeship, see Jeremy Dupertuis Bangs, *Pilgrim Edward Winslow: New England's First International Diplomat* (Boston: New England Historic Genealogical Society, 2004), 1–4, and George G. Wolkins, "Edward Winslow (O.V. 1606–11): King's Scholar and Printer," *Proceedings of the American Antiquarian Society at the Annual Meeting Held in Worcester* 60, no. 2 (1950): 235–66. Markham's text included two books, one on animal husbandry, the second a layperson's guide to medicine. See Gervase Markham, *The English Huswife, containing the Inward and Outward Vertues which Ought to be in a Complete Woman . . . A Worke very profitable and necessarie, gathered for the generall good of this kingdome* (London, 1615).
28. Winslow sometimes referred to Massasoit's village as Pokanoket; this term was also used to refer to the particular group of Wampanoags Massasoit led.
29. See *Relation or Journall,* 46.
30. Markham, *English Huswife,* 6–7.
31. Ibid., 7.
32. As Cohen has noted, this section "reads even today like a recipe: the goal of the recipe, the ingredients, the technique of preparation, the mode of serving, and even the pleased reaction of the eater are offered in sequence." Cohen, *Networked Wilderness,* 85.
33. See Roger Williams, *A Key into the Language of America: Or, An help to the* Language *of the* Natives *in that part of America, called New-England . . . By Roger Williams, of* Providence *in* New-England (London, 1643), 116.
34. Samson Occom, "Herbs and Roots (1754)," in *The Collected Writings of Samson Occom,*

Mohegan: Leadership and Literature in Eighteenth-Century America, ed. Joanna Brooks (Oxford: Oxford University Press, 2006), 46.

35. Gladys Tantaquidgeon, *Folk Medicine of the Delaware and Related Algonkian Indians* (Harrisburg: Pennsylvania Historical and Museum Commission, 1977), 75.
36. Gianna Pomata, "*Praxis Historialis:* The Uses of *Historia* in Early Modern Medicine," in *Historia: Empiricism and Erudition in Early Modern Europe,* ed. Gianna Pomata and Nancy G. Siraisi (Cambridge: MIT Press, 2005), 126.
37. Thomas Morton, *New English Canaan or New Canaan. Containing an Abstract of New England, Composed in three Bookes . . . written by Thomas Morton* (Amsterdam, 1637), 104.
38. Thomas Harriot, *A Briefe and True Report of the New Found Land of Virginia . . . By Thomas Harriot, seruant to the aboue named Sir Walter, a member of the Colony, and there employed in discouering* (Frankfurt, 1590), 29. Cristobal Silva also points out these connections, but he defines Tisquantum's account as a "counter-epidemiology," a story that posed "alternate explanations for the spread of disease." Silva argues that colonists appropriated these stories to serve imperial ends, so the appropriate context in which to consider them is not that of Native medical knowledge or history but rather colonial desires: "The central question when interrogating this scene thus becomes: What does this association mean for colonialism in New England?" See Cristobal Silva, *Miraculous Plagues: An Epidemiology of Early New England Narrative* (Oxford: Oxford University Press, 2011), 54 and 58.
39. See also Kathleen J. Bragdon, *Native People of Southern New England, 1500–1650* (Norman: University of Oklahoma Press, 1996), 184–85.
40. Frank Shuffelton argues that Tisquantum's "threats to loose the plague on the Indians and to bring war to them were . . . the claims of a would-be shaman." However, Shuffelton holds that neither Winslow nor Bradford understood the significance these claims held for the Wampanoags. Shuffelton, "Indian Devils and Pilgrim Fathers: Squanto, Hobomok, and the English Conception of Indian Religion," *New England Quarterly* 49, no. 1 (1976): 115.
41. Edward Johnson, *A History of New-England. From the English Planting in the Yeere 1628. untill the Yeere 1652 . . . With the Names of all their Governours, Magistrates, and Eminent Ministers* (London, 1654), 17. See also William A. Starna, "The Biological Encounter: Disease and the Ideological Domain," *American Indian Quarterly* 16, no. 4 (1992): 514.
42. Alexandir Whitaker, *Good Newes from Virginia . . . And a preface prefixed of some matters touching that Plantation, very requisite to be made known* (London, 1613), 25.
43. Dane Morrison, *A Praying People: Massachusett Acculturation and the Failure of the Puritan Mission, 1600–1690* (New York: Peter Lang, 1995), 14.
44. Gorges, *America Painted to the Life,* 27. See also Morton, *New English Canaan,* 132–33.
45. Bragdon, *Native People,* 150.
46. William Bradford, *Of Plimouth Plantation,* 99.
47. Most scholarship reproduces this focus. See Shuffelton, "Indian Devils and Pilgrim Fathers," 111–12, and Silva, *Miraculous Plagues,* 56–57.
48. *Oxford English Dictionary,* 2nd ed., s.v. "Possess," 3, 10, 10c.
49. Karen Ordahl Kupperman, *Indians and English: Facing Off in Early America* (Ithaca: Cornell University Press, 2000), 120.
50. Matt Cohen has argued convincingly that Winslow's cure of Massasoit enacted the colonists' ability to influence the flow of information and power in New England social

and political realms, a message that publishing *Good Newes* also communicated in transatlantic contexts. Cohen argues that Winslow's message was made all the more powerful by the "systemic noise" of herb gathering and cooking that he employed to make Massasoit's broth, actions that were gendered as female in both Wampanoag and English contexts. However, Cohen argues that Winslow's cure lacked the "manipulation of insects, colors, fire, or language" that marked shamans' practices. See Cohen, *Networked Wilderness,* 84. By contrast, I argue that Winslow's actions were presented and seen as similar to those of a *powah.* Even if Winslow performed a selective imitation of Native medical practices, *powahs'* statues and responsibility seem to have served both Winslow and the Wampanoags as a framework for understanding and interpreting his medical practices.

51. Morrison, *Praying People,* 57. On the appeal of Christianity in a French Jesuit context, see Starna, "Biological Encounter," 511–19.
52. On the differences between physic and medicine in the seventeenth century, see Harold J. Cook, "Physick and Natural History in Seventeenth-Century England," in vol. 24 of *Revolution and Continuity: Essays in the History and Philosophy of Early Modern Science,* ed. Peter Barker and Roger Ariew (Washington, DC: Catholic University of America Press, 1991), 63–80, and Harold J. Cook, "The New Philosophy and Medicine in Seventeenth-Century England," in *Reappraisals of the Scientific Revolution,* ed. David C. Lindberg and Robert S. Westman (Cambridge: Cambridge University Press, 1990), 397–435.
53. Winslow's "Consort" was John Hamden, an Englishman who lived only temporarily in New England and who was a member of the English Parliament in the 1640s. See Conrad Russell, "John Hampden (1595–1643)," *Oxford Dictionary of National Biography.*
54. See John Gerard, *The Herball, Or, Generall Historie of Plantes. Gathered by John Gerarde of London, Master in Chirvrgerie* (London, 1597), 1341. Gerard called sassafras the "ague tree."
55. Jacques Cartier, *The Voyages of Jacques Cartier,* ed. Henry Percival Biggar and Ramsay Cook (Toronto: University of Toronto Press, 1993), 80.
56. Nicolás Monardes, *Joyfull Newes Out of the Newe Founde World . . . Englished by Jhon Frampton, Marchant,* trans. John Frampton (London, 1577), fol. 46r.
57. Cartier, *Voyages of Jacques Cartier,* 80.
58. Keith Hutchison, "What Happened to Occult Qualities in the Scientific Revolution?," in *The Scientific Enterprise in Early Modern Europe: Readings from* Isis, ed. Peter Dear (Chicago: University of Chicago Press, 1997), 89. Hutchison argues that because occult virtues were insensible, they were also considered to be incorporeal (spiritual entities the senses could not perceive), unintelligible, and idiosyncratic, or specific (and thus not evidence of a general principle). On the difficulty distinguishing between preternatural and supernatural phenomena, see also Lorraine Daston, "Marvelous Facts and Miraculous Evidence in Early Modern Europe," *Critical Inquiry* 18, no. 1 (1991): 93–124.
59. Ibid.
60. Cartier, *Voyages of Jacques Cartier,* 80.
61. Williams, *Key into the Language,* 119–20.
62. Cushman, *Sermon Preached at Plimmoth,* A4r.
63. Ibid., 11.
64. José de Acosta, *The Naturall and Morall Historie of the East and West Indies . . . Written*

in Spanish by Joseph Acosta, *and translated into English by E.G.* (London, 1604), To the Reader.

65. Anthony Pagden, *The Fall of Natural Man: The American Indian and the Origins of Comparative Ethnology* (Cambridge: Cambridge University Press, 1986), 149.
66. Acosta, *Naturall and Morall Historie,* To the Reader.
67. See ibid., 327–590.
68. As Kupperman notes, the sacrifices Winslow described probably involved burning piles of wood, not children. See Kupperman, *Indians and English,* 114.
69. Pagden, *Fall of Natural Man,* 18.
70. Kupperman, *Indians and English,* 113.
71. James Axtell, *The European and the Indian: Essays in the Ethnohistory of Colonial North America* (Oxford: Oxford University Press, 1981), 307.
72. For just a few studies on the relations between civilization and Christianity, see Pagden, *Fall of Natural Man,* chap. 2; James Axtell, *The Invasion Within: The Contest of Cultures in Colonial North America* (Oxford: Oxford University Press, 1985), 131; and Richard W. Cogley, *John Eliot's Mission to the Indians before King Philip's War* (Cambridge: Harvard University Press, 1999), 7.
73. Winslow stated that the Plimouth colonists received news of this attack directly from Virginia, when Captain Francis May sailed from Plimouth to Virginia and back with news of the "bloody slaughter." See Winslow, *Good Newes,* Postscript. For an official account of the attack, see Edward Waterhouse, *A Declaration of the State of the Colony and Affaires in Virginia: With a Relation of the Barbarous Massacre in the Time of Peace and League, Treacherously Executed by the Natiue Infidels vpon the English, the 22 of March Last . . . And a Note of the charges of necessary prouisions fit for euery man that intends to goe to Virginia* (London, 1622).
74. Harriot, *Briefe and True Report,* 29.
75. See Axtell, *European and the Indian,* 305, and Drew Lopenzina, *Red Ink: Native Americans Picking Up the Pen in the Colonial Period* (Albany: SUNY University Press, 2012), 27.
76. English encroachment onto and dispossession of New England Natives' land following epidemics in 1633–34 also opened the way for English missionaries to preach to Natives whose sachems had submitted to the colonies' political authority. See Cogley, *John Eliot's Mission,* chap. 2.
77. David Silverman, *Faith and Boundaries: Colonists, Christianity, and Community among the Wampanoag Indians of Martha's Vineyard, 1600–1871* (Cambridge: Cambridge University Press, 2005), 10.
78. On the ways that Natives also shaped missionaries' message and its rhetorical and material forms, see Kristina Bross, *Dry Bones and Indian Sermons: Praying Indians in Colonial America* (Ithaca: Cornell University Press, 2004), 75, and Philip H. Round, *Removable Type: Histories of the Book in Indian Country, 1663–1880* (Chapel Hill: University of North Carolina Press, 2010).
79. Silverman, *Faith and Boundaries,* 24.
80. Shepard, *Clear Sun-Shine of the Gospel,* 26. Winslow played a key role in defining and communicating this message in English contexts, for he published three of minister John Eliot's tracts promoting his missions for the New England Algonquians. Winslow also obtained financial support for Eliot's missions from Parliament by arguing for and overseeing the formation of the Society for the Propagation of the Gospel. See Michael P.

Clark, introduction to *The Eliot Tracts: with Letters from John Eliot to Thomas Thorowgood and Richard Baxter*, by John Eliot (Westport, CT: Praeger, 2003), 11, and Bangs, *Pilgrim Edward Winslow*, 251–61.

81. Robert Boyle, a Fellow of the Royal Society, was also the president of the Society for the Propagation of the Gospel in Foreign Parts. For more on the interconnections between the Eliot missions and empirical science, see Sarah Rivett, *The Science of the Soul in Colonial New England* (Chapel Hill: University of North Carolina Press, 2011).
82. Ibid., 169.
83. Shepard, *Clear Sun-Shine of the Gospel*, 25.
84. Ibid., 26.
85. Henry W. Bowden and James P. Ronda, eds., *John Eliot's Indian Dialogues: A Study in Cultural Interaction* (Westport, CT: Greenwood Press, 1980), 36.
86. *The Glorious Progress of the Gospel, Amongst the Indians in New England . . . With an Appendix to the foregoing Letters, holding forth Conjectures, Observations, and Applications, by J.D. Minister of the Gospell* (London, 1649), 8.
87. Ibid.
88. John Eliot, *Tears of Repentance: Or, A Further Narrative of the Progress of the* Gospel *Amongst the Indians In New-England . . . Related by Mr.* Eliot *and Mr.* Mayhew, *two Faithful Laborers in that Work of the Lord* (London, 1653), C3r.
89. Ibid. Although the Martha's Vineyard Wampanoags did accept Christianity, they did so for a variety of reasons. Embracing Christianity allowed them to determine their relation to missionary Thomas Mayhew, but many Natives were also attracted to Christianity on a spiritual level. As David Silverman writes, even as they accepted Christianity, the Wampanoags "transformed Christianity into a bulwark for Wampanoag communities and an expression of their own culture." See Silverman, *Faith and Boundaries*, 13.
90. Matthew Mayhew, *The Conquests and Triumphs of Grace Being a Brief Narrative of the Success which the Gospel hath had Among the Indians of Martha's Vineyard (and the Places Adjacent) in New-England . . . Whereto is Added, An Account concerning the Present State of Christianity among the* Indians, *in other Parts of* New-England: *Expressed in the* Letters *of several Worthy Persons, best acquainted therewithal* (London, 1695), 29. On Massasoit's rejection of Christianity, see also Silverman, *Faith and Boundaries*, chap. 1.
91. Serge Gruzinski, *The Mestizo Mind: The Intellectual Dynamics of Colonization and Globalization*, trans. Deke Dusinberre (New York: Routledge, 2002), 33.
92. Ibid., 62.

3. African Testimony, Dangerous Communications, and Colonial Medical Knowledge in the 1721 Boston Inoculation Controversy

1. Patricia A. Watson, *The Angelical Conjunction: The Preacher-Physicians of Colonial New England* (Knoxville: University of Tennessee Press, 1991), 41.
2. William Douglass, *A Dissertation Concerning Inoculation of the Small-Pox . . . illustrated by sundry cases of the Inoculated* (Boston, 1730), 21.
3. Ibid.
4. On Mather and medicine, see Otho T. Beall, Jr. and Richard H. Shryock, *Cotton Mather, First Significant Figure in American Medicine* (Baltimore: Johns Hopkins University Press, 1954).

5. Margaret Humphreys Warner, "Vindicating the Minister's Medical Role: Cotton Mather's Concept of the *Nishmath-Chajim* and the Spiritualization of Medicine," *Journal of the History of Medicine* 26, no. 3 (1981): 279. On the inoculation controversy, see also Mitchell Breitwieser, "Cotton Mather's Pharmacy," *Early American Literature* 16, no. 1 (1981): 42–49; Louise A. Breen, "Cotton Mather, The 'Angelical Ministry,' and Inoculation," *Journal of the History of Medicine and Allied Sciences* 46 (1991): 333–57; Carla Mulford, "New Science and the Question of Identity in Eighteenth-Century British America," *Finding Colonial Americas: Essays Honoring J. A. Leo Lemay,* ed. Carla Mulford and David S. Shields (Newark: University of Delaware Press, 2001), 79–103; and Cristobal Silva, *Miraculous Plagues: An Epidemiology of Early New England Narrative* (Oxford: Oxford University Press, 2011), chap. 4.
6. See Humphreys Warner, "Vindicating the Minister's Medical Role," 279.
7. Simon Schaffer and Steven Shapin, *Leviathan and the Air-Pump: Hobbes, Boyle, and the Experimental Life* (Princeton: Princeton University Press, 1985), 39. On Douglass's education, see William R. Brock, *Scotus Americanus: A Survey of the Sources for Links between Scotland and America in the Eighteenth Century* (Edinburgh: Edinburgh University Press, 1982), 179.
8. James W. Schmotter, "William Douglass and the Beginnings of American Medical Professionalism: A Reinterpretation of the 1721 Boston Inoculation Controversy," *Historical Journal of Western Massachusetts* 6 (1977): 23.
9. David D. Hall, *Cultures of Print: Essays in the History of the Book* (Amherst: University of Massachusetts Press, 1996), 157.
10. Schmotter, "William Douglass and the Beginnings of American Medical Professionalism," 23.
11. Eric Richards, "Scotland and the Uses of the Atlantic Empire," in *Strangers within the Realm: Cultural Margins of the First British Empire,* ed. Bernard Bailyn and Philip D. Morgan (Chapel Hill: University of North Carolina Press, 1991), 91. See also Ned C. Landsman, *Scotland and Its First American Colony, 1683–1765* (Princeton: Princeton University Press, 1985), 263. Douglass had obtained his degrees at Leiden, Utrecht, and Edinburgh. Although Edinburgh would later become a highly regarded center for medical education, it did not yet possess this reputation in the early eighteenth century. See Brock, *Scotus Americanus,* 179. On colonial degeneration more generally, see John Canup, "Cotton Mather and 'Criolian Degeneracy,'" *Early American Literature,* 24, no. 1 (1989): 20–34; Ralph Bauer, *The Cultural Geography of Colonial American Literatures: Empire, Travel, Modernity* (Cambridge: Cambridge University Press, 2003); and the essays in Ralph Bauer and José Antonio Mazzotti, eds., *Creole Subjects in the Colonial Americas: Empires, Texts, Identities* (Chapel Hill: University of North Carolina Press, 2009).
12. The *Summary* was published in several volumes in 1749–1752 and again in 1760.
13. For example, the English translation of Sydenham's work promises "*short and clear Accounts of the Symptoms of most Diseases incident to Mankind, with succinct Histories of the Progress and Periods of many of 'em*" (A2v). See Thomas Sydenham, *The Compleat Method of Curing Almost all Diseases . . . Written in* Latin, *by Dr.* Thomas Sydenham, *And now faithfully Englished* (London, 1694). See also Kenneth Dewhurst, *Dr. Thomas Sydenham (1624–1689): His Life and Original Writings* (Berkeley: University of California Press, 1966), 62.
14. See Douglass, *The Boston News-Letter,* 17 July 1721, 3.
15. Ibid.
16. Ibid.

17. William Douglass, *The New-England Courant,* 7 August 1721, 1.
18. Ibid.
19. Ibid.
20. Ibid.
21. Douglass, *The Boston News-Letter,* 17 July 1721, 3.
22. Ibid.
23. William Douglass, *The New-England Courant,* 7–14 August 1721, 1.
24. Douglass, *The New-England Courant,* 7 August 1721, 1.
25. Douglass, "To the Author of the *New-England Courant,*" *The New-England Courant,* 7–14 August 1721, 1. The piece was published anonymously; Benjamin Franklin added authors' names by hand later. Massachusetts governor Samuel Shute declared war on the Abenakis in 1722. See Kenneth Silverman, ed., *Selected Letters of Cotton Mather* (Baton Rouge: Louisiana State University Press, 1971), 343.
26. Douglass, "To the Author of the *New-England Courant,*" *The New-England Courant,* 7–14 August 1721, 1.
27. See Richard B. Sheridan, *Sugar and Slavery: An Economic History of the British West Indies, 1623–1775* (Barbados: Caribbean Universities Press, 1974), 421.
28. John Williamson, vol. 2 of *Medical and Miscellaneous Observations, Relative to the West India Islands* (Edinburgh, 1817), 142. Hans Sloane commented on the communication of yaws from "Blacks to Whites" in 1707. See Hans Sloane, vol. 1 of *A Voyage to the Islands Madera, Barbados, Nieves, S. Christophers and Jamaica . . . Illustrated with The Figures of the Things describ'd, which have not been heretofore engraved; In large Copper-plates as big as the Life* (London, 1707), cxxvi.
29. See Richard B. Sheridan, *Doctors and Slaves: A Medical and Demographic History of Slavery in the British West Indies, 1680–1834* (Cambridge: Cambridge University Press, 1985), chap. 3.
30. Sheridan writes: "West Indian blacks reportedly continued the African practice of inoculating their children with yaws." See ibid., 87–88.
31. Henry Barham, *Hortus Americanus: Containing An Account of the Trees, Shrubs, and other Vegetable Productions of South-America and the West India Islands, and particularly of the Island of Jamaica . . . Respecting their Uses in Medicine, Diet, and Mechanics* (Kingston, 1714), 96. See also pages 60, 73, 87. Barham, like Douglass and Mather, was a member of the British Royal Society, throughout which his manuscripts circulated; it is thus likely that the colonists had access to his accounts of African medicine. Scholars have more recently noted that although many Europeans believed that yaws and syphilis were the same illness, the maladies have different properties. See, for one example, Sheridan, *Doctors and Slaves,* 83.
32. Barham, *Hortus Americanus* 96.
33. Sloane, vol. 1 of *Voyage to the Islands,* cxxvii.
34. John Quier, "An Account of the Success of Inoculation for the Small-Pox at Jamaica," in *Letters and Essays on the Small-pox and Inoculation . . . By different practitioners,* ed. D. Munro (London, 1778), 6.
35. William Hillary, *Observations on the Changes of the Air and the Concomitant Epidemical Diseases, in the Island of Barbadoes. To Which is Added A Treatise on the Putrid Bilious Fever, Commonly Called the Yellow Fever; And Such other Diseases as are Indigenous or Endemial, in the West India Islands, or in the Torrid Zone* (London, 1766), 341.
36. Ibid., 340. The linguistic attribution of "yaws" to Africa should not be treated as

conclusive evidence for an African origin for yaws, for Europeans often attributed medical practices to Africa in order to categorize them as foreign.

37. Bryan Edwards, vol. 2 of *History, Civil and Commercial, of the British West Indies: in Two Volumes* (London, 1793), 63.

38. Benjamin Moseley, *Medical tracts. I. On sugar. II. On the cow-pox. III. On the Yaws. IV. On Obi; or African Witchcraft . . . VIII. On prisons* (London, 1800), 187.

39. George Lyman Kittredge, ed., *Some Lost Works of Cotton Mather* (Cambridge: Cambridge University Press, 1912), 422.

40. Historians do not agree about the translation of "Guramantese," and there are consequently several theories about Onesimus's country of origin. Gordon W. Jones translates "Guramantese" to mean Coromantee and to refer to people from the Gold Coast of Africa. See Jones, ed. *The Angel of Bethesda by Cotton Mather* (Barre, MA: American Antiquarian Society, 1972), 350, n. 37. Eugenia W. Herbert suggests that "Guramantese" may be a "quaint" and imprecise term for black Africans but she also raises the possibility that the term is a reference to the "Kanuri-speaking people of the Central Sahara." See Herbert, "Smallpox Inoculation in Africa," *Journal of African History*, 16 (1975): 543. Donald R. Hopkins suggests that "Guramantese" may be translated "Gurumanche" to refer to people from "eastern Upper Volta rather than to the Garamantes of Fezzan, in southern Libya, as is often stated." See Hopkins, *The Greatest Killer: Smallpox in History*, 2nd ed. (Chicago: University of Chicago Press, 2002), 174.

41. James Bruce, vol. 6 of *Travels to Discover the Sources of the Nile, in the years 1768, 1769, 1770, 1771, 1772, & 1773 . . . To Which is Prefixed, A Life of the Author*, 3rd ed. (Edinburgh, 1813), 403.

42. Hopkins, *Greatest Killer*, 178. He adds that a 1776 letter from a French traveler on a slave ship described the practice of inoculation in Africa's interior, and he dates the presence of smallpox in Africa from 1085 BC, in Egypt. Ibid., 14.

43. See ibid., 164–80.

44. Philip D. Curtin, "Disease Exchange Across the Tropical Atlantic," in *Migration and Mortality in Africa and the Atlantic World, 1700–1900* (Burlington: Ashgate, 2001), 350. Curtin notes that the Fon of Dahomey also had a smallpox god. On Yoruba smallpox gods see also Anthony D. Buckley, "The God of Smallpox: Aspects of Yoruba Religious Knowledge," *Africa* 55, no. 2 (1985): 187–200.

45. Many of these deities survived the middle passage to the new world. See Robert Farris Thompson, *Flash of the Spirit: African and Afro-American Art and Philosophy* (New York: Random House, 1983), xv.

46. James Kirkpatrick, *The Analysis of Inoculation: Comprizing The History, Theory, and Practice of it: With an Occasional Consideration of the Most Remarkable Appearances in the Small Pocks* (London: 1754), 147.

47. Bruce, *Travels to Discover*, 403–4.

48. Theophus Smith, *Conjuring Culture: Biblical Formations of Black America* (New York: Oxford University Press, 1994), 5.

49. On the communal nature of medicine in West Africa, see James H. Sweet, *Domingos Álvares, African Healing, and the Intellectual History of the Atlantic World* (Chapel Hill: University of North Carolina Press, 2011), chap. 1.

50. See Herbert, "Smallpox Inoculation in Africa," 543.

51. On Mather's attempts to convert his slaves, see Kathryn S. Koo, "Strangers in the House of God: Cotton Mather, Onesimus, and an Experiment in Christian Slaveholding," *Proceedings of the American Antiquarian Society* 117, part 1 (2007): 143–75.

52. Cotton Mather, *Diary of Cotton Mather, vol. 2: 1709–1724* (New York: Frederick Ungar, 1957), 271.
53. Ibid., 272.
54. Ibid., 363.
55. Ibid.
56. Ibid., n.1.
57. See Koo, "Strangers in the House of God," 165–66.
58. For a different view of Onesimus, see Silva, *Miraculous Plagues,* 176.
59. Cotton Mather, *Some Account of What is said of Innoculating or Transplanting the Small Pox. By the Learned Dr. Emanuel Timonius, and Jacobus Pylarinus . . . To which are added, a few quaeries in answer to the scruples of many about the lawfulness of this method* (Boston, 1721), 9. Mather probably assured his readers that Africans were not conspiring to revolt in response to a recent slave revolt in New York. See Ira Berlin, *Many Thousands Gone: The First Two Centuries of Slavery in North America* (Cambridge: Belknap Press of Harvard University Press, 2005), esp. 190.
60. Steven Shapin, *A Social History of Truth: Civility and Science in Seventeenth-Century England* (Chicago: University of Chicago Press, 1994), 78.
61. Michel de Certeau, *Heterologies: Discourse on the Other,* trans. Brian Massumi (Minneapolis: University of Minnesota Press, 1986), 74. As de Certeau writes, the myth of this "illiterate" had existed since the fourteenth century and was developed in a number of histories and essays, of which Michel de Montaigne's *Of Cannibals* was only one. Ibid.
62. Ibid.
63. Mather, *Some Account,* 9. Colonists sometimes characterized their own speech as blundering in their writings to English natural philosophers, usually in "rhetorical gestures of self-validation." See Susan Scott Parrish, *American Curiosity: Cultures of Natural History in the Colonial British Atlantic World* (Chapel Hill: University of North Carolina Press, 2006), 118.
64. Cotton Mather, *The Negro Christianized. An Essay to Excite and Assist that Good Work, the Instruction of Negro-Servants in Christianity* (Boston, 1706), 25.
65. Anthony Pagden, "The Savage Critic: Some European Images of the Primitive," *The Yearbook of English Studies* 13 (1983): 40.
66. Mather, *Some Account,* 9.
67. Michel de Certeau, *The Writing of History,* trans. Tom Conley (New York: Columbia University Press, 1978), 224.
68. Thomas Tryon, *Friendly Advice to the Gentlemen-Planters of the East and West Indies In Three Parts . . . By Philotheos Physiologus* (London, 1684), 146.
69. Philippe Rosenberg, "Thomas Tryon and the Seventeenth-Century Dimensions of Antislavery," *William and Mary Quarterly* 3d. ser., 61, no. 4 (2004): 623. In 1684, Tryon had described slaves in nearly the same terms that Mather had used in *The Negro Christianized.* Tryon wrote: "Though I think it will be to as little purpose, as to go about to *wash thy Skin* White, to inform such dark *stupid Heathens* as you are." Although Mather does not mention Tryon as a source, these similarities suggest that the minister was familiar with Tryon's text and the practice of employing slaves as simple yet trustworthy witnesses. See Tryon, *Friendly Advice,* 152.
70. Tryon, *Friendly Advice,* 196.
71. Bauer, *Cultural Geography,* 145.
72. Silva, *Miraculous Plagues,* 172.

73. Barbara Shapiro, *Probability and Certainty in Seventeenth-Century England: A Study of the Relationships Between Natural Science, Religion, History, Law, and Literature* (Princeton: Princeton University Press, 1983), 246.
74. Murray Cohen, *Sensible Words: Linguistic Practice in England, 1640–1785* (Baltimore: Johns Hopkins University Press, 1977), 8.
75. Ibid., 11.
76. Hall, *Cultures of Print*, 161.
77. John Williams, *Several Arguments Proving, that Inoculating the Small Pox is Not Contained in the Law of Physick, either Natural or Divine, and Therefore Unlawful . . . And Also, a Short Answer to a Late Letter in the New England Courant* (Boston, 1721).
78. Sarah Rivett, *The Science of the Soul in Colonial New England* (Chapel Hill: University of North Carolina Press, 2011), 304.
79. Cohen, *Sensible Words*, 23.
80. Mather, *Some Account*, 9.
81. Cotton Mather, "Sentiments on the Smallpox Inoculated," in *Several Reasons Proving that Inoculating or Transplanting the Small Pox, is a Lawful Practice, and That It Has Been Blessed by God for the Saving of Many a Life* (Boston, 1721), 2.
82. Mather, *Some Account*, 8.
83. Ibid., 9.
84. Parrish, *American Curiosity*, 286.
85. Bauer, *Cultural Geography*, 4.
86. Mather, *Some Account*, 9.
87. Douglass, "To the Author of the *New-England Courant*," 1. For a different reading of this satire, through the lens of epidemiology, see Silva, *Miraculous Plagues*, 167.
88. Douglass, *Dissertation Concerning Inoculation*, 21.
89. Ibid.
90. Ibid.
91. William Douglass, *Inoculation of the Small Pox as practiced in Boston, Consider'd in a Letter to A—S—M.D. & F.R.S. in London* (Boston, 1722), 6–7.
92. Ibid., 7.
93. Ibid., 6.
94. John Locke, *An Essay Concerning Human Understanding. In Four Books* (London, 1690), 3.2.1.
95. See ibid., 3.5.1.
96. Cohen, *Sensible Words*, 27.
97. Locke, *Essay Concerning Human Understanding*, 3.2.2.
98. Douglass, *Dissertation Concerning Inoculation*, 21.
99. Douglass, *Inoculation of the Small Pox*, 11.
100. Ibid., 7.
101. Ibid.
102. Margot Minardi, "The Boston Inoculation Controversy of 1721–1722: An Incident in the History of Race," *William and Mary Quarterly* 3d. ser., 61, no. 1 (2004): 51. Minardi argues that Douglass's medical training predisposed him to take bodily characteristics such as skin color into account when evaluating medical evidence.
103. William Douglass, vol. 2 of *A Summary, Historical and Political, Of the First Planting, Progressive Improvements, and Present State of the* British *Settlements in North America . . . By William Douglass, M.D.* (Boston, 1760), 350.

104. Douglass, *Dissertation Concerning Inoculation,* 21.
105. Douglass, vol. 2 of *Summary, Historical and Political,* 350.
106. Ibid., vol. 1, 448.
107. Ibid., vol. 2, 350.
108. Ibid., vol. 1, 448.
109. Douglass, *Inoculation of the Small Pox,* A2r.
110. Ibid., 11.
111. Ibid., A2r.
112. Ibid., A2v.
113. On views of Scots in America, see Richards, "Scotland and the Uses of the Atlantic Empire."
114. Isaiah Greenwood, *A Friendly Debate; or, A Dialogue, Between Academicus; and Sawney & Mundungus, Two Eminent Physicians, About Some of their Late Performance* (Boston, 1722), 1.
115. Douglass, *Inoculation of the Small Pox,* 13.
116. Douglass, vol. 1 of *Summary, Historical and Political,* 161.
117. Ibid.
118. Ibid.
119. Ibid., vol. 2, 348. Interestingly, Mather makes a similar point in *Angel of Bethesda,* writing that Sydenham's method could not be "Strictly in all Points adher'd unto" in the colonies because of differences of seasons and climate. See Mather, *The Angel of Bethesda by Cotton Mather,* ed. Gordon W. Jones (Barre, MA: American Antiquarian Society, 1972), 98.
120. On Sydenham, see Dewhurst, *Dr. Thomas Sydenham (1624–1689).*
121. Douglass, vol. 1 of *Summary, Historical and Political,* 173.
122. Ibid.
123. Ibid.
124. Ibid.
125. Ibid., 161.
126. For example, Thomas Jefferson answered several queries from François Marbois, the secretary to the minister from France, by noting that they did not apply to America. See Jefferson, *Notes on the State of Virginia,* ed. Frank Shuffelton (New York: Penguin, 1998), query 3 and 10.
127. Douglass, vol. 1 of *Summary, Historical and Political,* 173.
128. Ibid., vol. 2, 406.
129. Cadwallader Colden, "Extract of letter from Cadwallader Colden, esq. to Dr. Fothergill, concerning the throat distemper," *The American Museum, or Repository of Ancient and Modern Fugitive Pieces, &c. Prose and Poetical, For January, 1788* 3, no. 1 (Philadelphia, 1788), 58–59.
130. James Kirkpatrick, *An Essay on Inoculation, Occasioned by the Small-Pox Being Brought into South Carolina in the Year 1738 . . . and a summary Relation of the principal Cases* (London, 1743), 47.

4. Obeah, Slave Revolt, and Plantation Medicine in the British West Indies

1. Jerome S. Handler and Kenneth M. Bilby, "On the Early Use and Origin of the Term 'Obeah' in Barbados and the Anglophone Caribbean," *Slavery and Abolition* 22, no. 2 (2001): 87.

2. On Tacky's Rebellion, see Orlando Patterson, *The Sociology of Slavery: An Analysis of the Origins, Development, and Structure of Negro Slave Society in Jamaica* (Rutherford: Fairleigh Dickinson University Press, 1969), 271; Michael Craton, *Testing the Chains: Resistance to Slavery in the British West Indies* (Ithaca: Cornell University Press, 1982); and Mavis C. Campbell, *The Maroons of Jamaica, 1655–1796* (Trenton, NJ: Africa World Press, Inc., 1990), 154–57. For primary sources on Tacky's Rebellion, see Edward Long, vol. 2 of *The History of Jamaica, Or, General Survey of the Antient and Modern State of that Island: with Reflections on its Situation, Settlements, Inhabitants... In Three Volumes* (London, 1774), 447–71; "The engrossed bill to remedy the evils arising from irregular assemblies of slaves and for preventing the practice of obeah," in *1760 Journals of the Assembly Jamaica* 245, no. 1 (16 December 1798): 173–246, and Bryan Edwards, vol. 2 of *History, Civil and Commercial, of the British West Indies: In Two Volumes* (London, 1793), 88–99.
3. On Grainger's medical education, see John Gilmore, *The Poetics of Empire: A Study of James Grainger's* The Sugar-Cane (London: Athlone Press, 2000), 5–9.
4. James Grainger, *The Sugar-Cane: A Poem* (London, 1764), vii. Future references to this text will appear parenthetically.
5. See William Earle, *Obi; or the History of Three-fingered Jack, In a Series of Letters from a Resident in Jamaica to his Friend in England* (London, 1800). Historians and anthropologists traditionally cited Edward Long's *History of Jamaica* and Edwards's *History, Civil and Commercial, of the British West Indies* as the first and most influential sources on obeah. As this chapter shows, however, Grainger's poem described obeah just after Tacky's Rebellion and before the later histories. See Roger Bastide, *African Civilizations in the New World*, trans. Peter Green (London: C. Hurst, 1967); Patterson, *Sociology of Slavery;* and George Eaton Simpson, *Black Religions in the New World* (New York: Columbia University Press, 1978).
6. Anthony Low, *The Georgic Revolution* (Princeton: Princeton University Press, 1985), 117–26.
7. Joseph Addison, "An Essay on Virgil's Georgics," vol. 1 of *The Works of the Right Honourable Joseph Addison, Esq.; In Four Volumes* (London, 1721), 249.
8. Low, *Georgic Revolution*, 142.
9. On the georgic revolution, see Low, *Georgic Revolution*, and Rachel Crawford, "English Georgic and British Nationhood," *English Literary History* 65, no. 1 (1998): 123–58.
10. See David S. Shields, *Oracles of Empire: Poetry, Politics, and Commerce in British America, 1690–1750* (Chicago: University of Chicago Press, 1990), 65. Shields suggests (p. 71) that colonial poets followed Virgil's *Georgics*, which depicted the "imposition of control upon nature, upon the newly conquered or colonized lands," more closely than they did neoclassical georgics by English poets. In addition, see George Ogilvie's "Carolina, or the Planter" (1776), which praises North American plantations by comparing the act of transforming uncleared land into cultivated fields to early colonists' attempts to civilize the wilderness. See Ogilvie, "Carolina, or the Planter," *The Southern Literary Journal Special Issue* (Chapel Hill: University of North Carolina Press, 1986), and Shields, *Oracles of Empire*, 64–65.
11. Virgil, "Georgics," in *The Works of Virgil: Containing His Pastorals, Georgics, and Aeneis ... Translated into English Verse; By Mr. Dryden*, trans. John Dryden, 2nd ed. (London, 1698), 4.10.
12. Ibid., 4.40.

13. Shields, *Oracles of Empire,* 73.
14. Ibid.
15. Shaun Irlam, "'Wish You Were Here': Exporting England in James Grainger's *The Sugar-Cane,*" *English Literary History* 68, no. 2 (2001): 391.
16. Ibid., 390.
17. Ibid., 392.
18. Ibid., 390.
19. In my focus on African views and uses of obeah, I depart from recent characterizations of the obeah man as the dangerous "inverted double" of the "Negro Doctor." As this chapter shows, enslaved Africans turned to obeah men as sources of power within the system of slavery, and obeah men put their expertise to purposes that Africans perceived as good and, sometimes, as evil. On the obeah man as the double of the "Negro doctor," see Christopher P. Iannini, *Fatal Revolutions: Natural History, West Indian Slavery, and the Routes of American Literature* (Chapel Hill: University of North Carolina Press, 2012), 47.
20. See Richard B. Sheridan, *Doctors and Slaves: A Medical and Demographic History of Slavery in the British West Indies, 1680–1834* (Cambridge: Cambridge University Press, 1985), 71.
21. James Grainger, "An Essay on the More Common West-India Diseases," in *On the Treatment and Management of the More Common West-India Diseases (1750–1802),* ed. J. Edward Hutson (Jamaica: University of the West Indies Press, 2005), 43, n. 70. The note is William Wright's.
22. Ibid. This comment is also Wright's. William Sells's taxonomy of slave diseases defines "Cachexies" as "bad habit of body." See Sells, *Remarks on the Condition of the Slaves in the Island of Jamaica* (London, 1823), 20.
23. Grainger, "Essay on the More Common West-India Diseases," 43, n. 70. Wright was probably inflating Grainger's status as the first practitioner to discover inoculation as a cure for yaws, since, as chapter 3 shows, African knowledge about inoculation had already been circulating throughout the Caribbean and North America by the 1760s.
24. Earle, *Obi; or the History of Three-Fingered Jack,* 136.
25. See Patterson, *Sociology of Slavery,* 193.
26. "Grenada and St. Christopher's," in *Report Of The Lords of the Committee of Council appointed for the Consideration of all Matters relating to Trade and Foreign Plantations; . . . and Concerning the Effects and Consequences of this Trade, as well in Africa and the West Indies, as to the General Commerce of this Kingdom* (London, 1789), 376.
27. Spooner was John Bourryau's (Grainger's patron) uncle and was married to Grainger's wife's sister. On Grainger's relation to Spooner, see Gilmore, *Poetics of Empire,* 14 and 18.
28. Similarly, the North American poet Joel Barlow added notes to his epic poem *The Columbiad,* in order to gloss unfamiliar words and to expand on his references to classical history. Unlike Grainger, however, Barlow felt that putting the notes at the end of the poem would facilitate ease in reading. He placed one note in the text, adding at that point: "This explanation seemed of such immediate importance for understanding the machinery of the poem, as to require its being placed here. The other notes, being numerous and some of them long, have been forced to yield to typographical elegance; and are placed at the end of the volume, with suitable reference to the passages to which they belong." See Barlow, *The Columbiad, A Poem* (Philadelphia, 1807), 28.
29. George Ogilvie's georgic, "Carolina, or the Planter," similarly employed footnotes to gloss unfamiliar words and to include information considered unsuitable for poetic verses. One

possible exception to the complementary relation between the notes and the poem in *The Sugar-Cane* occurs in Book 2, when Grainger describes the "bles'd apple Median climes produce" (2.131), which legendarily had properties that could "counteract / Dire spells, slow-mutter'd o'er the baneful bowl" (2.134–35). In the note to the verse on the "bles'd apple," Grainger admitted that authors disagreed regarding the identity of the apple but that this lack of knowledge was no concern, "for as spells cannot affect us, we are at no loss for antidotes to guard against them." See Grainger, *Sugar-Cane,* 62. Although the verses describe the spells that the apple counteracted, the notes stated that spells could not affect "us." Interestingly, the note falters over the same question that the note on obeah does: whether practices that worked by preternatural or supernatural causes had any effect and, if so, what effects they had. I address Grainger's statements about the effects of spells on colonists later in this chapter.

30. My reading of Grainger's account of obeah differs from that of Alan Richardson, who argues that Grainger's description "reflects the common attitude among West Indian planters," who laughed at slaves' magical-religious practices. By contrast, I argue that planters took obeah seriously, both as a threat to order on plantations and as a potentially useful medical practice. See Alan Richardson, "Romantic Voodoo: Obeah and British Culture, 1797–1807," in *Sacred Possessions: Voudou, Santeria, Obeah, and the Caribbean,* ed. Margarite Fernandez Olmos and Lizabeth Paravisini-Gerbert (New Brunswick, NJ: Rutgers University Press, 1997), 175.
31. Frank Palmeri, "The Satiric Footnotes of Swift and Gibbon," *The Eighteenth Century* 31, no. 3 (1990): 245–62.
32. Ibid., 245.
33. Ibid., 247. On supplementarity, see also Jacques Derrida, *Of Grammatology,* trans. Gayatri Chakravorty Spivak (Baltimore: Johns Hopkins University Press, 1976), esp. 144–64.
34. Palmeri, "Satiric Footnotes," 250.
35. Ibid., 247.
36. Sheridan, *Doctors and Slaves,* 77.
37. On absenteeism, see Elsa V. Goveia, *Slave Society in the British Leeward Islands at the End of the Eighteenth Century* (New Haven: Yale University Press, 1969), 108–9.
38. Edward Brathwaite, *The Development of Creole Society in Jamaica, 1770–1820* (Oxford: Clarendon Press, 1971), 162.
39. Griffith Hughes, *The Natural History of Barbados. In Ten Books* (London, 1750), 15–16.
40. Ibid., 15, n. 20.
41. Jerome S. Handler, "Slave Medicine and Obeah in Barbados, Circa 1650 to 1834," *New West Indian Guide* 74, no. 1 & 2 (2000): 70.
42. Ibid., 78.
43. Brathwaite, "The African Presence in Caribbean Literature," in *Slavery, Colonialism, and Racism,* ed. Sidney W. Mintz (New York: Norton, 1974), 75.
44. Bastide, *African Civilizations,* 60.
45. Ibid. See also page 101 on Creole Africans' uses of Obeah. For an opposing view of obeah as a "type of sorcery," see Patterson, *Sociology of Slavery,* 188.
46. Braithwaite, "African Presence," 74.
47. Ibid.
48. Edward Green, "Roles for Traditional African Healers in Mental Health Care," *Medical Anthropology* 4 (1980), quoted in Handler, "Slave Medicine," 66.

49. Ibid., 66–67.
50. Peter Kalm, vol. 1 of *Travels into North America; Containing its Natural History, and a Circumstantial Account of its Plantations and Agriculture in General . . . Enriched with a Map, several Cuts for the Illustration of Natural History, and some additional Notes*, trans. Johann Reinhold Forster (Warrington, 1770–71), 398–99.
51. Ibid., 400.
52. As Handler points out: "whites, and perhaps slaves as well, considered Obeah persons knowledgeable in making poisons from local flora." See Handler, "Slave Medicine," 65. On later uses of obeah to punish slaves perceived as causing harm or illness to the community, see Randy M. Browne, "The 'Bad Business' of Obeah: Power, Authority, and the Politics of Slave Culture in the British Caribbean," *William and Mary Quarterly* 3d. ser., 68, no. 3 (2011): 451–80.
53. Kalm, *Travels into North America*, 398.
54. Ibid., 400.
55. Bastide, *African Civilizations*, 90.
56. Ibid., 47.
57. Long, *History of Jamaica*, 451.
58. See ibid., 451–53.
59. Patterson, *Sociology of Slavery*, 261.
60. See ibid., 192.
61. James Lind, *An Essay on Diseases Incidental to Europeans in Hot Climates With the Method of Preventing their Fatal Consequences . . . To the Whole is Annexed, A Simple and Easy Way to Render Salt Water Fresh, and to Prevent a Scarcity of Provisions in Long Voyages at Sea* (London, 1768), 63–64.
62. Ibid., 146.
63. Ibid., 146–47.
64. Long, *History of Jamaica*, 279.
65. Ibid.
66. William Falconer, *Remarks on the Influence of Climate, Situation, Nature of Country, Population, Nature of Food and Way of Life, on the Disposition and Temper, Manners and Behaviour, Intellects, Laws and Customs, Form of Government, and Religion, of Mankind* (London, 1781), 8.
67. Ibid., 119.
68. John Brathwaite, "Replies to Queries in Report of the Lords of the Committee of Council . . . Concerning the Present State of the Trade to Africa," in House of Commons, London, Parliamentary Papers, 26, 1789, part 3, quoted in Handler, "Slave Medicine," 59.
69. Kurt Heinzelman, "Roman Georgic in the Georgian Age: A Theory of Romantic Genre," *Texas Studies in Literature and Language* 33, no. 2 (1991): 201.
70. Ibid.
71. James Boswell, vol. 2 of *The life of Samuel Johnson, LL.D. Comprehending an Account of his Studies and Numerous Works* (London, 1791), 29. Grainger mentions rats at several points in the poem, but he revised this particular line before publishing *The Sugar-Cane*.
72. Ibid., 29–30.
73. Samuel Johnson, *Critical Review*, Oct. 1764, in *Critical Opinions of Samuel Johnson*, arr. by Joseph Epes Brown (Princeton: Princeton University Press, 1926), 170.

74. James C. Riley, *The Eighteenth-Century Campaign to Avoid Disease* (Houndsmills: Macmillan, 1987), 13.
75. Ibid., 17–19. See also Lester S. King, *The Medical World of the Eighteenth Century* (Chicago: University of Chicago Press, 1958).
76. John Arbuthnot, *Essay Concerning the Effects of Air on Human Bodies* (London, 1733), 146. See also Lind, *Essay on Diseases,* and Thomas Trapham, *A Discourse of the State of Health In the Island of Jamaica. With a Provision Therefore Calculated From the Air, the Place, and the Water: The Customs and Manners of Living, &c.* (London, 1678).
77. Thomas Sydenham, "De Arte Medica," in *Dr. Thomas Sydenham (1624–1689): His Life and Original Writings,* ed. Kenneth Dewhurst (Berkeley: University of California Press, 1966), 82.
78. Juan Huarte, *The Examination of Mens Wits. In Which, by Discovering the Varietie of Natures, is Shewed for What Profession each One is Apt, and How Far He Shall Profit Therein . . . Englished out of his Italian, by R.C. Esquire,* trans. R.C. (London, 1594), 183.
79. Roxann Wheeler, *The Complexion of Race: Categories of Difference in Eighteenth-Century British Culture* (Philadelphia: University of Pennsylvania Press, 2000), 23–24.
80. Grainger, "Essay on the More Common West-India Diseases," 22.
81. Homi K. Bhabha, "The Other Question: Difference, Discrimination and the Discourse of Colonialism," in *Literature, Politics, and Theory,* ed. Francis Barker, Peter Hulme, Margaret Iversen, and Diana Loxley (London: Methuen, 1986), 156.
82. Ibid.
83. Ibid.
84. Grainger, "Essay on the More Common West-India Diseases," 33.
85. Ibid., 3.
86. Ibid., 6. See Thomas Sydenham, "Anatomie," in Dewhurst, *Dr. Thomas Sydenham,* 86.
87. Grainger, "Essay on the More Common West-India Diseases," 3.
88. Ibid., 11.
89. Ibid., 52.
90. Ibid. On the interconnections between slavery, sentiment, and antislavery discourses, see Philip Gould, *Barbaric Traffic: Commerce and Antislavery in the Eighteenth-Century Atlantic World* (Cambridge: Harvard University Press, 2003), esp. the introduction.
91. Shields, *Oracles of Empire,* 82.
92. See Goveia, *Slave Society,* 1–4.
93. Ibid., 71.
94. Goveia cites this system as the beginning of the sugar colonies' decline. See ibid., 1–4.
95. See Long, *History of Jamaica,* for an example of such perceptions, esp. 260–319.
96. As David Collins writes, "To the rules, herein recommended, for the increase of our gangs, by the natural means of procreation, no objection can possibly be made, as they are neither expensive, nor of difficult application." See David Collins, *Practical Rules for the Management and Medical Treatment of Negro Slaves, in the Sugar Colonies. By a Professional Planter* (London, 1803), 30.
97. Grainger, "Essay on the More Common West-India Diseases," 51.
98. See ibid., 51 and 11.
99. See ibid., 24.
100. Ibid., 8.

101. Long, *History of Jamaica,* 270.
102. Gilmore, *Poetics of Empire,* 287. The ceded islands included Grenada, Tobago, St. Vincent, and Dominica; Britain obtained them in 1763, as a result of defeating France in the Seven Years War. See J. R. Ward, *British West Indian Slavery, 1750–1834: The Process of Amelioration* (Oxford: Clarendon Press, 1988), esp. chap. 3. As Ward explains, the addition of these islands resulted in increased expenses for planters already part of the British Empire and new competitors for slaves and sugar.
103. See Gilmore, *Poetics of Empire,* 287–88, where he notes that the line is from the Roman playwright Terence.
104. Grainger, "Essay on the More Common West-India Diseases," 8.
105. See Hutson, *On the Treatment and Management,* 130, note on page 8.
106. Grainger, "Essay on the More Common West-India Diseases," 52.
107. On the ways in which antislavery discourses could liberate both African slaves and Europeans who participated in the slave trade, see Gould, *Barbaric Traffic,* 24.
108. Grainger, "Essay on the More Common West-India Diseases," 11.
109. Ibid., 53. On planters' debt, see Goveia, *Slave Society,* 108–10.
110. Grainger, "Essay on the More Common West-India Diseases," 6.
111. Ibid., 52.
112. Ibid., 11.
113. See Goveia, *Slave Society,* 32–38, 144, 190–202, and Ward, *British West Indian Slavery.*
114. John Williamson, vol. 1 of *Medical and Miscellaneous Observations, Relative to the West India Islands* (Edinburgh, 1817), 135.
115. Ibid.
116. Collins, *Practical Rules,* 152–53.
117. See Brathwaite, *Development of Creole Society,* 293: "In this way, the white Establishment hoped to justify its ways to God, the Humanitarians, perhaps the slaves themselves, and certainly to the men in the Colonial Office."
118. Williamson, *Medical and Miscellaneous Observations,* 98.
119. Ibid., 115.
120. Ibid., 116.
121. Ibid., 98.
122. Ibid.
123. Ibid., 140.
124. Contemporary anthropological studies often describe obeah as sorcery. See Handler and Bilby, "On the Early Use," 92, and Brathwaite, "African Presence," 75.
125. Handler and Bilby suggest that the word could have been a "variant or corruption of an Efik or Ibo word from the northeast or east of the Niger delta, which simply means 'Doctor.'" Moreover, they suggest that we might trace "obeah" to the Igbo word "dibia," meaning a doctor who combined herbal and sacred knowledge. See Handler and Bilby, "On the Early Use," 91.
126. Ibid., 93.
127. On post-slavery meanings of obeah, particularly the way in which obeah was redefined as fraud, see Diana Paton, "Obeah Acts: Producing and Policing the Boundaries of Religion in the Caribbean," *small axe* 28 (2009): 1–18, and the chapters in Paton and Maarit Forde, eds., *Obeah and Other Powers: The Politics of Caribbean Religion and Healing* (Durham: Duke University Press, 2012).
128. On "White Obi," see Earle, *Obi; or the History of Three-Fingered Jack,* 228.

129. Grainger, "Essay on the More Common West-India Diseases," 52.
130. See Srinivas Aravamudan, introduction to *Obi; or the History of Three-Fingered Jack,* by William Earle (Ontario: Broadview, 2005), 29.
131. Grainger, "Essay on the More Common West-India Diseases," 52.
132. Collins, *Practical Rules,* 258.
133. Ibid.
134. Brathwaite, *Development of Creole Society,* 293.
135. Bastide, *African Civilizations,* 103.
136. The literary evidence is supported by historical studies, as Handler and Bilby note: St. Kitts and Barbados, the first West Indian colonies to be settled and to develop sugar plantations "might have actually been the point of origin" for such interpretations. See Handler and Bilby, "On the Early Use," 98, n. 25.
137. Bastide, *African Civilizations,* 103.
138. Ibid.
139. See John Gabriel Stedman, "Narrative of a Five Years Expedition against the Revolted Negroes of Surinam," in *Stedman's Surinam: Life in an Eighteenth-Century Slave Society,* ed. Richard Price and Sally Price (Baltimore: Johns Hopkins University Press, 1992); and Maria Edgeworth, *Belinda* (London, 1801). See also Edgeworth, "The Grateful Negro" (London, 1804); Thomas Campbell, *The Pleasures of Hope* (Edinburgh, 1799); William Shepherd, "The Negro Incantation" (London, 1797); *A Description of Furibond; or Harlequin Negro* (performed 1807); Anonymous, *Poems, Chiefly on the Superstition of Obeah* (Jamaica, 1816); and Anonymous, *Hamel, the Obeah Man* (London, 1827). Candace Ward and Tim Watson argue that *Hamel* was written by Cynric R. Williams. See Cynric R. Williams, *Hamel, the Obeah Man,* eds. Candace Ward and Tim Watson (Ontario: Broadview, 2010). On these representations of obeah, see Richardson, "Romantic Voodoo," and Aravamudan, "Introduction."
140. James Thomson, *A Treatise on the Diseases of Negroes, As They Occur in the Island of Jamaica: with the Observations on The Country Remedies* (Jamaica, 1820), 8.
141. On the connections between capitalism, ideas of race, and sentimental discourses, see Gould, *Barbaric Traffic,* esp. his introduction.

5. *Drunkenness, Syphilis, and History in Samson Occom's Medical Writing*

1. See Patricia Fara, *Sex, Botany & Empire: The Story of Carl Linnaeus and Joseph Banks* (New York: Columbia University Press, 2003), 8–12, and Nicholas Thomas, "Licensed Curiosity: Cook's Pacific Voyages," in *The Cultures of Collecting,* ed. John Elsner and Roger Cardinal (London: Reaktion Books, 1997), 129.
2. The full title of Hawkesworth's compilation is *An Account of the Voyages Undertaken by the Order of his Present Majesty for Making Discoveries in the Southern Hemisphere . . . Illustrated with Cuts, and a great Variety of Charts and Maps relative to Countries now first discovered, or hitherto but imperfectly known* (London, 1773). The text was republished in 1774 in America as: *A New Voyage, Round the World, in the Years 1768, 1769, 1770, and 1771 . . . In Two Volumes: with Cutts and a Map of the whole Navigation* (New York: J. Rivington, 1774). I will refer to Hawkesworth's text by the American title, since it is the text Occom cites.
3. Occom's execution sermon for Moses Paul has been the focus of scholars interested in Occom's comments on alcohol abuse and racial stereotypes of Native Americans. See

Michael Elliott, "'This Indian Bait': Samson Occom and the Voice of Liminality," *Early American Literature* 29 (1994): 233–53; Sandra M. Gustafson, *Eloquence Is Power: Oratory & Performance in Early America* (Chapel Hill: University of North Carolina Press, 2000), 97–101; and Katy L. Chiles, "Becoming Colored in Occom and Wheatley's Early America," *PMLA* 123, no. 5 (2008): 1398–1417.

4. Moor's Charity School was named for Joshua Moor, who donated land for the school.
5. David Maccleur to Eleazar Wheelock, 30 June 1772, DCA 772380, Rauner Library, Dartmouth College, Hanover, NH.
6. On Occom's life, see Joanna Brooks, "'This Indian World': An Introduction to the Writings of Samson Occom," in *The Collected Writings of Samson Occom, Mohegan: Leadership and Literature in Eighteenth-Century America,* ed. Brooks (Oxford: Oxford University Press, 2006), 3–39.
7. Although the sermon is undated, it is possible to locate its writing in the mid-1770s, and certainly after 1774, for Occom cites the American edition of Hawkesworth's text, published in 1774. Brooks cites the sermon as undated when reproducing it in *Collected Writings,* but she suggests elsewhere that it was written in 1792. See Brooks, *Collected Writings,* 165.
8. Joanna Brooks, *American Lazarus: Religion and the Rise of African-American and Native American Literatures* (Oxford: Oxford University Press, 2003), 56.
9. See Lisa Brooks, *The Common Pot: The Recovery of Native Space in the Northeast* (Minneapolis: University of Minnesota Press, 2008).
10. Joanna Brooks, "'This Indian World,'" 32.
11. Carlos Fausto and Michael Heckenberger, "Indigenous History and the History of the 'Indians,'" in *Time and Memory in Indigenous Amazonia: Anthropological Perspectives,* ed. Fausto and Heckenberger (Gainesville: University Press of Florida, 2007), 13.
12. Samson Occom, "When he drowned his reason," in *Collected Writings,* 226. Further references to this text will appear parenthetically.
13. Samson Occom, "A Sermon, Preached at the Execution of Moses Paul, An Indian (1772)," in *Collected Writings,* 192.
14. Ibid., 192–93.
15. Ibid.
16. Ibid., 192.
17. Ibid.
18. Ava Chamberlain, "The Execution of Moses Paul: A Story of Crime and Contact in Eighteenth-Century Connecticut," *New England Quarterly* 77, no. 3 (2004): 421.
19. Samuel Danforth, *The Woful Effects of Drunkenness. A Sermon Preached at Bristol, Octob. 12. 1709 When Two Indians,* Josias *and* Joseph, *Were Executed for Murder Occasioned By the Drunkenness Both of the Murthering and Murthered Parties* (Boston, 1710), 18.
20. Ibid., 19. Danforth's account of alcohol's physiological effects paralleled medical practitioners' understanding of alcohol's effects on the body. For example, the physician Benjamin Rush wrote: "Spirits in their first operation are stimulating upon the system. They quicken the circulation of the blood, and produce some heat in the body. Soon afterwards, they become what is called sedative, that is, they diminish the action of the vital powers, and thereby produce languor and weakness." See Rush, *An Inquiry Into the Effects of Spirituous Liquors on the Human Body. To Which is Added, a Moral and Physical Thermometer* (Boston, 1790), 2.
21. Danforth, *Woful Effects,* 31.

22. Ibid.
23. Ibid., 19.
24. Ibid.
25. Jonathan Edwards, *Memoirs of the Rev. David Brainerd, Missionary to the Indians on the Borders of New-York, New-Jersey, and Pennsylvania: Chiefly Taken from His Own Diary . . . Including His Journal, Now for the First Time Incorporated With the Rest of His Diary, In a Regular Chronological Series* (New Haven: S. Converse, 1822), 233–34.
26. William A. Hunter, ed., *John Hays' Diary and Journal of 1760, Pennsylvania Archaeologist* 24 (1954), 75. Peter Mancall records that a Moravian missionary wrote that "when [an Indian] is drunk, he looks like the Devil." See Mancall, *Deadly Medicine: Indians and Alcohol in Early America* (Ithaca: Cornell University Press, 1995), 87.
27. Edwards, *Memoirs of the Rev. David Brainerd,* 219.
28. Ibid., 233.
29. In fact, Natives did incorporate alcohol into spiritual ceremonies and rituals of hospitality, mourning, and healing. Colonists, however, viewed such incorporations as more evidence that Natives were naturally inclined to use diabolic practices. See Mancall, *Deadly Medicine,* 68–79.
30. Samuel Kirkland, "Samuel Kirkland to John Rodgers," June 20, 1772, Samuel Kirkland Correspondence (1765–1793), Hamilton College, Burke Library, Clinton, NY.
31. Ibid.
32. Peter Chester to the Earl of Dartmouth, June 4, 1774, in vol. 8 of *Documents of the American Revolution, 1770–1783, Transcripts 1774,* ed. K. G. Davies (Dublin: Irish University Press, 1975), 127–28.
33. Eleazar Wheelock, *A Continuation of the Narrative of the* Indian *Charity-School, in Lebanon, in Connecticut; from the Year 1768, to the Incorporation of it with* Dartmouth-*College, and Removal and Settlement of it in Hanover, In the Province of New-Hampshire, 1771* (1771), 23. As Hilary Wyss points out, such rhetoric "emphasizes that Natives must be brought under English political domination to attain salvation. The primary rationalization for English domination is the assumption that Natives are innately flawed." See Wyss, *Writing Indians: Literacy, Captivity, and Redemption* (Amherst: University of Massachusetts Press, 2000), 129.
34. See Chamberlain, "Execution of Moses Paul," 420–21. It had long been customary among colonists to drink alcoholic beverages rather than water, which was often perceived as (and often was) unsafe or unhealthy. Such everyday drinking usually involved hard cider or beer rather than the rum that contained higher alcohol content and that traders exchanged with Native Americans.
35. Mancall, *Deadly Medicine,* 172.
36. Kirkland, "Samuel Kirkland to John Rodgers."
37. Ibid.
38. Wheelock, *A Plain and Faithful Narrative of the Original Design, Rise, Progress and Present State of the* Indian *Charity-School At Lebanon, in Connecticut* (Boston, 1763), 25.
39. Chamberlain, "Execution of Moses Paul," 421.
40. Ibid.
41. Roxann Wheeler, *The Complexion of Race: Categories of Difference in Eighteenth-Century British Culture* (Philadelphia: University of Pennsylvania Press, 2000), 299.
42. Ibid., 298.
43. Kirkland, "Kirkland to John Rodgers."

44. These new conceptions of Natives' identity and mental capacity paradoxically circulated during the revivals known as the Great Awakening, which emphasized the work of grace in individuals' souls, including those of Natives and Africans. Although ministers expressed new interest in Natives' and Africans' experience of grace, they also failed to revise beliefs that Natives and Africans were barbaric, worshiped the devil, and possessed inherently inferior mental faculties. For example, ministers such as Jonathan Edwards defined Natives as ideal witnesses of the work of grace on the soul, but he and other ministers insisted that they themselves had to do the interpretive work of discovering the signs of grace on Native souls. See Sarah Rivett, *The Science of the Soul in Colonial New England* (Chapel Hill: University of North Carolina Press, 2011), chap. 6. On attitudes regarding Natives and Africans during the Great Awakening more generally, see Joanna Brooks, *American Lazarus,* chap. 1, and Gustafson, *Eloquence Is Power,* chap. 2.
45. The debate concerning the origins of syphilis began in the late fifteenth century and continues today. Spanish historians claimed that the disease had been brought back to Europe by several of Columbus's men who had sexual relations with Native women. Others blamed King of France Charles VIII's siege of Naples for spreading the disease throughout Europe; in this way, it became known as the French disease, even after the Italian physician Fracastoro coined the name "syphilis" for it. Finally, some medical practitioners argued that the pox was a new form of leprosy spread by Jews who were displaced from Spain and Portugal. See Fracastoro, *Syphilis: Or, a Poetical History of the French Disease . . . now Attempted in English by N. Tate* (London, 1686). Recent studies of syphilis and its origins include: Claude Quetel, *History of Syphilis,* trans. Judith Braddock and Brian Pike (Baltimore: Johns Hopkins University Press, 1990); Alfred W. Crosby, *The Columbian Exchange: Biological and Cultural Consequences of 1492* (Westport, CT: Greenwood Press, 1972), chap. 4; Brenda J. Baker and George J. Armelagos, "The Origin and Antiquity of Syphilis: Paleopatholgical Diagnoses and Interpretation," in vol. 26 of *Biological Consequences of the European Expansion, 1450–1800,* ed. Kenneth F. Kiple and Stephen V. Beck (Variorum: Ashgate, 1997), 1–35; and Amy G. Carmichael, "Syphilis and the Columbian Exchange: Was the New Disease Really New?," *The Great Maritime Discoveries and World Health,* ed. Mário Gomes Marques and John Clue (Lisbon: Escola Nacional de Saude Publica Ordem dos Medicos Instituto De Sintra, 1991), 187–200.
46. A "Mr. John Sarjeant, of Stockbridge" and a "Dr. Serjeant, at Stockbridge" are listed among the publisher James Rivington's subscribers, suggesting that both the elder and younger Sergeants had copies of Hawkesworth's text. See Hawkesworth, vol. 1 of *New Voyage,* 2. John Sargeant, Jr. established a ministry at New Stockbridge, where he and Occom disagreed about which of them should serve as the town's primary minister. See Joanna Brooks, *Collected Writings,* 137, n. 152 and 377, n. 229. Occom frequently mentions staying with the Sergeants while on his travels. See Brooks, *Collected Writings,* 324, 355, 377, 378–80, 386, 403.
47. Joseph Banks, vol. 1 of *The Endeavour Journal of Joseph Banks, 1768–1771,* ed. J. C. Beaglehole (Sydney: Angus & Robertson Ltd, 1962), 375. Hawkesworth included elements of both Cook's and Banks's explanations of the origin of the venereal disease that infected the Tahitians, but he relied most heavily on the structure and content of Banks's journal.
48. Hawkesworth, vol. 1 of *New Voyage,* 145.

49. On the Black Legend, see Margaret R. Greer, Walter D. Mignolo, and Maureen Quilligan, eds., *Rereading the Black Legend: The Discourses of Religious and Racial Difference in the Renaissance Empires* (Chicago: University of Chicago Press, 2008).
50. Hawkesworth, vol. 1 of *New Voyage,* 145.
51. Ibid., 145–46. Wallis explored the Pacific in 1766.
52. John Astruc, vol. 1 of *A Treatise of the Venereal Disease, in Six Books; Containing An Account of the Original, Propagation, and Contagion of this Distemper in General . . . now translated into* English *by William Barrowby, M.B.* (London, 1737), 103.
53. Ibid.
54. Ibid., 102.
55. Ibid., 103.
56. Ibid., 102.
57. Ibid., 104.
58. Ibid., 103.
59. Ibid.
60. Gonzalo Fernández de Oviedo y Valdés, "The Hystorie of the Weste Indies," in *The Decades of the Newe Worlde or West India Conteynyng the Nauigations and Conquestes of the Spanyardes, with the Particular Description of the Moste Ryche and Large Landes and Ilandes lately Founde in the West Ocean . . . Wrytten in the Latine Tounge by Peter Martyr of Angleria, and Translated into Englysshe by Rycharde Eden* (London, 1555), 183v. Spanish historians carefully disproved ancient writers such as Aristotle, who claimed the Torrid Zone was uninhabitable, by admitting that America's climate was hot but arguing that its heat was not detrimental to Europeans' health.
61. José de Acosta, *The Naturall and Morall Historie of the East and West Indies . . . Written in Spanish by Joseph Acosta,* and translated into English by *E.G.* (London, 1604), 101.
62. James I, *A Covnter-Blaste to Tobacco* (London, 1604), B1v.
63. Oviedo, "Hystorie of the Weste Indies," 208r.
64. Amerigo Vespucci, *The Letters of Amerigo Vespucci and Other Documents Illustrative of his Career,* trans. Clements R. Markham (London: Hakluyt Society, 1894), 8.
65. Ibid., 9.
66. Ibid., 46.
67. Although later colonial writers would describe Native women as modest, they also referenced fifteenth- and sixteenth-century accounts of Native women's sexual passion. See Rebecca Lush, "The 'Other' Woman: Early Modern English Representations of Native American Women, 1579–1690" (PhD diss., University of Maryland, 2011).
68. Gonzalo Fernández de Oviedo y Valdés, *Natural History of the West Indies,* ed. Sterling A. Stoudemire (Chapel Hill: University of North Carolina Press, 1959), 88–89. Stoudemire's edition includes sections of the *Natural History* omitted by Richard Eden, the sixteenth-century translator and editor of Oviedo's work.
69. Amélia A. B. de Ricon-Ferraz, "An Early Work on Syphilis: The Diaz de Ysla's Treatise on the 'Serpentine Disease' of Hispaniola Island," in *Great Maritime Discoveries,* 205.
70. Bartolomé de Las Casas, vol. 5 of *Historia de las Indias* (Madrid, 1875–76), quoted in Andrew F. Downing, "Were the Sailors of Columbus the First European Syphilitics?," *The Boston Medical and Surgical Journal* 175 (1916): 520.
71. Nicolás Monardes, *Joyful Newes out of the Newe Found World . . . Whereunto are added three other bookes treating of the Bezaar stone, the herb escuer conera, the properties of iron and steele in medicine, and the benefit of snow,* trans. John Frampton (London, 1580), fol. 10v–11r.

72. Ibid., fol. 10v. Charles Manning and Merrill Moore explain: "Because syphilis was considered by many to have come from America, it was only natural, according to the medical thought of the day, that its cure should be found there." See Manning and Moore, "Sassafras and Syphilis," *New England Quarterly* 9, no. 3 (1936): 474. Anna Foa argues that the "Indians continued to be blamed for syphilis for two fundamental reasons: first, the diffusion of a cure containing guaiac wood found in the Antilles, which made contemporaries think by analogy that because the remedy had been found beyond the ocean, the sickness had also originated there; second, the elaboration already completed of the *topos* of the Indian as Other." See Foa, "The New and the Old: The Spread of Syphilis (1494–1530)," trans. Carole C. Gallucci, in *Sex and Gender in Historical Perspective: Selections from "Quaderni Storici,"* ed. Edward Muir and Guido Ruggiero (Baltimore: John Hopkins University Press, 1990), 32.
73. John Jossleyn, *An Account of Two Voyages to New-England . . . a Large Chronological Table of the Most Remarkable Passages, From the First Discovering of the Continent of America, to the Year 1673* (London, 1674), 131.
74. Ibid. William Eamon shows that a number of marvelous tales and stereotypes of Native Americans supported arguments for the New World origin of syphilis, including the claim that the Natives were cannibals whose savage practices ensured that they became ill with venereal disease. See Eamon, "Cannibalism and Contagion: Framing Syphilis in Counter-Reformation Italy," *Early Science and Medicine* 3, no. 1 (1998): 11.
75. Daniel Webb, *A General History Of The Americans, Of Their Customs, Manners, And Colours An History Of The Patago, Selected From M. Pauw, By Daniel Webb, Esq.* (Rochdale, UK, 1806), 28. On theories of syphilis and metropolitan bias regarding America, see Foa, "New and the Old," 28, and Francisco Guerra, "The Dispute over Syphilis: Europe versus America," *Clio Medica* 13, no. 1 (1978): 39–61.
76. Oviedo, "Hystorie of the Weste Indies," 188r.
77. Webb, *General History,* 11.
78. Ibid., 17–18.
79. Marie E. McAllister, "Stories of the Origin of Syphilis in Eighteenth-Century England: Science, Myth, and Prejudice," *Eighteenth-Century Life* 24, no. 1 (2000): 28.
80. As scholars have shown, some colonists developed theories that difference was innate in order to protest European theories of colonial degeneration and to argue that the environment had no influence on them. See Ralph Bauer, "The Hemispheric Genealogies of 'Race': Creolization and the Cultural Geography of Colonial Difference across the Eighteenth-Century Americas," in *Hemispheric American Studies,* ed. Robert Levine and Caroline Levander (New Brunswick: Rutgers University Press, 2007), 36–56.
81. "London Evening Post: London, 29 August 1771," in *A Voyage to the Great South Sea Completed: How England learned of Cook's return in 1771,* ed. John Currey (Malvern: The Banks Society, 2006), 44.
82. Ibid., 46. In 1778, John Reinhold Forster echoed these comments when writing of his voyage to Tahiti with Cook: "we are now certain, that there is hardly a country to be found, where the young unmarried females are allowed such a latitude as at O-Taheitee and its neighborhood in admitting a variety of young males, and abandoning themselves to various embraces without derogating from their character. . . . It is therefore no wonder that in a hot climate, in a libidinous nation, inclined to leprosy and its various branches, a disease should pullulate, which may become contagious only by

cohabitation." See Forster, *Observations Made During a Voyage Round the World on Physical Geography, Natural History, and Ethic Philosophy. Especially on . . . The Human Species* (London, 1778), 491–92.

83. "General Evening Post, London, 27 July 1771," in *Voyage to the Great South Sea,* 39. On sexual contacts on Cook's three voyages and Tahitian conceptions of sexual activity, see Margaret Jolly, "Desire, Difference, and Disease: Sexual and Venereal Exchanges on Cook's Voyages to the Pacific," in *Exchanges: Cross Cultural Encounters in Australia and the Pacific,* ed. Ross Gibson (Sydney: HHT Publications, 1977), 186–217.
84. See Banks, *Endeavour Journal,* 375.
85. Hawkesworth, vol. 1 of *New Voyage,* 53.
86. Ibid., 130.
87. Ibid., 146.
88. Banks, *Endeavour Journal,* 375.
89. Ibid., 334.
90. Tim Fulford, Debbie Lee, and Peter J. Kitson, *Literature, Science, and Exploration in the Romantic Era: Bodies of Knowledge* (Cambridge: Cambridge University Press, 2004), 13.
91. Mary Louise Pratt, "Scratches on the Face of the Country; Or, What Mr. Barrow Saw in the Land of the Bushmen," *Critical Inquiry* 12, no. 1 (1985): 120–21.
92. Ibid.
93. Johannes Fabian, *Time and the Other: How Anthropology Makes Its Object* (New York: Columbia University Press, 1983), 73.
94. Ibid.
95. See Fulford, *Bodies of Knowledge,* 13.
96. Hawkesworth, vol. 1 of *New Voyage,* 145.
97. Beth Fowkes Tobin, *Colonizing Nature: The Tropics in British Arts and Letters, 1760–1820* (Philadelphia: University of Pennsylvania Press, 2005), 163.
98. Ibid., 165.
99. Hawkesworth, vol. 1 of *New Voyage,* 146.
100. Londa L. Schiebinger, *Plants and Empire: Colonial Bioprospecting in the Atlantic World* (Cambridge: Harvard University Press, 2004), 224.
101. As Sandra M. Gustafson points out, Occom defined sobriety as a "political [and] spiritual gesture, demonstrating the rational self-control that European colonists insisted was impossible for Indians, an argument they used to justify land theft, displacement, and extermination." See Gustafson, *Eloquence Is Power,* 97.
102. Occom, "Moses Paul," in *Collected Writings,* 192.
103. Samson Occom, "Journal 6: November 21, 1765–July 22, 1766," in *Collected Writings,* 267.
104. Kirkland, "Kirkland to John Rodgers."
105. Samson Occom, " 'The Most Remarkable and Strange State Situation and Appearence of Indian Tribes in This Great Continent' (1783)," in *Collected Writings,* 59.
106. Ibid.
107. Gladys Tantaquidgeon, *Folk Medicine of the Delaware and Related Algonkian Indians* (Harrisburg: Pennsylvania Historical and Museum Commission, 1972), 5. Tantaquidgeon was a Mohegan anthropologist and herbal specialist.
108. Ibid.
109. Anne-Christine Taylor, "Sick of History: Contrasting Regimes of Historicity in the

Upper Amazon," in *Time and Memory,* 153–54. On Natives' "sense of sin as a collective experience of hardship overlapping and intermingled with the deprivations of colonialism," see Joanna Brooks, "Hard Feelings: Samson Occom Contemplates His Christian Mentors," in *Native Americans, Christianity, and the Reshaping of Early America's Religious Landscape,* ed. Joel W. Martin and Mark A. Nicholas (Chapel Hill: University of North Carolina Press, 2010), 32.

110. Samson Occom, "'Thou Shalt Love Thy Neighbor as Thyself' Luke 10:26–27 (May 13, 1787?)," in *Collected Writings,* 206.

111. Ibid., 202.

112. Ibid., 206.

113. Ibid.

114. Ibid.

115. Occom, "'Most Remarkable and Strange State Situation,'" 59.

116. Ibid., 58.

117. Occom, "'Thou Shalt Love Thy Neighbor as Thyself,'" in *Collected Writings,* 201–2.

118. As Joanna Brooks has pointed out, Occom and other Natives recognized correspondences between elements of New Light Christianity that circulated in the revivals known as the Great Awakening and their traditional beliefs, and they "adapted the teachings, customs, and forms of New Light Christianity to develop new venues for spiritual revitalization among Native people" and opportunities for self-governance. See Brooks, "Indian World," 36. On nativist movements more generally, see Gregory Evans Dowd, *A Spirited Resistance: The North American Indian Struggle for Unity* (Baltimore: Johns Hopkins University Press, 1992).

119. On signs of grace and empirical methodologies, see Rivett, *Science of the Soul,* chap. 6.

120. Occom, "Tuesday, Novr 8," in *Collected Writings,* 309. See also Occom's journal entry "Febr 10, 1785": "At Mr Josiah Maples in eveng and there was a great many People and attention becoming Rational Creatures." *Collected Writings,* 288.

121. Occom, "Tuesday, Novr 8," 309.

122. On the performative nature of words, see Charles L. Briggs, *Competence in Performance: The Creativity of Tradition in Mexicano Verbal Art* (Philadelphia: University of Pennsylvania Press, 1988), esp. 1–24, and J. L. Austin, *How to Do Things with Words,* 2nd ed., ed. Marina Sbisá and J. O. Urmson (Cambridge: Harvard University Press, 1975).

123. See Occom, "'In Christ, He is a New Creature,' 2 Corinthians 5:17 (July 13, 1766)," in *Collected Writings,* 174.

124. Occom, "Moses Paul," in *Collected Writings,* 191.

125. Bleeding was a common European and colonial medical practice, but reports of Native medical practices include "cupping procedures," with which a practitioner would draw an offending object and fluids out of the patient's body. See Virgil J. Vogel, *American Indian Medicine* (Norman: University of Oklahoma Press, 1970), 129.

126. Occom, "Saturday, Octr 13," in *Collected Writings,* 380–81.

127. Ibid., 381.

128. Samson Occom, "Herbs and Roots (1754)," in *Collected Writings,* 47.

129. Samson Occom, "Monday, July 16," in *Collected Writings,* 373.

130. Ibid.

131. Occom, "Moses Paul," in *Collected Writings,* 191.

132. Tantaquidgeon, *Folk Medicine,* 2.

133. Ibid.
134. See Brooks, *Collected Writings,* 42.
135. Tantaquidgeon, *Folk Medicine,* 12.
136. Pratt, "Scratches on the Face," 120.
137. Robert Allen Warrior, *Tribal Secrets: Recovering American Indian Intellectual Traditions* (Minneapolis: University of Minnesota Press, 1995), 124.
138. Ibid., 122. Elsewhere, I discuss intellectual sovereignty as displayed in Occom's herbal. See Kelly Wisecup, "Medicine, Communication, and Authority in Samson Occom's Herbal," *Early American Studies* 10, no. 3 (2012): 541–66.
139. Warrior, *Tribal Secrets,* 122.
140. Thomas Bender, "Introduction: Historians, the Nation, and the Plenitude of Narratives," in *Rethinking American History in a Global Age,* ed. Thomas Bender (Berkeley: University of California Press, 2002), 9.
141. Ibid.
142. Ibid.
143. Paul Cohen, "Was There an Amerindian Atlantic? Reflections on the Limits of a Historiographical Concept," *History of European Ideas* 34, no. 5 (2008): 394. See also Amy Turner Bushnell, "Indigenous America and the Limits of the Atlantic World, 1493–1825," in *Atlantic History: A Critical Appraisal,* ed. Jack P. Greene and Philip D. Morgan (Oxford: Oxford University Press, 2008), 191–221; James Sidbury and Jorge Cañizares-Esguerra, "Mapping Ethnogenesis in the Early Modern Atlantic," *William and Mary Quarterly* 3d. ser., 68, no. 2 (2011): 181–208; as well as responses to Sidbury and Cañizares-Esguerra, including: Claudio Saunt, "The Indians Old World," ibid., 215–18; and Pekka Hämäläinen, "Lost in Transitions: Suffering, Survival, and Belonging in the Early Modern Atlantic World," ibid., 219–23.
144. On Native Americans who traveled to Britain, see Alden T. Vaughan, *Transatlantic Encounters: American Indians in Britain, 1500–1776* (Cambridge: Cambridge University Press, 2006).

Conclusion

1. The same narrative of lagging and inferiority characterized the historiography of early American medicine. See Raymond Phineas Stearns, *Science in the British Colonies of America* (Urbana: University of Illinois Press, 1970).
2. William Spengemann, *A New World of Words: Redefining Early American Literature* (New Haven: Yale University Press, 1994), 49.
3. See, for just a few examples, David S. Shields, *Oracles of Empire: Poetry, Politics, and Commerce in British America, 1690–1750* (Chicago: University of Chicago Press, 1990); Spengemann, *A New World of Words;* Ralph Bauer, *The Cultural Geography of Colonial American Literatures: Empire, Travel, Modernity* (Cambridge: Cambridge University Press, 2003); Susan Scott Parrish, *American Curiosity: Cultures of Natural History in the Colonial British Atlantic World* (Chapel Hill: University of North Carolina Press, 2006); and Christopher P. Iannini, *Fatal Revolutions: Natural History, West Indian Slavery, and the Routes of American Literature* (Chapel Hill: University of North Carolina Press, 2012). The work of Joseph Roach and Paul Gilroy is also key to the shift from national to transnational, transatlantic, and hemispheric perspectives. However, although Roach and Gilroy emphasize not only European perspectives but also the

experiences and histories of the Africans and (in Roach's case) the Native Americans who shared the Atlantic with European colonists, early Americanists have not always adopted this emphasis when drawing on Black and circum-Atlantic frameworks. Moreover, Roach and Gilroy primarily focus on relations between Europeans and Natives or Africans, occluding colonists who were born or settled in the Americas from these encounters. See Paul Gilroy, *The Black Atlantic: Modernity and Double Consciousness* (Cambridge: Harvard University Press, 1993), and Joseph Roach, *Cities of the Dead: Circum-Atlantic Performance* (New York: Columbia University Press, 1996).

4. On these efforts, see, for just a few examples, Sandra Gustafson, "American Literature and the Public Sphere," *American Literary History* 20, no. 3 (2008): 465–78, and Lisa Brooks, *The Common Pot: The Recovery of Native Space in the Northeast* (Minneapolis: University of Minnesota Press, 2008).
5. Birgit Brander Rasmussen, *Queequeg's Coffin: Indigenous Literacies and Early American Literature* (Durham: Duke University Press, 2012), 142.
6. On studying a "deeper historical past," see Neil Safier, "Global Knowledge on the Move: Itineraries, Amerindian Narratives, and Deep Histories of Science," *Isis* 101, no. 1 (2010): 141–42.
7. Eric Slauter, "History, Literature, and the Atlantic World," *Early American Literature* 43, no. 1 (2008): 169. Slauter argues that a "trade gap"—not only methodological differences but also uneven interchange between historians and literary scholars (privileging historians)—characterizes the relation between early American historical and literary studies.
8. Ibid., 154.
9. As Justine S. Murison has explained, a new "somatic emphasis of eighteenth- and nineteenth-century psychology responded to the theological need to cordon off the soul from disease." The result was that the nerves, rather than sinful or immoral behavior, were seen as the origin of disease. Illness was considered to be "shaped by the social and physical environment rather than . . . lodged in a 'deep' conception of the self." See Murison, *The Politics of Anxiety in Nineteenth-Century American Literature* (Cambridge: Cambridge University Press, 2011), 2. As Murison points out, these conceptions of the body and especially of the nervous system contributed to defining the citizens of the United States.
10. On bodies as mechanical entities, see Colleen E. Terrell, "'Republican Machines': Franklin, Rush, and the Manufacture of Civic Virtue in the Early Republic," *Early American Studies* 1, no. 2 (2003): 100–132. For histories of early national medicine, see John Duffy, *From Humors to Medical Science: A History of American Medicine,* 2nd ed. (Urbana: University of Illinois Press, 1993), and Lester Snow King, *Transformations in American Medicine: From Benjamin Rush to William Osler* (Baltimore: Johns Hopkins University Press, 1991).
11. The first medical school was founded in Philadelphia in 1766. See Duffy, *From Humors to Medical Science,* 32–34.
12. *Wetu* is the Wampanoag word for house. On this shift from classificatory to clinical medical science, see Michel Foucault, *The Birth of the Clinic: An Archaeology of Medical Perception,* trans. A. M. Sheridan Smith (New York: Vintage, 1975).
13. James Engell, *The Creative Imagination: Enlightenment to Romanticism* (Cambridge: Harvard University Press, 1981), viii. On early Americans' embrace of the imagination

and its powers, as well as their attempts to ensure that its use remained virtuous, see Edward Cahill, *Liberty of the Imagination: Aesthetic Theory, Literary Form, and Politics in the Early United States* (Philadelphia: University of Pennsylvania Press, 2012).

14. Bruno Latour, *We Have Never Been Modern*, trans. Catherine Porter (Cambridge: Harvard University Press, 1993), 41.
15. Ibid., 103.
16. On this shift, see Roxann Wheeler, *The Complexion of Race: Categories of Difference in Eighteenth-Century British Culture* (Philadelphia: University of Pennsylvania Press, 2000), esp. 252–53.
17. Ibid., 252.
18. Benjamin Rush, *An Oration, Delivered February 4, 1774, Before the American Philosophical Society, Held at Philadelphia . . . By Benjamin Rush, M.D. Professor of Chemistry in the College of Philadelphia* (Philadelphia: American Philosophical Society, 1774), 60.
19. Edward Long, vol. 2 of *History of Jamaica . . . Or, General Survey of the Antient and Modern State of that Island: with Reflections on its Situation, Settlements, Inhabitants . . . In Three Volumes* (London, 1774), 381.
20. Roxann Wheeler makes the point that slavery and conceptions of race emerged together, though, she argues, not in a "one-to-one correspondence nor at the same pace." See Wheeler, *Complexion of Race*, 287. On the connections between conceptions of Natives' inferiority and U.S. national identity, see Susan Scheckel, *The Insistence of the Indian: Race and Nationalism in Nineteenth-Century American Culture* (Princeton: Princeton University Press, 1998). On the connection between the acquisition of Native land and definitions of Natives as savages, see Colin G. Calloway, *The American Revolution in Indian Country: Crisis and Diversity in Native American Communities* (Cambridge: Cambridge University Press, 1995).
21. David Collins, *Practical Rules for the Management and Medical Treatment of Negro Slaves, in the Sugar Colonies. By a Professional Planter* (London, 1803), 22.
22. Thomas Jefferson, *Notes on the State of Virginia*, ed. Frank Shuffelton (New York: Penguin, 1999), 147.
23. The imagination—and the degree to which Africans possessed it—became a key point in arguments for and against slavery. Antislave trade and abolitionist arguments were often founded on the claim that Africans did indeed comprehend their enslavement and experience great mental and physical suffering. However, many proslavery advocates and abolitionists alike held that mental faculties differed among different peoples. See for example, Julie Ellison, *Cato's Tears and the Making of Anglo-American Emotion* (Chicago: University of Chicago Press, 1999), chap. 4, and Wheeler, *Complexion of Race*, 254.
24. Jefferson, *Notes on the State of Virginia*, 64.
25. Ibid.
26. See, for just a few examples, George Washington, "Third Annual Address, Oct. 25, 1791," in vol. 1 of *A Compilation of the Messages and Papers of the Presidents, 1789–1902*, ed. James D. Richardson (Washington, DC: Bureau of National Literature and Art, 1897): 102–6; Thomas Jefferson, "To Governor William H. Harrison, Washington, February 27, 1803," in vol. 9 of *The Writings of Thomas Jefferson, Definitive Edition*, ed. Albert Ellery Bergh (Washington, DC: Thomas Jefferson Memorial Association, 1905), 368–74; Lydia Maria Child, *Hobomok: A Tale of Early Times* (Boston, 1824), and Catharine Maria Sedgwick, *Hope Leslie: or Early Times in the Massachusetts* (New York,

1827). See also the documents in Francis Paul Prucha, ed., *Documents of United States Indian Policy,* 3rd ed. (Lincoln: University of Nebraska Press, 2000).

27. As Hilary E. Wyss shows, Natives did face "unforgiving institutions" in the boarding schools, but the schools also "provided an avenue through which Natives could use their hard-won literacy skills for their own purposes, to forge alliances and build their own communities." See Wyss, *English Letters and Indian Literacies: Reading, Writing, and New England Missionary Schools, 1750–1830* (Philadelphia: University of Pennsylvania Press, 2012), 5.
28. On this scrutiny, see Joanna Brooks, "'This Indian World': An Introduction to the Writings of Samson Occom," in *The Collected Writings of Samson Occom, Mohegan: Leadership and Literature in Eighteenth-Century America,* ed. Brooks (Oxford: Oxford University Press, 2006), 19.
29. Robert Warrior, *The People and the Word: Reading Native Nonfiction* (Minneapolis: University of Minnesota Press, 2005), 7.
30. See Katy L. Chiles, "Becoming Colored in Occom and Wheatley's Early America," *PMLA* 123, no. 5 (2008): 1407, and Wheatley, "On Imagination," in *Phillis Wheatley: Complete Writings,* ed. Vincent Carretta (New York: Penguin, 2001), line 43. Chiles analyzes Wheatley's discussion of blackness and genius not through environmental theories about the imagination and its association to hot climates but by noting that Apollo was god of sun, poetry, and music. Meanwhile, John C. Shields traces connections between Wheatley's writings on the imagination and European philosophers and poets. See Shields, *Phillis Wheatley and the Romantics* (Knoxville: University of Tennessee Press, 2010). On Wheatley's representation of the imagination, see also Ellison, *Cato's Tears,* 114–22.
31. Wheatley, "On Imagination," lines 19–22.
32. Ibid., 13.
33. William Apess, "Eulogy on King Philip," in *A Son of the Forest and Other Writings,* ed. Barry O'Connell (Amherst: University of Massachusetts Press, 1997), 107.
34. Ibid., 108.

INDEX

KELLY WISECUP is an assistant professor of early American literature at the University of North Texas. She has held research fellowships at the Newberry Library and the John Carter Brown Library, and her articles have appeared in *Early American Literature, Early American Studies, Studies in Travel Writing, and the Southern Literary Journal.*